Essential Midwifery Practice:
Intrapartum Care

Essential Midwifery Practice: Intrapartum Care

Edited by

Denis Walsh
RM, MA, PhD

Soo Downe
RM, BSc, PhD

WILEY-BLACKWELL

A John Wiley & Sons, Ltd., Publication

Blackwell Publishing was acquired by John Wiley & Sons in February 2007. Blackwell's publishing programme has been merged with Wiley's global Scientific, Technical, and Medical business to form Wiley-Blackwell.

Registered office
John Wiley & Sons Ltd, The Atrium, Southern Gate, Chichester, West Sussex, PO19 8SQ, United Kingdom

Editorial offices
9600 Garsington Road, Oxford, OX4 2DQ, United Kingdom
2121 State Avenue, Ames, Iowa 50014-8300, USA

For details of our global editorial offices, for customer services and for information about how to apply for permission to reuse the copyright material in this book please see our website at www.wiley.com/wiley-blackwell.

Library of Congress Cataloging-in-Publication Data
Intrapartum care / edited by Denis Walsh, Soo Downe.
p. ; cm. – (Essential midwifery practice)
Includes bibliographical references and index.
ISBN 978-1-4051-7698-9 (pbk. : alk. paper) 1. Midwifery. I. Walsh, Denis, 1955- II. Downe, Soo.
[DNLM: 1. Delivery, Obstetric – methods. 2. Labor, Obstetric. 3. Midwifery – methods.
WQ 415 E78 2010]
RG950.A2I+ 2010
618.2 – dc22
2009024487

A catalogue record for this book is available from the British Library.

Set in 10/12.5pt Palatino by Laserwords Private Limited, Chennai, India

Printed and bound in Malaysia by KHL Printing Co Sdn Bhd

1   2010

Contents

Contributors

Tricia Anderson (1961–2007)
Former Senior Lecturer in Midwifery
Bournemouth University
Independent Midwife Practitioner
(all-round brilliant person who sadly died during the gestation
of this book)

Sarah Buckley
Author and General Practitioner
Email: sarahjbuckley@yahoo.com

Soo Downe
Professor of Midwifery Studies
Midwifery Studies Research Unit
University of Central Lancashire
Email: sdowne@uclan.ac.uk

Debra Erikson-Owens
Doctoral Student
University of Rhode Island College of Nursing Kingston
Email: deri7917@postoffice.uri.edu

Jenny Hall
Senior Lecturer in Midwifery
Faculty of Health & Social Care
University of the West of England
Email: halltribe@blueyonder.co.uk

Nicky Leap
Professor of Midwifery Practice Development & Research
Centre of Midwifery, Child & Family Health
University of Technology Sydney
Email: nicky.leap@uts.edu.au

Rosemary Mander
Professor of Midwifery
School of Health
University of Edinburgh
Email: rmander@staffmail.ed.ac.uk

Chris McCourt
Professor of Anthropology and Women's Health
Centre of Research in Midwifery & Childbirth
Faculty of Health & Human Sciences
Thames Valley University
Email: chris.mccourt@tvu.ac.uk

Judith Mercer
Clinical Professor
College of Nursing
University of Rhode Island
Email: jme3053u@postoffice.uri.edu

Mary Nolan
Professor in Perinatal Education
The University of Worcester,
Email: mlnolan@aned.fsnet.co.uk

Holly Powell Kennedy
Professor of Midwifery Yale School of Nursing
Yale University
Email: holly.kennedy@yale.edu

Verena Schmid
Midwife, Founder of *Donna e Donna-Il Giornale delle Ostetriche*
Florence
Email: verena@dinonet.it

Mary Stewart
Research Midwife
National Perinatal Epidemiology Unit
University of Oxford
Email: mary.stewart@npeu.ox.ac.uk

Gill Thompson
Research Assistant
University of Central Lancashire
Email: gill.thomson@blueyonder.co.uk

Denise Tiran
Director, Expectancy Ltd
London
Email: root@expectancy.co.uk

Denis Walsh
Associate Professor in Midwifery
University of Nottingham
Email: denis.walsh@ntlworld.com

Introduction

Denis Walsh

This book is an attempt to bring together experts in their respective fields to place in one volume, for the first time, a comprehensive examination of normal birth practice. A glance through the Contents pages will reveal the variety of perspectives included here. Soo and I wanted to capture, as far as we could, a holistic overview of the current state of knowledge and skills in the wonderful complexity of labour and birthing. At the risk of overstating the significance of this particular era of childbirth practice, we both feel a sense of crisis confronting advocates of physiological birth. All over the planet, there appears to be an exorable drift towards a technocratic model of birthing (Davis-Floyd 1992) and a marginalisation of the low-tech, non-hospital birth.

These chapters are intended to feed the soul of women, midwives and other childbirth activists who still champion the experience of drug-free, normal labour and vaginal birth.

In Chapter 1, I give an overview of the recent history and trends in intrapartum practice and the philosophical models they are predicated on. Soo Downe then examines the historical legacy of these models in greater depth by explicating the struggle over 'ways of knowing' in childbirth. She contextualises the debate around childbirth in broader theories of complexity and constructionist influences of the postmodern era we live in.

In Chapter 3, Mary Nolan brings us up to date with the challenges facing childbirth education. Adult learning styles must be adopted if education is to be effective. The challenge of preparing childbearing women realistically for the institutional birth environment most will encounter is elaborated on before Nolan concludes by championing education as a tool for change.

Change is a central focus to the next two chapters on birth environment and labour rhythms. Both are undergoing reform, though mostly in birth centres and home-birth settings. These still only represent around 5% of births in the Western world, but their usage is increasing slowly as policy makers strive to address soaring Caesarean sections rates. Getting the birth environment right so that women can reconnect with an ancient nesting instinct and accepting that normal labour rhythms vary from woman to woman may reduce rates.

Judith Mercer and Debra Erikson-Owens discuss the exciting new developments around the third and fourth stage of labour, highlighting the significance of the intact cord after birth and the conditions necessary for early post-natal bonding.

Against these clinical and environmental factors, Holly Powell Kennedy, Nicky Leap and the late Tricia Anderson stress the importance of attitude to the birth process in their inspiring thoughts on midwifery presence. Linked to this is a need to view labour pain in a new way as Rosemary Mander discusses in Chapter 8. She concludes that labour pain can be transformatory.

Denise Tiran, the UK midwifery expert on complementary therapies takes us through their relevance and application to labour care in the next chapter before Verena Schmidt and Soo Downe in Chapter 10 overview unusual labours that are usually classed as abnormal. They believe that many such births can be normalised with the appropriate skills.

Gill Thompson, a psychologist, shares her important research with women who experienced traumatic births followed by healing births and tries to tease out the key elements that enable some women to refer to birth as a 'peak experience'. This is followed by one of the international authorities on childbirth hormones, Sarah Buckley, who addresses the rarely examined area of labour and sexuality.

Jenny Hall has had a long-standing interest in the spirituality of birth and brings her wisdom in this area in Chapter 13. In another under-researched area, Jenny discusses the relevance of the spirituality to contemporary childbirth.

Midwifery organisational models for intrapartum care is the specialist field of Chris McCourt, one of the original researchers on the One-to-One Midwifery Model at Queen Charlottes in London. She brings her depth of knowledge to this vexed field with a clarity and vision. Mary Stewart edited the visionary book on feminist perspectives on childbirth (Stewart 2004) and brings aspects of this thinking up to date in the penultimate chapter.

Soo Downe gathers up the interconnecting and overlapping threads of all chapters in an articulation of a vision for birth in the 21st century in the final chapter. Utilising her well-known application of salutogenesis, she makes a clarion call for all stakeholders in maternity care to work together to transform how birthing is done on our planet for the benefit of mothers, babies and families.

Soo and I hope this book becomes an important contribution to knowledge around intrapartum care and a source of inspiration and challenge for those who read it. As Suzanne Arms, the long-term childbirth advocate from the United States reminds us,

How we care for women and babies in the hours around birth makes a difference for the rest of their lives . . .

References

Davis-Floyd R (1992) *Birth as an American Rite of Passage*. London, University of California Press.

Stewart M (2004) *Pregnancy, Birth and Maternity Care: Feminist Perspectives*. London, Elsevier Science.

Chapter 1
Evolution of Current Systems of Intrapartum Care

Denis Walsh

This chapter provides a brief overview of the recent history of labour care and the predominant influences that have impacted on it. It includes a discussion of different models and approaches, reflected in trends around the place of birth and the evidence underpinning this. The roles of maternity-care professionals and of birth technologies are seminal in intrapartum care's recent history and will be critically reviewed. The chapter closes with speculation on what the future influences are likely to be.

Introduction and history

It may seem a little far-fetched to link ancient Greek philosophy to current labour care practices but the legacy of Greek thought around the understanding of the mind and body is relevant to these deliberations. Plato is credited with originating the dualism of mind–body split which posited the mind as superior (Rauchenstein 2008). This legacy in western thought has resulted in a suspicion of bodily processes as liable to error and breakdown. The mind needs to govern the body to prevent this from happening. Reproduction has suffered under this belief for millennia, both in relation to sexual behaviour and childbirth (Christiaens & Bracke 2007). Both have been cast as base and potentially errant behaviours and experiences. In the context of labour, the unfolding of physical expression should therefore be subject to rational planning and ongoing monitoring and regulation. It is easy to see how the body physiology becomes reduced to mechanical functioning within this paradigm.

The suspicion of parturition has been aided and abetted by another historical-cultural belief deeply embedded in western societies that can again be traced backed to Greek and Roman times – patriarchy (Longman 2006). This holds that social structures and especially power in the public sphere privileges men. Patriarchal beliefs and values, it could be argued, preceded mind–body dualism as it was men who propagated such ideas. In fact the history of western philosophy could be recast as a 'male only' mediated history (Zergan 2005). Patriarchy imposes control of men over women, especially in the public sphere and this has been played out in the recent history of childbirth where man midwives and subsequently male obstetricians oversaw many of the trends in the medicalisation of childbirth and the evolution and regulation of the midwifery profession (Donnison 1988).

Both patriarchy and dualism largely ignored childbirth until the Enlightenment period commenced in the 17th century when both the ideas and practices around childbirth began to migrate from the private, domestic sphere and enter the public domain (Fahy 1998). The Enlightenment saw an explosion in scientific advances, including the understanding of the human body. The accompanying rapid industrialisation saw the emergence of a wealthy middle class with disposable income. The emerging profession of man midwives saw an opportunity to profit from this wealth by offering childbirth services (Donnison 1988).

Prior to this, lay midwives and traditional birth attendants had provided support in childbirth, probably since the beginning of human evolution (Rosenberg & Trevathan 2002). Socrates' mother was a midwife and midwives are mentioned a number of times in ancient texts like the Bible. In the 17th century in the West, they continued to offer care to a huge majority of poor women but began to be excluded from the wealthy as male midwifery spread (Donnison 1988).

With the advent of inventions like the forceps by the Chamberlain family and pain-relieving drugs, and the rise of state provision for health care, childbirth was rapidly being viewed as belonging in the public sphere, overseen by accredited professionals. This heralded a drawn out battle for midwifery to be recognised as a profession in its own right with each country writing its own history of this struggle (Donnison 1988; Rhodes 1995).

Medicalisation of childbirth

Childbirth practitioners in the Western world in the 21st century are inevitably influenced by the conditions of practice we are exposed to and the kind of education and training we have had. For the vast majority of midwives that means a 'surveillance' orientation to care in labour. Surveillance is premised, as Foucault argued, on a dominant discourse of what should happen so that the one doing the surveying, is judging whether what is under observation complies with a preordained order (Foucault 1979). Foucault argued powerfully that dominant discourses regulate public behaviours by imposing a particular reading (knowledge) of what should happen. One such discourse is the medicalisation of childbirth (Van Teijlingen *et al*. 2000). An illustration of the power of this discourse is the fact that labour is divided into three stages that entirely reflect a professional nomenclature (Walsh 2007). Each is required to be framed in chronological time that may bear little resemblance to narrative accounts by women. The pervasiveness of labour stages and their timing is illustrated by the ubiquity of the partograms in maternal labour records across most of the world.

By far the most potent marker of medicalisation is the ever-increasing rates of Caesarean section, especially over the last decade (Johanson *et al*. 2002). The rises have not been accompanied by improving maternal and perinatal mortality, which begs the question of whether the Caesareans were necessary. The normalisation of Caesarean birthing has reached a point where, in the United States, an active debate exists as to whether Caesarean delivery should be a choice for women (Maier *et al*. 2000). The Caesarean issue raises another consequence of medicalisation – the attendant morbidities for mother and babies. Both Johanson *et al*. (2002) in Britain and Barros *et al*. (2005) in Brazil have raised concerns in this area. In Brazil, the 'modernisation' of maternity services has resulted in such high rates of intervention that a counter movement (REHUNA, Movement for the Humanisation of Birth 2008) has arisen to humanise birthing practices.

Backlash

Across the western world a backlash against the discourse of medicalisation is gathering momentum. This is being led by an alliance of consumer groups, midwives and other childbirth professionals challenging orthodoxies like hospital birth for all and the routine application of technologies like continuous fetal monitoring (Goer 2004). They have been successful in some countries in reducing episiotomy and artificial rupture of membrane rates but not in lowering Caesarean rates. Arguably, they have been more successful in addressing infrastructure and policy issues in maternity services such as the development of a vibrant midwifery profession and installing a woman-centred ethos to maternity care policy (Hirst 2005; DH 2007).

A woman-centred ethos is fleshed out with recurrent themes of choice, information and continuity appearing in policy documents on maternity services across the western world over the past 25 years (DH 1993; Declerq *et al*. 2002; Roberts *et al*. 2002). These themes have prompted the exploration of different midwifery models of working like teams, caseloads and group practices in addition to redressing the bias to acute services in maternity services (Page 1995). Continuity schemes like these are generally based in primary care. Consumer action has also stimulated more social science research and from the late 1980s onwards, alternative models of care began being hypothesised (Kirkham 2004).

Models of childbirth

Jordan (1983) was the first to suggest that cultural determinants constructed birth in contrasting ways in different settings but it was left to Davis-Floyd (1992) to conceptualise these variations as models of childbirth. She framed the medicalisation of birth as a technocratic model and a midwifery approach as holistic model. She delineated a number of values and beliefs which she believed typified attitudes and practices within each model and these have become a useful heuristic device in much of the literature since (Wagner 2001; Walsh & Newburn 2002). The debate around models is explicit in the midwifery and sociological childbirth literature but almost entirely absent from medical journals, though it is known that obstetricians and midwives conflict over what each considers to be the appropriate care of labouring women (Reime *et al.* 2004). There is still clearly a need for greater dialogue between the two professional groups, challenging though that is likely to be, given the historical imbalance of power between them.

The literature around models of birth runs a significant risk of essentialising the characteristics of contrasting beliefs when inter-relationships and practices in context do not reflect this. There are plenty of exceptions to the rule where obstetricians endorse normality and midwives favour intervention. Recent literature on the meaning of natural or normal birth demonstrates that neither is a self-evident state, which is revealed when all trappings of medicalisation are stripped away (Mansfield 2008). Instead, Mansfield argues that each is accomplished by enacting particular social practices which she suggests are related to activity during birth, preparation before birth and social support.

No one would argue that either a medical or social model of birth could be applied with consistency to every birth, depending on which model was favoured by the principal actors. Purists on both sides would agree that there may be a place for elements of each in certain births. Even the elective Caesarean choice can be undertaken in a women-centred, holistic way and, from time to time, natural labours require medical interventions. Davis-Floyd *et al.* (2001) argues for a postmodern midwife who can seamlessly traverse between social and technocratic models but that transition often requires a geographical movement between home or birth centre and hospital. Does working and birthing in different settings hinder or help the provision of intrapartum care? The next section examines this issue.

Place of birth debate

Nowhere has the divide over place of birth been more evident than in the United Kingdom. Against a backdrop of a long history of home-birth provision by midwives, recent wholesale hospitalisation of birth has prompted argument and counter-argument around the interpretation of evidence (Gyte & Dodwell 2007; Steer 2008). Though epidemiological research is very reassuring about the safety of home birth, when the National Institute for Health and Clinical Excellence (NICE) intrapartum guideline was being formulated in 2007, different members of the guideline group could not agree on the weighting of evidence around home-birth transfers (Gyte & Dodwell 2007). One of the consumer representatives resigned in protest at the way some of the professionals on the group had admitted evidence that was clearly not robust enough. It was as though their deeply held beliefs about the risks of home birth won out over a dispassionate consideration of the evidence.

It is now acknowledged by the most influential sources of evidence that there is no risk-based justification for requiring the birth of all women in hospital and, furthermore, that women should be offered an explicit choice when they become pregnant over where they want to have their baby (Enkin *et al.* 2000). Tew (1998) argues that the perinatal mortality rate for planned home birth is actually better at home than in hospital, though she is reliant on retrospective analysis of data. Nevertheless, her scholarship has been in-depth and meticulous. Most experts agree that it would be almost impossible to undertake a prospective randomised controlled trial in this area because of the large numbers required to establish statistical significance on perinatal mortality and because it is a topic that most women are not neutral about (Devane *et al.* 2004; Fullerton & Young 2007). In other words, they may be reluctant to be randomised to either hospital or home.

Apart from the recent NICE Intrapartum Guideline (NICE 2007), the most comprehensive recent review of the home-birth research literature was undertaken by Fullerton and Young (2007) and included 26 studies from many parts of the developed world. The conclusions were that the 'studies demonstrate remarkably consistency in the generally favourable results of maternal and neonatal outcomes, both over time and among diverse population groups.' (p. 323) The outcomes were also favourable when viewed in comparison to various reference groups (birth centre births, planned hospital births).

It is important to note that randomised controlled trials have demonstrated clear benefit in a number of associated elements of the home-birth 'package of care'. These include continuity of care during labour and birth (Hodnett *et al.* 2007) and midwife-led care (Hatem *et al.* 2008), both of which are probably universal aspects of home-birth provision.

Though official UK-government policy up to the present is to offer women a choice about the place of birth, the national home-birth rate is still only about 2% compared with 25% in the early 1960s (The Information Centre 2006). Despite the rhetoric of choice, there are plenty of anecdotal stories of women being discouraged from choosing the home-birth option.

Home birth has been described by Cheyney (2008) as 'systems-challenging praxis' because it is such a countercultural choice in the western world. Both women and midwives have to challenge powerful discourses of safety, authoritative obstetric knowledge and professional hegemony to secure their choice of home birth. What was exciting about her findings of women choosing home birth in the United States was the narrative of personal empowerment that was a consequence of their choice. Many spoke of inhabiting the metaphysical place of 'labourland' where they uncovered and experienced the power of birth that left them in awe.

There are no randomised controlled trials and generally a paucity of good quality research on free-standing birth centres or midwifery-led units. Walsh and Downe's (2004) structured review found these environments lowered childbirth interventions but methodological weaknesses in all studies made conclusions tentative at best. Stewart *et al.*'s (2005) commissioned review reached similar conclusions. However, this model has still been endorsed by the Department of Health (2007) in the Maternity Matters Report and this may reflect policy thinking that free-standing birth centres would be unlikely to have worse outcomes than home birth as a similar profile of women use both.

Regarding integrated birth centres or alongside midwifery-led units, evaluations have shown no statistical difference in perinatal mortality and encouraging results regarding the reduction in some labour interventions (Hodnett *et al.* 2005). Debate has continued to rage over the noted non-significant trend in some of the studies of higher perinatal mortality for first-time mothers (Fahy 2005; Tracy *et al.* 2007). This is unlikely to be resolved until contextual studies exploring the interface at transfer or clinical governance arrangements or the impact of contrasting philosophies is examined in depth.

All of which underlines the need for robust, prospective, multi-method studies which separate out modes of care from types of birthing centre and this is now being addressed by the birthplace study being conducted by the National Perinatal Epidemiology Unit (NPEU 2008).

Qualitative literature on home birth and free-standing birth centres highlight two other aspects of care in these settings. These are to do with how temporality is enacted and how smallness of scale impacts on the ethos and ambience of care. The regulatory effect of clock time is much less in evidence both at home and in birth centres. Labour rhythms rather than labour progress tend to be emphasised by staff and there is usually greater flexibility with the application of partograms. Part of the reason for this lies in the absence of an organisational imperative to 'get women through the system' (Walsh 2006a). Small numbers of women birthing mean less stress on organisational processes and a more relaxed ambience in the setting. This appears to suit women and staff well. It also appears to be attuned to labour physiology, which inherently manifests biological rhythms based on hormonal pulses of activity, rather than regular clock-time rhythms (Adams 1995).

Home birth and birth centres have enormous potential to expand as currently they provide 4% or less of all births across the western world (Walsh 2007a). This represents a tiny proportion of all suitable births. Estimates of what proportion of women might take up this option vary from 15% (Wagner 2006) to 80% (Arms 1999). Within the United Kingdom, there is evidence that long-standing integrated birth centres birth around 25% of all births from their catchment areas (Walsh 2006b).

Contemporary challenges

Current issues for intrapartum care are divergent depending on whether one is considering the Western world or the developing world. For the latter, the spectre of unacceptable perinatal and maternal mortality continues to dominate the agenda. Yet even here, strategies to address the problem have to be more than replicating high-tech Western-style maternity hospitals. Arguable poverty is the greatest killer of all in these contexts, but as Ronsmans and Graham (2006) comment, the statistics defy simplistic analysis and the identification of linear cause and effect. Multiple interventions are required to address a complex phenomenon, including the provision of midwifery care to remote areas.

In the west, morbidity rates are on the rise in some countries, primarily related to private provision of maternity care where financial incentives reward intervention (Block 2007). Governments are vexed by the problem of how to incentivise non-intervention as the Payment by Results formulae in England illustrates (O'Sullivan & Tyler 2007). As one would expect intuitively, midwifery-led care of low-risk women is cheap (Tracy & Tracy 2003) with clear reductions in consumables. It is likely that the imperative to provide one-to-one care in labour will drive alternative service provision as this is always more complex to address in large maternity hospitals. What is emerging in the western world is the rationalisation of perinatal services by the creation of tertiary centres of excellence forming a hub for local midwifery-led units or birth centre and home birth (Maternity & Newborn Working Party 2007). This model is likely to increase the numbers of birth centres and midwifery-led units and will be welcomed by service users and midwives.

This will contribute positively to addressing the trend to increasing medicalisation of birth but this phenomenon is fed by a number of powerful discourses including the techno-rationalist age, risk and professional power (Walsh 2006b). Techno-rationalism proffers that science is progressive and altruistic, and holds an optimistic view of technology (Lauritzen & Sachs 2001). It is challenging for an anthropological approach to childbirth to have credibility, competing for women's hearts and minds, when up against such a ubiquitous and pervasive alternative. In what other context of our lives would we embrace pain as part of 'rites of passage' transition? In what other context would we reject the use of technology in favour of traditional skills? This is why preserving the anthropological alternative in out-of-hospital birth settings is so crucial. It is unlikely that these frontiers will ever be rolled back in hospital where professional vested interest in maintaining them is strong. In the hospital context, technologies application in treating pathology is appropriate and beneficial but in childbirth its attendant iatrogenic effects have undermined this intent. In addition, the integration of technologies with labour care in the context of institutional hospitals has tended to dehumanise the birth experience (Kitzinger 2006).

Sensitivity to the user voice in maternity care is also driving reform, especially around choice and options for birth. As in broader health, the rise and rise of what are now called 'experts by experience' (Preston-Shoot 2007), is requiring service providers to move beyond tokenism in user consultation to planning services and evaluations with them. This is beginning to challenge professional and managerial power as a number of stories of resisting closures of birth centres illustrate (Walsh 2006a).

Conclusion

The future is uncertain regarding trends in intrapartum care. The postmodern era that we are moving into is characterised by choice, eclecticism and a suspicion of grand narratives that propose to answer all the questions (Walsh 2007b). Both technocratic birth and natural birth are childbirth versions of a grand narrative. Neither can claim complete jurisdiction over the vagaries of the childbirth experience, though both have an appropriate context of application. There will continue to be ongoing tension over their respective claim on the care and practices in childbirth.

References

Adams B (1995) *Timewatch: The Social Analysis of Time*. Cambridge, Polity Press.

Arms S (1999) *Birthing the Future*, available from http://www.suzannearms.com/OurStore/ (accessed 02/08).

Barros F, Victoria C, Barros D *et al.* (2005) The challenge of reducing neonatal mortality in middle-income countries: findings from three Brazilian birth cohorts in 1982, 1993, and 2004. *Lancet* 365: 847–54.

Block J (2007) *Pushed: The Painful Truth about Childbirth and Modern Maternity Care*. Los Angeles, De Capo Life Long Books.

Cheyney M (2008) Homebirth as systems-challenging praxis: knowledge, power, and intimacy in the birthplace. *Qualitative Health Research* 18(2): 254–67.

Christiaens W, Bracke P (2007) Does a referral from home to hospital affect satisfaction with childbirth? A cross-national comparison. *BMC Health Services Research*, http://www.biomedcentral.com/content/pdf/1471-2393-7-26.pdf. (accessed 12/08).

Davis-Floyd R (1992) *Birth as an American Rite of Passage*. London, University of California Press.

Davis-Floyd R, Cosminsky S, Leigh Pigg S (eds) (2001) Daughters of time: the shifting identities of contemporary midwives. A special triple issue of *Medical Anthropology* 2–3: 4.

Declerq E, Sakala C, Corry M, Applebaum S, Risher P (2002) *Listening to Mothers: Report of the First National US Survey of Women's Childbearing Experiences*. New York, Maternity Center Association.

Department of Health (1993) *Changing Childbirth: Report of the Expert Committee on Maternity Care*. London, HMSO.

Department of Health (2007) *Maternity Matters: Choice, Access and Continuity of Care in a Safe Service*. London, DH.

Devane D, Begley C, Clarke M (2004) How many do I need: basis principles of sample size calculation. *Journal of Advanced Nursing* 47(3): 297–302.

Donnison J (1988) *Midwives and Medical Men*. London, Historical Publications.

Enkin M, Kierse M, Renfrew M, Neilson J (2000) *A Guide to Effective Care in Pregnancy and Childbirth*. Oxford, Oxford University Press.

Fahy K (1998) Being a midwife or doing midwifery? *Australian Midwives Journal* 11(2): 11–6.

Fahy K (2005) Safety of Stockholm birth centre study: a critical review. *Birth* 32(2): 145–50.

Foucault M (1979) The eye of power. In Gordon C (ed) *Power/Knowledge*. Brighton, Harvester Press.

Fullerton J, Young S (2007) Outcomes of planned home birth: an integrative review. *Journal of Midwifery and Women's Health* 52: 323–33.

Goer H (2004) Humanising birth: a global grassroots movement. *Birth* 31(4): 308–14.

Gyte G, Dodwell M (2007) Safety of planned home birth: an nct review of the evidence. *New Digest* 40: 1–10.

Hatem M, Hodnett ED, Devane D, Fraser WD, Sandall J, Soltani H (2008) Midwifery-led versus other models of care delivery for childbearing women. (Protocol) *Cochrane Database of Systematic Reviews* (4).

Hirst C (2005) *Rebirthing: Report of the Review of the Maternity Services in Qld.* Brisbane, Qld.

Hodnett ED, Downe S, Edwards N, Walsh D (2005) Home-like versus conventional institutional settings for birth. *The Cochrane Database of Systematic Reviews* (4).

Hodnett E, Gates S, Hofmeyr G, Sakala C (2007) Continuous support for women during childbirth. *The Cochrane Database of Systematic Reviews* (3).

The Information Centre (2006) *NHS Maternity Statistics England 2004–2005*, available online: www.ic.nhs.uk (accessed December, 2008).

Johanson R, Newburn M, Macfarlane A (2002) Has medicalisation of childbirth gone too far? *British Medical Journal* 321: 892–5.

Jordan B (1983) *Birth in Four Cultures: A Cross-Cultural Investigation of Childbirth in Yucatan, Holland, Sweden and the United States.* Montreal, Eden Press.

Kirkham M (2004) *Birth Centres: A Social Model for Maternity Care.* London, Books for Midwives Press.

Kitzinger S (2006) *Birth Crisis.* Abingdon, Routledge.

Lauritzen S, Sachs L (2001) Normality, risk and the future: implicit communication of threat in health surveillance. *Sociology of Health and Illness* 23(4): 497–516.

Longman P (2006) The Return of Patriarchy. Foreign Policy Magazine, March 1, 1–3.

Maier B, Lechner M, Akmanlar-Hirscher G, Staudach A (2000) Caesarean section on demand: medical and ethical challenges. *International Journal of Obstetrics and Gynaecology* 70(1): 52.

Mansfield B (2008) The social nature of natural childbirth. *Social Science and Medicine* 66: 1084–94.

Maternity & Newborn Clinical Working Party (2007) *Review of London Maternity Services*, available from: http://www.yorksandhumber.nhs.uk/Library/Communications/Darzi/London%20Maternity%20and%20Newborn%20Working%20Group%20Report.pdf (accessed March, 2008).

National Perinatal Epidemiology Unit (2008) *Birthplace Study.* http://www.npeu.ox.ac.uk/birthplace (accessed March, 2008).

NICE (2007) *Intrapartum care: Care of Healthy Women and their Babies During Childbirth.* London, NHS.

O'Sullivan S, Tyler S (2007) Payment by results: speaking in code. *Midwives* 10(5): 241.

Page L (1995) *Effective Group Practice in Midwifery: Working with Women.* London, Blackwell Science.

Preston-Shoot M (2007) Whose lives and whose learning? Whose narratives and whose writing? Taking the next research and literature steps with experts by experience. *Evidence and Policy* 3(3): 343–59.

Rauchenstein T (2008) *New Dualism.* http://www.newdualism.org/papers/T.Rauchenstein/mbd.htm (accessed October, 2008).

REHUNA (2008) *Statement on the Humanisation of Birth*. http://www.rehuna. org.br/ (accessed October, 2008).

Reime B, Klein M, Kelly A, Duxbury N, Saxell L (2004) Do maternity care provider groups have different attitudes towards birth? *BJOG: An International Journal of Obstetrics and Gynaecology* 111: 1388–93.

Rhodes P (1995) *A Short History of Clinical Midwifery: The Development of Ideas in the Professional Management of Childbirth Cheshire (Books for Midwives)*, Hale.

Roberts C, Algert C, Peat B, Tracy S, Douglas I (2002) Trends in labour and birth interventions among low-risk women in an Australian population. *Australia and New Zealand Journal of Obstetrics and Gynaecology* 42(2): 176–81.

Ronsmans C, Graham W (2006) Maternal survival 1. Maternal mortality: who, when, where and why. *The Lancet* 368: 1189–200.

Rosenberg K, Trevathan W (2002) Birth, obstetrics and human evolution. *BJOG: An International Journal of Obstetrics and Gynaecology* 109(11): 1199–206.

Steer P (2008) How safe is home birth? Editors Choice. *BJOG, An International Journal of Obstetrics and Gynaecology* 115(5): i–ii.

Stewart M, McCandlish R, Henderson J, Brocklehurst P (2005) *Report of a Structured Review of Birth Centre Outcomes, 2004*. Oxford, National Perinatal Epidemiology Unit, University of Oxford.

Tew M (1998) *Safer Childbirth? A Critical History of Maternity Care*. London, Chapman & Hall.

Tracy S, Dahlen H, Caplice S *et al*. (2007) Birth centres in Australia: a national population-based study of perinatal mortality associated with giving birth in a birth centre. *Birth* 34(3): 194–201.

Tracy S, Tracy M (2003) Costing the cascade: estimating the cost of increased obstetric intervention in childbirth using population data. *BJOG: An International Journal of Obstetrics and Gynaecology* 110(8): 717–24.

Van Teijlingen E, Lowis J, McCaffery P, Porter M (2000) *Midwifery and the Medicalisation of Childbirth: Comparative Perspectives*. London, Nova Medical.

Wagner M (2001) Fish can't see water: the need to humanize birth. *International Journal of Gynaecology and Obstetrics* 75: S25–S37.

Wagner M (2006) *Born in the USA: How a Broken Maternity System Must be Fixed to Put Women and Children First*. London, University of California Press.

Walsh D (2006a) Subverting assembly-line birth: childbirth in a free-standing birth centre. *Social Science and Medicine* 62(6): 1330–40.

Walsh D (2006b) Risk and normality in maternity care. In Symon A (ed) *Risk and Choice in Childbirth*. London, Elsevier Science.

Walsh D (2007a) *Improving Maternity Service. Small is Beautiful: Lessons for Maternity Services from a Birth Centre*. Oxford, Radcliffe Publishing.

Walsh D (2007b) A birth centre's encounters with discourses of childbirth: how resistance led to innovation. *Sociology of Health and Illness* 29(2): 216–32.

Walsh D, Downe S (2004) Outcomes of free-standing, midwifery-led birth centres: a structured review of the evidence. *Birth* 31(3): 222–9.

Walsh D, Newburn M (2002) Towards a social model of childbirth: part 1. *British Journal of Midwifery* 10(8): 476–81.

Zergan J (2005) *Patriarchy, Civilisation and the Origins of Gender*. http://www. insurgentdesire.org.uk/patriarchy.htm (accessed March, 2008).

Chapter 2
Debates about Knowledge and Intrapartum Care

Soo Downe

Introduction

The following exchange between Humpty Dumpty and Alice may, at first glance, just seem to be a childish nonsense:

> 'When I use a word,' Humpty Dumpty said, in rather a scornful tone, 'it means just what I choose it to mean – neither more nor less.'
> 'The question is,' said Alice, 'whether you can make words mean so many different things.'
> 'The question is,' said Humpty Dumpty, 'which is to be master – that's all.'
>
> (Carroll 1994)

However, beyond the children's story, Lewis Carroll was raising important issues about what words mean and, therefore, about the kind of knowledge that counts, and the way the world is perceived and understood, by both societies and individuals. As Humpty Dumpty so insightfully noted, the most important thing to know in trying to understand a society and how it operates is 'which is to be master'. In Jordan's terms, this is determined by whose knowledge is authoritative:

> the power of authoritative knowledge is not that it is correct, but that it counts
>
> (Jordan 1997, p. 58)

This chapter explores the changing nature of authoritative knowledge in childbirth, and the way this might impact on service delivery and decision-making.

Ways of seeing childbirth

As Jordan has noted elsewhere 'Birth is *everywhere socially marked and shaped*' (Jordan 1993). Most cultures and individuals appear to recognise that childbirth is a transforming event, both for an individual, and for a society. In many communities across the world, the events of pregnancy and birth are still marked by formal rites of passage (Grimes 2000). These rites note that first birth, in particular, changes the mother (and father) fundamentally, both in terms of the social role they adopt, and in their physical, emotional and psychological outlook on life. Also for birth, formal rites of passage operate in life-changing events such as coming of age, marriage (or pair bonding) and death. They tend to separate the individual from their cultural norms, and to expose them to dangerous or frightening events. This causes the individual to have to draw on inner resources they did not know they had, as they do battle with unknown forces and deal with difficult or dangerous situations they have never encountered before, in a so-called liminal, or 'betwixt and between' state of being. If the individual triumphs, they complete the rite of passage, and re-enter the community in their new role.

Most high-resource societies in which midwives work no longer have these formal rites of passage. However, birth is an undeniably life-changing event. Even without a formal way of framing it, women who are actively experiencing childbirth usually encounter stages of fear, liminality, hard and painful work, and triumph. Some of the positive consequences of this are explored further in other chapters in this book. In post-industrial late modern societies, childbirth is governed by institutional ritual and expectations, which define the way it should be conducted, who should be present, and even the type of physical experiences the women (and their partners) should undergo (Kitzinger 1987). For example, since the 1970s, childbirth activists have claimed that the rituals of removing women's clothes, forcing them to shower, undertaking perineal shaves, and administering enemas were all processes designed to strip women of their autonomy, making them ready to receive the administrations of the maternity care system at the time (Arms 1975; Kitzinger 1987; Gaskin 1990). This can be seen as a classic rite of passage process, even if the formal biomedical justification (at the time) was the reduction of infection for mother and baby.

The underpinning rationale used for these rites of passage events demonstrated the prevailing epistemology and ontology of the time and the culture in which they apply. Epistemology refers to the nature of knowledge – how we (choose to) know what we know. Ontology refers to the nature of reality: what we perceive things to be. The next section addresses some of the epistemological and ontological systems that have been in operation in the maternity services in many countries of the world in recent history.

Framing of childbirth as a religious duty

Until the early 20th century, much of the formal history we have on childbirth comes from medical practitioners, and not from women or midwives. Between the late 19th and early 20th centuries in most of the Western word, philosophical ideas were beginning to migrate from a largely religious (usually Christian) ideology, that saw pain in labour as a God-given trial that should be endured, towards a biological process that could be understood through the science of observation and deduction from the natural world. An example of this difference in ontological understanding is provided by the debate in the United Kingdom and the United States about pain relief in labour at this time in history, when pharmacological methods were just beginning to be developed.

An article published in 1846 in the Boston Surgical and Medical Journal (Bigelow 1846) reports on a demonstration of the efficacy of inhaled ether by William Morton, a dentist. Bigelow reported that ether had been used orally since the beginning of the 19th century, but that the inhalation method had been viewed with some suspicion, despite accounts of its successful use in animals as early as 1816. Dr Crawford Long, reporting in the Southern Medical Journal in 1849, claims its first use in a surgical operation in 1842, and backs this up with an affidavit from the patient involved (Long 1849). However, despite the increasing acceptance of ether as an anaesthetic in the surgical field, the use of pharmacological pain relief in maternity care was slow to develop. A number of authors have examined the initial resistance to, and gradual acceptance of, pharmacological agents for the relief of pain in childbirth (Caton 1970; Farr 1980; Zuck 1991). These authors suggest that resistance to the introduction of such analgesia was based on three grounds: religious opposition to interference with 'God-given' pain; moral objections to the presumed effects of ether in rousing women's sexual passions; and medical concerns, both that pain is therapeutic in indicating excessive interference, and in causing improved healing, and that the use of narcotic agents caused morbidity and mortality to mother and fetus. It certainly seems to be likely that the general reluctance amid the emerging profession of obstetrics to chloroform and ether was rooted in society's attitude to the pain of childbirth, which was that it was a natural trial that should be borne as part of the lot of women. Connor and Conner quote the following which illustrates this point:

> No female for whom I have any regard shall, with my consent, inhale chloroform. I look upon its exhibition as pandering to the weakness of humanity, especially the weaker sex.
>
> (Connor & Connor 1996)

Movement towards (and away from) scientific medicine

However, the simple division between God and nature, doctor and patient, and men and women that is suggested by the analysis above is misleading. From the early 1900s, discoveries such as penicillin and acceptance of the importance of hygiene began to change maternal and infant mortality rates, but women were still desperate for improvements in their experience of childbirth. The foundation of the National Birthday Trust in 1928 was prompted by concerns of influential women about the lack of access of working class women to obstetric care, and to pain relief in labour. The Trust lobbied successfully to increase such access, and their intervention popularised, and made accessible, the minnitt apparatus for delivering nitrous oxide and oxygen to labouring women, both at home and in hospital (Beinart 1990; Caton 1996). The pressure group, the Association for Improvements in Maternity Services (AIMS), was formed in 1960, initially to increase access for women to hospital beds (Durward & Evans 1990). This continued some of the work that had been undertaken by the Women's Co-operative Guild maternity campaign (Lewis 1990). Paradoxically, 4 years earlier, the National Childbirth Trust was formed, to promote 'natural' ways of approaching childbirth, following the work of the obstetricians Dick Read and Lamaze (Kitzinger 1990). There was, therefore, an interesting dichotomy prevailing – some activists were seeking an increase in access to the perceived advantages of a medicalised hospital environment, while others were attempting to minimise the use of drugs in labour.

The development of pain relief in labour was simultaneously championed and opposed both by doctors, and women of all classes. Happlin (1997) concurs with Leavitts' (1986) analysis of the potential for women to set the childbirth agenda, and states that

> many leaders of the twilight-sleep movement were suffragists and women's rights leaders. Twilight-sleep represented women's control over birth decisions.

However, most of the agents available at that time did not have specific analgesic properties beyond their amnesic effect, and there was an increasing recognition in the obstetric literature that they had harmful side-effects, particularly relating to haemorrhage and the effect on respiration for the baby. Elam (1943) noted that the Royal College of Obstetrics and Gynaecology, in a report in 1936, had not approved the use of either paraldehyde or chloroform. This left very few agents, none of which had any specific anaesthetic effect. As John Elam goes on to claim:

> ... anaesthesia and analgesia in obstetrics is not only a medical problem, but a sociological one.

Within 25 years of this statement, views about the meaning of childbirth pain had changed radically. Most hospitals administered inhalation analgesia, many used narcotics and opiates, and the consensus of opinion was swinging towards the development of techniques such as epidural analgesia. The prevailing ontology of childbirth had changed in a generation, and, to use Kuhn's term, the post-industrial 'normal science' (Kuhn 1970) of observation, measurement and objective enquiry began to form the basis of formal, institutional maternity care provision in many parts of the world.

Positivist science in the ascendancy

The concept of (logical) positivism, or objectivism, began to be developed by the so-called 'Vienna Circle' in the 1920s (Crotty 1998). The philosophy spread widely over the next few decades. Its basic epistemology was that knowledge about the world can only be developed by observational evidence of what things are, and how they work, and that this evidence can best be obtained by mathematical deduction and theorising. Some of the principles of the theory were challenged as it dispersed. Most notably for this chapter, Karl Popper disputed the (ontological) assumption that, if we look hard enough and long enough, we will eventually gather enough information to verify how the world is, once and for all. Popper proposed that we can only ever get close to this truth, and that the way to do this was to propose a hypothesis, then try to falsify it (Popper 1959). As each theory is found to have flaws, a better and more precise theory can be proposed. This is the basic philosophy of basic biological science, and of the randomised controlled trial (RCT), both of which are dominant (but by no means universal) ways of finding out about pregnancy and childbirth in late modern societies.

Once established as a profession, the authority of medical practitioners to dictate the application of new clinical techniques was largely unquestioned by external agencies. There is, however, convincing evidence that internal challenges relating to particular techniques have always been prevalent, as examples in maternity care have demonstrated (Arney 1982; Tew 1990; Loudon 1992; Chamberlain *et al.* 1993; Graham 1997). Practice usually developed through trial and error, anecdotes and sharing of case studies (Bromley 1986). However, even influential individuals, such as the American obstetrician DeLee, were called upon by colleagues to provide objective, positivist evidence for more radical claims (Graham 1997, p. 49). The development of the RCT as applied to health care issues was a consequence of this increasing concern to find out if health care practices were really effective at the level of populations (Meinert 1986). The RCT was a revolution in the design, collection and analysis of data. It was borrowed from the design of experiments undertaken by agriculturists. It is based on the logic that if you rule out anything that might affect an outcome, then introduce the one element that you want to test for some of those in the experiment, but not for others, you will find out if the new element works or not. Any other element that is introduced (such as culture, gender, the state of mind of the participants, or the beliefs of the practitioners about the intervention) is seen as 'noise' that gets in the way of finding the true answer to the question under investigation. Randomising people to either the intervention or the control group allows both known and unknown 'noise' to be controlled for. To those who believed that universal truths were there to be discovered, this new technique promised answers to the vexed problem of what works in health care.

The challenge from interpretivists and constructionists

The argument against logical positivism as the sole epistemology for health care is that it over-simplifies human experience. Humans are influenced by society and culture, and not just by the biological and physical elements around them. At the same time as positivist positions were gaining dominance in the science of health, those studying the social world of human culture were drawing on alternative positions, such as constructionism and interpretivism (Crotty 1998). These researchers held that people make sense of the world through social interaction and language, and not just by observing and relating to objects and events in the physical world. In this way of seeing, the same physical things and events are interpreted very differently by different individuals, depending on their cultural and social history. Anthropologists and sociologists were early adopters in this field of largely qualitative research. These groups developed methodological approaches like ethnography (focused on culture), grounded theory (focused on the generation of new theories to understand social situations) and approaches based in the philosophy of phenomenology (focused on the meaning-making of individuals). Their methods included interviews, focus groups, and observational fieldwork.

The difference between so-called objective (positivist) and subjective (interpretivist/constructionist) positions is more than methodological. For some, it was deeply political. For example, feminists and ethnic activists were quick to appreciate the value of the phenomenological approach (Phoenix 1990; Fisher & Embree 1999). Their critique was that the so-called objectivity of 'normal' (positivist) science was in fact a creation of the dominant Western (white, middle class, male, heterosexual, Christian) society. Attention to the cultural and personal dimensions of knowing allowed those outside this culture to finally make their voices heard (Phoenix 1990, pp. 92–3). Other marginalised groups have also seized on qualitative research as a way of gaining a voice. These include midwives and childbearing women (Kitzinger 1976; Kirkham 1987; Hunt & Symonds 1995).

For some philosophers and researchers, the two ontological positions described above are impossible to reconcile: either there is a *truth* waiting to be found, or there is not (Lincoln & Guba 1985). However, over the last couple of decades, there has been something of reconciliation between these two positions.

Bringing it all together

Since the early 1980s philosophers and researchers have begun to focus on the potential combination of positivist and more constructed positions, and on both qualitative and quantitative research ways of seeing. Bryman (1988) noted that different problems may need different methods:

> Rather than the somewhat doctrinaire posturing of a great deal of the literature dealing with the epistemological leanings of quantitative and qualitative research, there should be a greater recognition in discussions of the ... need to generate good research ... The critical issue is to be aware of the appropriateness of particular methods (or combinations of methods) for particular issues
>
> (Bryman 1988, p. 173)

Acceptance of the value of mixed methods has become increasingly evident (Daly & McDonald 1992). Proposals have come from researchers in fields as diverse as occupational therapy (Short-DeGraff & Fisher 1993) and maternity care (Oakley 1992). More recently, there has been a move to so-called 'realist research' that seeks to find out 'what works, for who, in what circumstances' (Pawson *et al.* 2005). This is a clear move towards the particular needs of individuals in their cultural, social and historical environments, and away from knowledge that is developed with large populations, and then applied in clinical practice to all individuals, regardless of their particular circumstances. Indeed, even the architects of evidence-based medicine held that

> Evidence-based medicine (EBM) is the integration of best research evidence with clinical expertise and patient value ... when these three elements are integrated, clinicians and patients form (an) ... alliance which optimises clinical outcomes and quality of life ...
>
> (Sackett *et al.* 2002)

Despite the continuing dominance of health care protocols and guidelines based on randomised trial data, there is some evidence that the more relative approach to knowledge for health care is becoming more mainstream (Wilson *et al.* 2001). The recent National Institute for Health and Clinical Excellence (NICE) guidelines for ante- and post-natal mental health use individual stories alongside more formal studies, to illustrate the fact that each person must be treated in their particular social and culture context, with an understanding of their personal life history (NICE 2007).

Oakley (1992) in reviewing the theoretical, philosophical and procedural basis of the Social Support and Mothering trial, offers a good example of a way forward. She illustrates the false dichotomy implicit in rejection of one or other technique, as she states:

> Science and knowledge are socially produced: that is, they are subject to the very influence of social processes and practicalities that their common-sense representations would dismiss as quite beyond their frames of references.
>
> (Oakley 1992, p. 335)

In an earlier paper relating to the same study (Oakley 1989) she succinctly argued the case for a common, value-free conceptualisation of the fundamental philosophy of research (and, by extension, of the kind of formal knowledge that should be used in health care). She claims that the tension between techniques such as randomisation and informed consent, or attention to protocol and clinical need, can be overcome, and the essential value of the RCT as a replicable, sound piece of evidence in guiding care can be matched with a participant-centred approach to the running of the trial. Oakley's study illustrates her hypothesis that the methodological debates are not mutually exclusive. She suggests the following factors in creating a 'non-dichotomous discourse of knowledge':

1. there is no single right way to present an enquiry . . . .
2. the standpoint of the researcher is critical . . . it is the failure to understand and explicate this that is dangerous, not the obverse
3. the primary goal of scientific research is not knowing but understanding . . .
4. experimental research . . . is possible . . . within the social sciences . . . .
5. such research . . . demands . . . attention to the standpoint of all those who take part in it . .
6. the knowledge demand for quantifiable data . . . must be combined with the understanding to be obtained by attention to subjective narrative . . .

7. it is out of the dialectic between the two that research findings are produced, and within which they are located ...

(Oakley 1989, p. 344–5)

Alternative explanations for childbirth processes, including complexity theory

In 1972, Archie Cochrane, then director of the Medical Research Council Epidemiology Unit, published a seminal book, entitled '*Effectiveness and Efficiency*' (Cochrane 1972). This put forward the apparently simple view that 'all *effective* treatment must be free' (my emphasis). Its implication was revolutionary in that it proposed by default that ineffective treatment should not be free. This agenda has become central to governmental thinking over the last decade. The problem arises in trying to define what is effective. This is not merely a matter of asking 'does it work', but, fundamentally, of deciding what should be evaluated, how this should be done, and how the results should be interpreted. More recently, Murray Enkin, one of the architects of the Cochrane Collaboration has confessed:

> This paper ... was conceived during an era of medical authoritarianism, born in a time of nascent ... family-centered maternity care, matured in a period of enthusiastic (but not unquestioning) homage to evidence-based obstetrics, and culminated in a reluctant but comforting acceptance of uncertainty ... it is, to use an ancient word I only recently learned, a clinamen, a swerve, a point of intellectual revision ...
>
> (Enkin *et al.* 2006)

There are echoes here of Ralph Pawson's Realist Research position mentioned (Pawson *et al.* 2005). Enkin's recent position also seems to be influenced by the growing sense that many scientific truths that have been taken for granted for most of the last 200 years are facing serious challenges, both by the recognition of the value of alternative positions noted above, and by the new science of complexity and chaos (Soloman 1985; Gleick 1998; Kernick 2002; Sweeney & Griffiths 2002). In outline, this science is based on the findings of thermodynamics. It recognises that many natural events are not linear. In a classic example, if water is heated, it will not heat up gradually at regular intervals, but it will suddenly move from not-boiling to boiling. It reaches a kind of 'tipping point' after which it changes state completely. Climate change is the most dramatic example of chaos theory in action. Models that predict that change will happen gradually over decades have had to be re-written as it seems that a tipping point has been reached after which melting happens much quicker than linear models would predict (Hasselmann 1999).

Complexity models are slightly different from chaotic ones. As in chaos models, complexity theory holds that most systems (the body, the weather, the heart, global finance) are highly interconnected, in a web-like manner, as networks. This means that messages, physical effects, and beliefs can travel exponentially through these networks, so that changes to systems do not need each person or element to link with everyone else directly. The internet is a clear example of this. Change can happen almost instantaneously in this kind of system. Chaos is the point reached when complex systems tip out of balance much more quickly and completely than might be expected, move from one state (for example, not boiling) to a completely new one (boiling).

This kind of understanding means that many of the formal ways of knowing that worked well when the world was less well-networked no longer seem to be so efficient. This is important for maternity care. As Downe and McCourt (2008) have observed, theories of complexity and chaos provide a different way of seeing how pregnancy and childbirth work, and particularly how they work for women who do not fit the 'norms' generated by linear research models. These newer ways of seeing allow for labour and birth as a process with its own rhythms (see Chapter 5) or cycles (see Chapter 10) governed by non-linear processes, such as the pulsatile cycles that govern hormonal activity.

The clear example of this in action is the woman who seems to be progressing slowly, who then suddenly seems to become extremely restless and distressed, declaring she wants to push (or, commonly, that she wants an epidural). Often, if the woman is supported over this transitional phase, the baby is born soon after. In this case, a tipping point has been reached in the neurohormonally interconnected network of the woman's body, and she moves rapidly from one state (early labour) to another (expulsive contractions). If this process is judged linearly, she seems to be completely out of control, as the partogramme would indicate that she could not possibly be ready to push. This reading leads to interference and a disruption of the labour process, usually through the administration of an epidural. If labour is seen as a complex dynamic process, the alternative reading that labour is progressing normally can be used, and the woman can be supported over the chaos of transition and into the hard and productive work of pushing. A number of the chapters in this book provide more discussion of these kinds of situations, informed by newly emerging knowledge about the impact of networked bodily systems, and neurohormonal feedback loops that operate under hormonal influence. These kinds of analysis of biological processes are likely to become more mainstream, as medical academics are increasingly willing to think in terms of complex systems:

> Health can only be maintained (or re-established) through a holistic approach that accepts unpredictability and builds on subtle emergent forces within the overall system.
>
> (Wilson *et al.* 2001)

An emerging approach to capturing more individualised experience is the collection of stories, or narratives. The next section examines this trend.

Knowledge from narratives and personal histories

In contrast to the kind of knowledge arising from randomised controlled trials, and even from formal qualitative research methods, such as ethnography and phenomenology, there is a growing interest in the highly individual and personal knowledge and insights that arise from story telling and narrative. Stories have always featured in midwifery practice: these include the tales told of a particularly difficult or unusual case at handovers, or in the staff room, and the 'did you hear' stories that come second and third hand from colleagues and friends. Tina Koch has written extensively in this area in the field of nursing. She noted that:

> Nursing work's wealth is found in the intensely personal, highly emotional, often brutal stories of everyday life as lived by clients and witnessed by nurse practitioners
>
> (Koch 1998)

These stories influence the conversations held between colleagues and with service users. In turn, the reality created by sharing the stories generates meaning. For example, stories of a woman who suffered a catastrophic haemorrhage at home birth may influence a whole team of caregivers against home-birth choices for women. These caregivers then tell the story to the women they come across, who then tell it to their friends, thus creating a local 'reality' that home birth is unsafe. This narrative reality can become a clinical reality if a lack of home-birth experience means that clinicians are not sure how to conduct such births safely. Conversely, if the conversation is changed, and positive stories of home birth are told, the reality of home birth locally can be completely transformed. Recognising the power of stories to organise experience,

Polkinghorne (1988) refers to narrative as 'a kind of organizational scheme expressed in story form'.

Beyond this point, and taking a constructivist approach, some would hold that hearing other people's stories makes their account and therefore their lives real, and that this provides a moral compass for the person doing the hearing:

> Being narratible implies value and attributes reality ... stories give legibility ... lives come from somewhere and they are going somewhere ... hearing the moral impulse in others' stories enables us to become part of their struggle to re-enchant a disenchanted world.
>
> (Frank 2002)

Practically, in maternity care hearing women's stories may provide important clues as to how they face childbirth, what their family history is, and what their hopes, fears and expectations are. If this accounting is limited to the tick boxes on a standard booking form, the account will only tell of those items of risk that population-based studies prompt us to ask about. This is stripped-down account of this particular woman's life. The bare nature of such accounts is in itself a risk, as it misses the opportunity for the woman to give her full story, that may contain hints and clues about risks, personal beliefs and cultures and, indeed salutogenic factors (see Chapter 16) that may materially affect her particular pregnancy, labour, and post-partum journey. In this case, the nature of knowledge is highly relative and particular. It is equally as meaningful for this woman in this pregnancy and labour as the research evidence generated by formal quantitative or qualitative research studies.

Conclusion: towards an ontology for childbirth in the 21st century

As Merry has said in considering the implications of complexity science:

> uncertainty, unpredictability, complexity and chaos are a natural, legitimate, necessary, inescapable aspect of reality, and will never go away
>
> (Merry 1995)

There is no evidence of a clear and consistent approach to childbirth taken by women or by clinicians at any one time or place. It appears that a number of discourses have always run in parallel to each other, with clinical practice shifting depending on which group has the strongest voice at any one time. The current rhetoric of choice would tend to suggest that all these competing ideologies could comfortably co-exist in contemporary maternity care. Such an assumption ignores the fact that this choice is to be exercised within a powerful hierarchy by those with the least control – the service users. This inability to make choice happen is illustrated by research which has examined the general lack of attention to women's voices (Belenky *et al.* 1986), and the specific effect of class on women's conceptions of childbirth, and consequent overt or covert choices (Nelson 1983; MacIntosh 1988). Such analyses illustrate that there are fundamental flaws in assumptions about the kind of choices women may make. The issue is even more complex when the model actually applied in many cases is based on professional interpretations of optimum childbirth which conflict with women's interpretations (Nelson 1983) despite high-profile governmental edicts designed to maximise 'women centred care'.

As Salsburg (1990) observes,

> There is no 'correct' (approach). Scientific reasoning consists of attempts to fit the complexities of reality into models useful for the organisation of observations ... some fit for the time being until we can find one that fits better, or until the lack of fit begins to trouble us. But we must always recognize that we fit our observations to very arbitrary models, and we must be prepared to abandon a model if it leads to nonsense.
>
> (Salsburg 1990, p. 296)

Following Rose (1983), the preferred ontological and epistemological stance for maternity care might be one based on *'hand brain and heart'*. This would lead to an approach in which

- equal value is given to a range of ways of knowing, including personal narrative;
- all stakeholders are engaged and respected;
- knowledge gained is of value to service users;
- the results obtained are always weighed up against the signs of health in the individual, even if this does not fit standard 'norms';
- the family and personal story of the woman is explored and taken seriously;
- decisions are based on the above, and on the values of the service user and the skills of the practitioner.

Knowledge and understanding from this perspective values well-designed studies from the whole range of possible perspectives and marries that with the wisdom gained from experience in both the expert practitioner, and the labouring woman and her birth companions. It is a knowledge that recognises the complex interconnectivity between the woman's personal and family history, society, culture, beliefs and expectations, her unique biophysical profile and responses, and the skills, experience, values and beliefs of those who support her in labour. It is also a perspective that recognises the knowledge that can be gained by a caring response that has been termed *love*, in its form of *caritas*. This response is engaged, empathetic, and mutually rewarding. It is explored in more detail as a form of 'prescencing' in Chapter 7.

In order to support women through the rite of passage that is childbirth, caregivers need to engage with and weigh up knowledge from a wide range of epistemological perspectives, and based on a range of ontological positions. Maybe at last we have moved on from Humpty Dumpty's position a little bit – words mean what we make them mean, but, in a postmodern age, we do not have to decide which is the master. We do, however, need to pay close attention to women, and to the way we negotiate knowledge with them. Maybe, again, Hilary Rose has a solution for the future:

> Where Bacon's origin story for science spoke of the intimate connection of knowledge and power, the feminist critique of science . . . has spoken of the danger of knowledge without love . . .
>
> (Rose 1994)

References

Arms S (1975) *Immaculate Deception: A New Look at Women and Childbirth*. Bantom Books, New York.

Arney WR (1982) *Power and the Provision Of Obstetrics*. London, University of Chicago press.

Beinart J (1990) Obstetric analgesia and childbirth. In Garcia J, Kilpatrick R, Richards M (eds) *The Politics of Maternity Care: Services for Childbearing Women in Twentieth Century Britain*. Oxford, Clarendon Paperbacks, 116–32.

Belenky M, Clinchy B, Goldberger N, Tarule J (1986) *Women's Ways of Knowing*. New York, Basic Books.

Bigelow HJ (1846) Insensibility during surgical operations produced by inhalation. *Boston Medical and Surgical Journal* 35: 16p.

Bromley DB (1986) *The Case Study Method in Psychology and Related Disciplines*. New York, John Wiley & Sons.

Bryman A (1988) *Quantity and Quality in Social Research*. London, Routledge.

Carroll L (1994) (first published 1872) *Through the Looking Glass (Chapter VI: Humpty Dumpty)*. London, Penguin Classics.

Caton D (1970) July obstetric anesthesia: the first ten years. *Anesthesiology* 33(1): 102–9.

Caton D (1996) Who said childbirth is natural? *Anesthesiology* 84(4): 955–63.

Chamberlain G, Wright A, Steer P (1993) *Pain and its Relief in Childbirth: The Results of a National Survey Conducted by the National Birthday Trust*. Edinburgh, Churchill Livingston.

Cochrane AL (1972) *Effectiveness and Efficiency: Random Reflections on Health Services*. London, Nuffield and Provincial Hospitals Trust.

Connor H, Connor T (1996) Did the use of chloroform by Queen Victoria influence its acceptance in obstetric practice? *Anaesthesia* 51: 955–7.

Crotty M (1998) *The Foundations of Social Research: Meaning and Perspective in the Research Process*. London, Sage Publications.

Daly J, McDonald I (1992) The problem as we saw it. In Daly J, McDonald I, Willis E (eds) *Researching Health Care: Designs, Dilemma, Disciplines*. London, Tavistock Routledge.

Downe S, McCourt C (2008) From being to becoming: reconstructing childbirth knowledges. In Downe S (ed) *Normal Birth, Evidence and Debate*. Oxford, Elsevier.

Durward L Evans R (1990) Pressure groups and maternity care. In Garcia J, Kilpatrick R, Richards M (eds) *The Politics of Maternity Care: Services for Childbearing Women in Twentieth Century Britain*. Oxford, Clarendon Paperbacks, 256–73.

Elam J (1943) Anaesthesia and analgesia in obstetrics from the viewpoint of the general practitioner. *Journal of Obstetrics and Gynaecology of the British Empire* 50(2): 120–7.

Enkin MW, Glouberman S, Groff P, Jadad AR, Stern A; Clinamen Collaboration (2006) Beyond evidence: the complexity of maternity care. *Birth* 33(4): 265–9.

Farr AD (1980) Early opposition to obstetric anaesthesia. *Anaesthesia* 35: 896–907.

Fisher L, Embree L (eds) (1999) *Feminist Phenomenology*. Boston, Kluwer.

Frank A (2002) Why study people's stories? The dialogical ethics of narrative analysis. *International Journal of Qualitative Methods* 1(1): 1–20.

Gaskin IM (1990) *Spiritual Midwifery*, 3rd edition. Summertown, Book Publisher Company.

Gleick J (1998) *Chaos: The Amazing Science of the Unpredictable*. London, Vintage.

Graham ID (1997) *Episiotomy; Challenging Obstetric Interventions*. Abingdon, Blackwell Science.

Grimes RL (2000) *Deeply into the Bone: Reinventing the Rites of Passage*. California, University of California Press.

Happlin S (1997) *Women and Obstetrics - The Loss of Childbirth to Male Physicians*. On-line journal http://www.gatech.edu/nar/win95/shira.html.

Hasselmann K (1999) Climate change: linear and nonlinear signatures. *Nature* 398: 755–6.

Hunt S, Symonds A (1995) *The Social Meaning of Midwifery*. London, MacMillan Press Ltd.

Jordan B (1993) *Birth in Four Cultures: A Cross-Cultural Investigation of Childbirth in Yucatan, Holland, Sweden and the United States*. Champaign, Waveland Press.

Jordan B (1997) Authoritative knowledge and its construction. In Davis-Floyd RE, Sargent CF (eds) *Childbirth and Authoritative Knowledge: Cross-Cultural Perspectives*. Berkley, University of California Press, 55–79.

Kernick D (2002) The demise of linearity in managing health services: a call for post normal health care. *Journal of Health Services Research and Policy* 7: 121–4.

Kirkham MJ (1987) *Basic supportive care in labour: interaction with and around labouring women*. Unpublished PhD thesis, University of Manchester.

Kitzinger S (1976) Effects of induction on the mother–baby relationship. *Practitioner* 217(1298): 263–7.

Kitzinger S (1987) *The Experience of Childbirth*, 5th edition. Middlesex, Penguin Books.

Kitzinger J (1990) Strategies of the early childbirth movement: a case study of the national childbirth trust. In Garcia J, Kilpatrick R, Richardson M (eds) *The Politics of Maternity Care: Services for Childbearing Women in Twentieth Century Britain*. Oxford, Clarendon Paperbacks, 92–115.

Koch T (1998) Story telling: is it really research? *Journal of Advanced Nursing* 28(6): 1182–90.

Kuhn TS (1970) *The structure of scientific revolutions*. Chicago, Chicago University Press.

Leavitt JW (1986) *Brought to Bed: Childbearing in America 1750 to 1950*. New York, Oxford University Press.

Lewis J (1990) Mothers and maternity practices in the twentieth century. In Garcia J, Kilpatrick R, Richards M (eds) *The Politics of Maternity Care: Services for Childbearing Women in Twentieth Century Britain*. Oxford, Clarendon Paperbacks, 15–29.

Lincoln YS, Guba EG (1985) *Naturalistic Inquiry*. Newbury Park, Sage Publications.

Long CW (1849) An account of the first use of sulphuric ether by inhalation as an anaesthetic in surgical operations. *Southern Medical and Surgical Journal* 5: 12.

Loudon I (1992) *Death in Childbirth: An International Study of Maternal Care and Maternal Mortality, 1800–1950*. Oxford, Clarendon Press.

MacIntosh J (1988) Models of childbirth and social class: a study of 80 working class primigravidae. In Robinson S, Thompson AM (eds) *Midwives, Research and Childbirth*, Vol. 1. London, Chapman & Hall, 189–214.

Meinert CL (1986) *Clinical Trials; Design, Conduct and Analysis*. Oxford, Oxford University Press.

Merry U (1995) *Coping with Uncertainty: Insights from the New Science of Chaos, Self-Organization and Complexity*. New York, Praeger.

Nelson MK (1983) Feb working-class women. *Middle-class Women, and Models of Childbirth Social Problems* 30(3): 284–97.

NICE (2007) CG45 Antenatal and Postnatal Mental Health: Full Guideline, available from: http://www.nice.org.uk/Guidance/CG45/Guidance/pdf/English (accessed 10/02/09).

Oakley A (1989) Who's afraid of the randomized controlled trial? Some dilemmas of the scientific method and "good" research practice. *Women and Health* 15(4): 25–59.

Oakley A (1992) Eve in the garden of health research. In Oakley A (ed) *Social Support and Motherhood: A Natural History of a Research Project*, Chapter 4. London, Blackwell, 76–92

Pawson R, Greenhalgh T, Harvey G, Walshe K (2005) Realist review – a new method of systematic review designed for complex policy interventions. *Journal of Health Services Research and Policy* 10(Suppl 1): 21–34.

Phoenix A (1990) Social research in the context of feminist psychology. In Burman E (ed) *Feminists and Psychological Practice*, Chapter 6. London, Sage Publications.

Polkinghorne DE (1988) *Narrative Knowing and the Human Sciences*. New York, State University of New York Press.

Popper K (1959) *The Logic of Scientific Discovery*. New York, Harper and Row.

Rose H (1983) Hand, brain, and heart: a feminist epistemology for the natural sciences. *Signs: Journal of Women in Culture and Society* 7: 73–90.

Rose H (1994) *Love Power and Knowledge Towards a Feminist Transformation of the Sciences*. Cambridge, Polity Press.

Sackett DL, Straus SE, Richardson WS, Rosenberg W, Haynes RB (2002) *Evidence Based Medicine. How to Practice and Teach EBM*. Edinburgh, Churchill Livingstone.

Salsburg D (1990) Hypothesis versus significance testing for controlled clinical trials: a dialogue. *Statistics in Medicine* 9: 201–11.

Short-DeGraff M, Fisher AG (1993) A proposal for diverse research methods and a common research language. *American Journal of Occupational Therapy* 47(4): 295–7.

Soloman A (1985) The emerging field of psychoneuroimmunology: advances. *Journal of the Institute for the Advancement of Health* 2: 6–19.

Sweeney K, Griffiths F (2002) *Complexity and Healthcare, an Introduction*. Oxford, Radcliffe Medical Press.

Tew M (1990) *Safer Childbirth? A Critical History of Maternity Care*. London, Chapman and Hall.

Wilson T, Holt T, Greenhalgh T (2001) Complexity science: complexity and clinical care. *British Medical Journal* 323(7314): 685–8.

Zuck D (1991) Early opposition to obstetric anaesthesia. *Anaesthesia: Correspondence* 6(5): 538–43.

Chapter 3
Childbirth Education: Politics, Equality and Relevance

Mary Nolan

Introduction: towards a political and social ideology of childbirth education

Childbirth education has, in the past, been a catalyst for change in women's thinking about childbirth and in the delivery of maternity care. Books such as Grantley Dick-Read's (2005) 'Childbirth without Fear', Marjorie Karmel and Karmel's (2005) book which publicised the ideas of Fernand Lamaze, 'Thank you, Dr. Lamaze', Frederick Leboyer's (2000) 'Pour une Naissance sans Violence', and Michel Odent's (1985) 'Entering the World: the demedicalization of childbirth' were at once political, social and spiritual commentaries on the status of women, the treatment of children, patriarchy in medicine and the kind of society that was being constructed through 20th-century birthing practices. Luke Zander commented at a meeting of the National Childbirth Trust in the early 1990s that if only we could get birth right, we might be well on the way to getting society right.

Why did these doctor-philosophers turned social activists – all of them, interestingly, men – consider birth to be so important? Is it that they could see from their position within the medical profession that the outcome of doctors' controlling birth was not the enhanced safety of women and their babies, but the denigration of women and the commodification of babies? Did their integrity as doctors cause them to ask whether current practice in obstetrics was compatible with their Hippocratic oath: first and foremost do no harm? Perhaps like Marsden Wagner (1994) some years later, they saw that the 'birth machine' was running amok. In India and China today, ultrasound technology has enabled female fetuses to be identified early in pregnancy. In the past 20 years, it is estimated that between 6 and 10 million pregnancies involving female fetuses have been terminated

(Toomey 2007). In affluent nations, Cardiotocograph (CTG) devices have played a major part in boosting Caesarean section rates, and the mega-million dollar market in infant formula is, at least in part, responsible for the fact that every 30 seconds a baby dies from unsafe bottle feeding (http://www.babymilkaction.org/).

Where giving birth is not a rite of passage, considered by society to be of huge significance in the life of a woman and her family, education for birth is not likely to be given high priority. When women are seen merely as carriers of a fetus whose value is assessed in accordance with a social or religious agenda over which the women themselves have no influence, educating them about birth may be seen as irrelevant or even undesirable. And while women in the United Kingdom may be told by the government that they have choices around their maternity care, it is interesting to observe that education for birth has nonetheless declined rapidly in recent years (Nolan 2008). When education is withdrawn from a particular group, it might be argued that oppression will follow (Freire 1972).

There are all sorts of reasons why National Heath Service (NHS) trusts in the United Kingdom may have taken the decision to cut back on childbirth preparation classes – shortage of cash, shortage of midwives, poor uptake of classes, prioritisation of other services more highly valued by the medical profession (regular first and second trimester antenatal visits; repeated pregnancy scans; antenatal screening and diagnosis) – but whatever the official reasons, the outcome is that one half of society, characterised solely by its female gender, is often deprived of accurate information about an event that the majority of that 50% will experience at some point in their lives.

Freire's (1972) 'Pedagogy of the Oppressed' is eloquent in its exegesis of how education can function either as an instrument by which the people are kept in subjugation or as an instrument of their freedom. The history of oppression in various parts of the world during the 20th century demonstrates the controlling power of education – in Maoist China; in Nazi Germany; in various South American dictatorships. Antenatal education can be an agent for a patriarchal model of birth or it can create opportunities for 'maternal literacy' and empowerment which will impact on the way in which the future citizens of the country are born and brought up.

If antenatal education is so important for women, why is the uptake of classes often very poor? The easy, cost-cutting answer is to say that women do not want such classes. However, it is only necessary to walk into any antenatal clinic in the land and ask the pregnant women there if they want to know what having a baby is like to find out that they most certainly do. Women are desperate to learn, but they will not buy into classes that do not tell them about how their bodies really work as opposed to how hospitals work, or which do not address their individual needs (Ho & Holroyd 2002).

In his book 'Evidence-based Care for Normal Labour and Birth', Denis Walsh (2007) mentions how weary he has become of defending home birth against attacks on its safety. I feel the same when I repeatedly find myself challenging people who say that there is no evidence that antenatal classes make any difference to what happens to women during labour. The poverty of research into childbirth education is scandalous (Nolan 2005). What research has been done (with some honourable exceptions mentioned later) reflects a medical agenda which, in the case of childbirth education, has attempted to correlate mere attendance at classes with the number of interventions experienced in labour. Few researchers have been interested in the philosophy underpinning childbirth educators' approach to classes – how their attitudes towards birth may infiltrate what and how they teach. There has been little or no description in the literature of the nature of the educational interventions assessed: whether the teacher assumed the role of expert or of co-learner; whether the parents participated in and created their own learning, or whether they were treated as 'empty vessels' in keeping with traditional pedagogy. Researchers have always assumed that midwives are skilled in creating effective learning opportunities for adult learners. This is by no means certain. Many excellent midwives acknowledge that their training as educators has been minimal or non-existent. In addition, many have never had the opportunity to debrief their own births or the births of the women they have cared for, making it potentially difficult for them to allow women attending classes the freedom to make the choices that are right for them.

Why have the fruits of many years of research into adult education and how humans learn, had, by and large, so little impact on childbirth education? Why is it that childbirth education has not manifested the dynamism of other adult learning packages, continuing to teach women to conform to a system of birth that has proved inflexible to the individuality of women and the unpredictability of labour? In my own research conducted in the mid-1990s (Nolan 1999), I was struck by how many of the childbirth educators I interviewed wanted to *tell* women about labour and birth. They wanted to *give* them information. Facts and figures were prominent in the classes I observed and heard about. Women learned that the latent phase of labour lasts until 4 cm dilatation. The cervix has to open to 10 cm before the baby can be born. Progress in labour should be at the rate of 1 cm per hour. The birthing pool cannot be used before the woman is 5 cm dilated. The midwife will perform an internal examination every 4 hours. Eating is not allowed after 6 cm. And so on. I am regularly asked by fathers attending classes whether midwives use a tape measure to measure the cervix. The mathematical approach to birth has certainly infiltrated the popular consciousness! And this being the case, classes which *tell* women and their partners what happens, and quote *statistics* about labour and birth, are merely reflecting childbirth as it is. They are not functioning as Freire's catalyst for change.

It is therefore hardly surprising that women's most consistent complaint about their antenatal classes, when they look back on them following the birth of their babies, is that they were unrealistic (McKay *et al.* 1990; Spiby *et al.* 1999; Nolan 2005). They say classes did not prepare them for an experience which had nothing to do, as far as they were concerned, with measurements and statistics. What they felt in their bodies – the relentlessness of the process of giving birth, its power, the altered states of consciousness; for some of them, the spiritual sense of oneness with a procreative universe – none of that had been conveyed in the classes they had attended. Even the pain so often mentioned by childbirth educators, or deliberately not mentioned, had not been quite what they had been led to expect. The intensity of contractions was beyond, and ultimately quite different from what they would describe as pain in their everyday lives.

Perhaps because it is so hard to talk about birth realistically, Michel Odent eschewed antenatal classes altogether in his clinic at Pithiviers. He chose simply to bring groups of pregnant women together to share meals and to sing – to create a harmony and an intimacy of female understanding which would support the women in the experience they were all soon to go through. I have much sympathy with this viewpoint, although in a world dominated by the media and the internet, I think women do need accurate information if only to correct what they have learned so wrongly from television and various (irresponsible) websites.

Antenatal education and adult education: learning in small groups

Knowles (1984) wrote that adult education should assist the learner to achieve a more profound adulthood, a greater understanding of the direction of her or his life, and a sense of increased control over personal and political decision-making. It should respect, value and build on the richness of the life experiences of every adult and acknowledge adults' right to determine what they need to know and how they can best come to know it. By definition, therefore, adult education is likely to be an enterprise carried on in small groups (Daines *et al.* 2004). It is at this very first hurdle that so many of the antenatal classes being offered in the United Kingdom today, fall.

The rationale for providing education for adults in small groups has been rehearsed many times. Some adults approach any educational setting with extreme caution. They may have painful memories of school, of humiliation, of failure, and of intimidation by other pupils, intentional or otherwise. If they are young parents, these memories may be very fresh; if they are older, they may have become prejudices which operate blindly when any opportunity for participating again in education becomes available. For some adults, their overwhelming recollection of school is of boredom and of the irrelevance of what they were taught.

Many adult learners are therefore cautious. Gather together eight pregnant couples for the first session of an antenatal course and observe their body language. Some appear defensive, arms crossed, legs crossed, turned slightly away from the group leader. Some may fiddle with notebooks, wondering anxiously if they should take notes. There is probably a general expectation that the course will be led by the person at the front, and that they, as the learners, will be passive. Conversation may be muted, if indeed there is any at all. Is it permitted to speak while the teacher is in the room?

Rewriting all of this so that the class becomes a meeting of equals, between knowledgeable adults embarking on a life-changing experience unique to each of them, is the challenge of antenatal education. To elicit and then work to the agenda which is relevant to the group can only be done if numbers in the group are small. Asking questions in a public forum is difficult for most people, let alone discussing their fears and expectations around one of the most intimate events of their lives. The childbirth educator must work hard to help the group 'perform'. However, get beyond the defensive body language and there is gathered together a group of learners who have perhaps never been so keen to learn in their lives.

The purpose of having a small group is not so that the childbirth educator can talk more easily to the parents, but so that the parents can talk more easily to each other. The childbirth educator is not part of this group of becoming parents. She needs the humility to accept that she is forever an outsider. Her role is not as a buddy for the parents, but to enable the parents to become friends with each other. The literature (Vehvilainen-Julkunen 1993; Tarkka & Paunonen 1996; Ho & Holroyd 2002) is clear that what most parents want primarily from their antenatal classes is to make friends (see Box 3.1).

Ho and Holroyd's (2002) beautifully designed and highly insightful exploration of antenatal classes in Hong Kong contains one sad little footnote where the researchers relate how some of the women who participated in their focus groups came to them afterwards and thanked them for giving them the chance to get to know each other. They had hoped to make friends at their antenatal classes, but as these had consisted on average of 50 people, that had been impossible. They had volunteered to take part in the research because they thought it was a 'good' thing to do and had been amply rewarded by making friends with other pregnant women whose babies were due at the same time as theirs.

Box 3.1

Kate was very nervous at the first antenatal class. When invited to introduce herself to the group, she said little about her pregnancy, seeming almost to dismiss it as of no importance. She was far more keen to explain that she was new to the town, having moved only a few weeks previously from a distant part of the country. She returned to this theme several times during the class. At the coffee break, she came to the childbirth educator and told her laughingly, but with her real pain scarcely concealed, that she had no friends in the area. During the classes, she worked almost too hard to get to know the other women. Fortunately, they were tolerant of what might have been construed as her intrusiveness, and Kate finally relaxed in their company. During the 2-day course, the group of women became close. Kate found herself receiving invitations to meet them in town, to attend aquanatal sessions with them, and to meet at their houses after the babies were born. By the end of the second day, she was focused on her pregnancy again, and secure enough to give her attention to the coming birth.

Antenatal education: the realism agenda

Helping people to make friends is really not that difficult, especially when they have something as momentous in common as having a baby. Creating for and with them a realistic impression of labour and birth is a far greater challenge.

Labour is an overwhelmingly physical experience that takes place anatomically, largely in the woman's pelvis. It is also an experience in which women can reach the depths of despair and terror and the heights of joy and triumph. Some would say there is a spiritual dimension where women experience a sense of connectedness with the whole of life. Whatever the nature of the experience, it is not one in which talking plays a great part. Indeed, for labour to flow, it is important that the higher cognitive centres remain quiescent, so that the primitive brain stem can release in abundance the hormones that stimulate and harmonise it.

Yet the dominant mode of communication in antenatal classes is talk, be that the childbirth educator giving information, or the parents asking questions, and perhaps engaging in discussion. Educators may not portray the physicality of labour, or help parents acquire physical skills for working with the forces of labour, because they find it embarrassing, or think that the parents will find it embarrassing. And parents may collude with the teacher to avoid working with their bodies rather than their minds to understand labour and birth.

The childbirth educator's philosophy of birth and her feelings about the purpose of antenatal education will also be influential. It may be that her own experience of having a baby is one of being delivered rather than giving birth. She may have no belief in women's ability to birth their babies. What she has seen of hospital practice may have persuaded her that not only is it pointless to set women up for an experience that the labour suite environment will not allow, but also unkind and unethical. She may simply be so ill at ease with her own body that she does not want to draw attention to it by demonstrating to women how they might work with theirs to manage contractions.

Yet when women start to work with their bodies, trying out different comfort positions for first stage, practising slow rhythmical breathing, receiving back massage, rocking their pelvis, and lunging to achieve asymmetrical positions that help the baby move downwards through the pelvis, they start to ask very different questions from the ones they were asking when they were passively looking at the pictures in the Birth Atlas. They ask practical questions:

- How many pillows are there in the delivery room? Do I need to take some of my own?
- How can I be upright if I'm being monitored?
- Is there enough space to use different positions in the delivery room? How can I make more space?

And they start, of their own accord, to challenge:

- Why do you always see women on TV lying on their backs in labour?
- Can I get in the bath at home if I'm in early labour, even if I might not be 5 cm dilated?
- You can be mobile if you have certain epidurals, can't you?

In my experience, men in particular are eager to discuss the contradiction between what they are being taught in an active birth class and what they have heard from friends and seen in the media. They enjoy learning about the mechanics of labour, the construction of the pelvis and how to optimise the space available within it, and become very keen to assist their partners to remain upright and mobile. This is why I like teaching mixed groups because the men are almost invariably staunch allies of straightforward vaginal birth!

Being realistic about the unpredictability of the course of labour is not helped by fixed agendas for classes. I know it is very difficult for midwives who may take only one session in a series to be flexible about what topics they cover. However, presenting parents with a course outline which runs

Week 1: Labour and birth
Week 2: Pain relief
Week 3: Infant feeding
Week 4: Post-natal life

does not help them to understand labour, birth and parenting as a continuum. The 'Pain Relief' session invariably means information on gas and air, Transcutaneous electrical nerve stimulation (TENS), pethidine and epidurals, thus leading parents to believe that drugs and gadgetry are the only 'real' ways of managing pain in labour. Similarly (although not under discussion in this chapter) separating 'infant feeding' from 'post-natal life' is like separating the warp from the weft. Do so and the fabric falls apart. Feeding the baby cannot be divorced from the experience of post-natal life.

I much prefer an agenda which is as fluid as labour itself. It develops as the parents wish it to develop and by virtue of its own logic, a logic which may change according to the individuals who are attending the classes. Within each class, realism is enhanced by avoiding the strong temptation to give prescriptive answers to questions which parents would very much like to have prescriptive answers for – a question such as, 'When should we come into hospital?' How do we help parents make their *own* decision about this nerve-wracking issue? How do we be realistic and help them understand that there is no 'right time' but only the right time for them? I can make two suggestions.

The first way is to wean parents off their fierce desire to commit to the idea of a cervix opening according to metric measurements. I am indebted to Sara Wickham who made me realise how unhelpful the rigid plastic chart is with cut-out circles measuring from 1 to 10 cm. She considers that this teaching aid is complicit with a medical model of labour wherein women's bodies are expected to behave in a predictable manner. She herself demonstrates how far the cervix has to open in order for a fully grown baby to be born by asking the mothers to spread the fingers of one hand and span the distance between the base of the thumb and little finger with the other. That span will vary from woman to woman, and the feel of the flesh of the hand conveys the suppleness of the cervix far more realistically than rigid plastic. This makes it perhaps easier for parents to accept that labour is a natural process and unique to each woman; so judging when to come into hospital is also an individual thing which they can decide for themselves by assessing their physical and emotional comfort, rather than trying to make a decision based on times (length and frequency of contractions) and measurements (dilatation of the cervix).

I also take parents on a mental tour of their homes to help them think about how they will labour in their own environment.

Shut your eyes for a moment, and relax . . .

Which is your favourite room at home?

Walk round it in your mind. What do you see in the room? Is there a window? What can you see out of it? What furniture is there? Are there pictures? Is the room a mess or is it tidy?

Is there an object that you particularly like in the room?

Now think about having a contraction in this room. What would you lean on? How would you make yourself comfortable?

If you are the mother's supporter, how would you help to make her comfortable in the room you are thinking of?

Imagine the contraction. How intense is it? Do you feel safe in this room?

When you have the next contraction, will you stay in the same position and comfort yourself in the same way?

Will you do something different to help the mother?

What about moving to another room? . . .

And so on. The idea is to help parents rehearse a situation that they may not even have considered, namely spending some time at home in labour before coming to hospital. I have no research-based evidence to prove that this is effective, but women have told me after the birth of their babies that they had felt very comfortable at home when labour started because they 'knew what to do' and could relax.

Preparing parents to manage the realities of the hospital delivery suite means encouraging flexibility in terms of using the room in which they find themselves. Given that most antenatal classes are held in locations which are neither very comfortable nor very like a delivery room, they provide a useful teaching aid for learning how to manage strange and less than ideal birthing environments. In classes, I do not always provide comfort aids such as balls, pillows, mats and soft chairs. Instead, we consider how the women would manage if they had to labour in the particular room we are currently in. They try supporting themselves using window-sills, tables and chairs, curling up on the floor and secreting themselves in nooks and crannies where they can find privacy. Their partners get used to the idea that they, too, will have to be active in labour, adjusting their own position to suit the woman's. Then we move to looking at pictures of the delivery rooms at the local hospitals, and work out how they can be adapted to facilitate an active labour in which the woman can feel in control.

The following idea was developed by one of my students to help parents think about how the environment of birth might affect the woman's ability to labour effectively. The group is split into four smaller groups, two male and two female (if this is an antenatal course for couples). Paper and felt-tips are handed out. Each group is allocated one of the following tasks; no group knows what the others are working on.

(a) Draw a room in which you could carry out a seduction. (men's group)
(b) Draw a room in which you would not feel comfortable making love. (men's group)
(c) Draw a delivery room in a hospital. (women's group)
(d) Draw a room in which you would like to give birth. (women's group)

After one class produced drawings, the parents were then asked to pair the drawings according to which seemed the most similar. This was not difficult; they put a) and d) together and b) and d). A discussion then ensued about how an environment in which you would make love is also an environment in which you could give birth (soft furnishings; gentle lights; music); and an environment which would not enable relaxed love-making had strong similarities to delivery rooms in hospital (people around; TV/monitoring screens; bright lights; no soft furnishings). A vigorous discussion about home versus hospital as place of birth ensued, including how parents could modify and make the best use of the hospital environment.

An essential aspect of realism in antenatal classes is helping parents to understand the multi-dimensional nature of birth – that there are physical, emotional and spiritual aspects intertwined – and that it is an intense and 'earthy' process. The language educators use is very important in this respect. To describe labouring women as 'ladies' seems to me to collaborate with the disempowerment of women. My image of the strength of women in labour is best represented by Epstein's sculpture 'Genesis'. Here the physical strength, the determination and the fecundity of women are wonderfully merged. Nor is the baby an 'it'; this is to reduce him to what midwifery textbooks sometimes describe as 'the passenger', a noun which belongs to the masculine world of transport. However laborious, the baby needs to be described as 'he or she'. I try hard to avoid talking about 'the birth canal', after being deeply impressed by Sheila Kitzinger's (1998) incisive article, written 10 years ago, in which she exposed the invidious nature of language and imagery in the world of childbearing. A vocabulary for pain can be learned from the work of Melzack and Wall (1994) who documented the words people use to describe their lived experiences of pain, including labour. The words women used to describe period pains were the same as they used to describe contractions, i.e. 'cramping' and 'aching' which enables the educator to relate the unknown experience of labour to an experience with which most of the women in the antenatal group will be very familiar. Equally interesting in Melzack's and Wall's research was that people described the pain of cancer or other serious illness as 'constant', yet this word was never selected by women in relation to labour. Instead, they chose 'rhythmical'. Their preferred word for the overall experience of pain in labour was 'intense'. Women find it helpful to be told about these different notions of pain, and especially to understand that contractions come in waves with breaks in between. Finally, on the subject of appropriate language for antenatal classes, it is vital to stress that women are not 'delivered'; they give birth. The gift of life is given by the woman to her child.

Labour is part of a continuum flowing from the end of pregnancy through to the birth of the baby. The late Tricia Anderson declared that she did not believe in the three stages of labour because 'they bear no relation to women's experiences' (Anderson 2007, p. 54). Labour is part of the continuum of most women's lives. The understanding and skills to cope with it develop out of women's understanding of their bodies gleaned over a lifetime. The young girl from the East End of London whom Dr. Grantly Dick-Read (1890-1959) attended in the early hours of a winter's morning, laboured instinctively, not in accordance with ideas received from elsewhere about how women behave in labour. She so impressed Dick-Read that he wrote his landmark book on childbirth education entitled *Childbirth without Fear* (first published 1944). Escott *et al.*'s work (2004) on women's pre-existing coping strategies is very important here. She shows how the skills which women use to manage contractions in labour are the ones they have used all their lives for coping with discomfort and pain. They are

- focusing away from the pain;
- using different positions;
- slow controlled breathing;
- holding something tightly;
- massage;
- warmth;
- distraction;
- vocalising.

Escott *et al.* (2004) also discuss 'positive reframing', a tool to help women with a tendency to catastrophise their fear of labour by replacing negative thoughts ("This hurts and it's going to get worse and I will never be able to give birth to this baby . . . .'') with positive ones that stress their capacity to complete the task in hand. So, for example, the woman may make empowering statements to herself, linked with a rhythmical breathing pattern. On the in-breath, she says to herself, "I can . . . ." and on the heavy out-breathe, she thinks, "do this". This kind of positive affirmation has certainly been found helpful by women whom I have taught. Practising positions, relaxed breathing and positive reframing in classes also helps women's birth companions to view labour as a process well within the physical and emotional capability of the women they are supporting.

Conclusion: creating a critical mass through maternal health literacy

Antenatal education should aim to set labour in the context of everyday life. This is difficult (and some might argue, misleading) because labour generally happens outside that context for most women – outside their homes where small comforts and complete freedom make aches, pains and distress more bearable. It may be that helping women and their partners to think about how difficult it is to draw on their familiar resources in a delivery suite can assist in the creation of that critical mass of maternity care consumers which is necessary in order to change the contemporary British way of birth. Education for adults must, at least occasionally, move people out of their comfort zone. If the aim of antenatal education is to foster maternal health literacy (a phrase I like very much because we consider literacy to be a basic human right, and for women to be literate about their childbearing health should therefore also be a basic right), there will be moments of revelation for class participants when they become uncomfortably aware that they have accepted certain ideas unquestioningly (see Box 3.2).

Box 3.2

At the end of the class, the leader asked each member of the group to share one thing they had learned or that had struck them during the session. Everybody took this very seriously, but none more so than Azeem who told the group, in troubled tones, that until today, he had genuinely thought that women should give birth flat on their backs with their feet in stirrups and that it was for babies' good that they were held upside down and smacked vigorously on their bottoms to make sure they were alive. Nobody laughed. Many simply nodded.

Helping women and men learn how to question is fundamental to antenatal classes and provides them with a skill which they can use in their encounters with the health service for the rest of their lives. One way of doing this is the use of the acronym BRAN:

Can you tell me what the Benefits are of doing this?	B
Are there any Risks?	R
What Alternative courses of action could we consider?	A
What if I decided to do Nothing?	N

To ask questions of health professionals demands self-confidence as well as a mindset which deems it acceptable to question people who are 'the experts'. The concept of partnership in care and shared decision-making (let alone the more advanced concept of the professional giving the requisite technical information to the woman and then standing back and letting her make decisions independently – see Collins *et al.* 2007: Chapter 3) is unfamiliar to many childbearing women. It may be completely new to women who come from a culture or domestic situation in which they are disempowered, or who perceive that they lack social status in relation to midwives and doctors, or who speak little English. Is the content of this chapter therefore irrelevant to these women?

I do not believe so. Patient participation in decision-making is the next stage in the evolution of health care services in the United Kingdom. The health service has changed dramatically in the 60 years of its existence; it must continue to do so if it is to serve the needs of a dynamic democracy. At present, it may be that few people are ready for patient partnership, fearing the responsibility that it entails. This does not mean that educators should not start to open up new horizons to adult consumers of health care services. It is vital in a world where women continue to experience gender discrimination (Global Gender Gap Report 2007) that a vision of equality should inform adult education in an affluent country which will, rightly or wrongly, be considered by many others to be a showcase for optimum care. Individuals will access the content of a challenging antenatal class at the level that is right for them. The thrill of antenatal education is that it can be a catalyst for change because helping women understand how to work with their bodies in order to realise their full potential to give birth to their babies, is also to empower them.

References

Anderson T (2007) Last word: stages of labour: bunkum! *The Practising Midwife* 10 (8): 54.

Collins S, Britten N, Ruusuvuori J, Thompson A (2007) *Patient Participation in Health Care Consultations: Qualitative Perspectives.* Berkshire, McGraw Hill/Open University Press.

Daines J, Daines C, Graham B (2004) *Adult Learning, Adult Teaching*, 3rd edition. Cardiff, Welsh Academic Press.

Dick-Read G (2005) *Childbirth Without Fear: Principles and Practice of Natural Childbirth*, 4th editions. London, Pinter & Martin.

Escott D, Spiby H, Slade P, Fraser RB (2004) The range of coping strategies women use to manage pain and anxiety prior to and during first experience of labour. *Midwifery* 20: 144–56.

Freire P (1972) *Pedagogy of the Oppressed*, Translated by Myra Bergman Ramos. New York: Herder and Herder.

Global Gender Gap Report (2007) online, *World Economic Forum are the Authors and Global Gender gasp 2007 Education*. http://www.weforum.org/en/initiatives/gcp/Gender%20Gap/index.htm (accessed July, 2008).

Ho I, Holroyd E (2002) Chinese women's perceptions of the effectiveness of antenatal education in the preparation for motherhood. *Journal of Advanced Nursing* 38 (1): 74–85.

Karmel M, Karmel A (2005) *Thank you Dr Lamaze*. London, Pinter & Martin.

Kitzinger S (1998) Sheila Kitzinger's letter from Europe: the caesarean epidemic in Great Britain. *Birth* 25 (1): 56–8.

Knowles M (1984) *Andragogy in Action: Applying Modern Principles of Adult Learning*. London, Jossey-Bass.

Leboyer F (2000) *Pour une Naissance Sans Violence*. Paris, Seuil.

McKay S, Barrows T, Roberts J (1990) Women's views of second stage labor as assessed by interviews and videotapes. *Birth* 17 (4): 192–8.

Melzack R, Wall PD (1994) *Textbook of Pain*. London, Churchill Livingstone.

Nolan M (1999) *Empowerment and Antenatal Education*. Unpublished PhD, University of Birmingham.

Nolan M (2005) Childbirth and parenting education: what the research says and why we may ignore it. In Nolan M, Foster J (eds) *Birth and Parenting Skills: New Directions in Antenatal Education*. Edinburgh, Churchill Livingstone, 1–16.

Nolan M, (2008) *Survey of Antenatal Classes in the UK: July to August: 2007 What Women Liked and What they Disliked about their Antenatal Classes*. The Practising Midwife 11 (2): 32–6.

Odent M (1985) *Entering the World: The Demedicalisation of Childbirth*. London, Penguin Books.

Spiby H, Henderson B, Slade P (1999) Strategies for coping with labour: does antenatal education translate into practice? *Journal of Advanced Nursing* 29 (2): 388–94.

Tarkka MT, Paunonen M (1996) Social support and its impact on mothers' experiences of childbirth. *Journal of Advanced Nursing* 23: 70–5.

Toomey C (2007) Gender Genocide. The Sunday Times Magazine. Aug 26, 34–43.

Vehvilainen-Julkunen K (1993) Empowering clients in parenthood education. *Journal of Clinical Nursing* 2: 257–60.

Wagner M (1994) *Pursuing the Birth Machine: The Search for Appropriate Birth Technology*. Camperdown, ACE Graphics.

Walsh D (2007) *Evidence-based Care for Normal Labour and Birth*. London, Routledge.

Chapter 4
Birth Environment

Denis Walsh

Introduction

In Chapter 1, the evidence on place of birth was discussed in relation to home, free-standing and alongside birth centres or midwifery-led units (MLU's) and consultant maternity hospitals. What was not addressed in that discussion was the context and culture of each of these settings and what potential impact that has on the birthing process. In this chapter, context and culture of differing birth settings will be examined critically. In the literature there is a tendency towards a dualistic analysis of birth settings, so that home and birth centres are constructed as encouraging normal/natural birth and hospitals as predisposing to labour and birth interventions. Depending on one's philosophy of birth, these effects are construed as either positive or negative. Research reveals these settings as more complex than this superficial rendering with a number of factors interacting to construct a 'pro' or 'anti' normal birth outcome. Among these are the physical elements of the space including the décor and ambience, the social relations within the space and the attitudes to labour of the key players in the space.

In the past 20 to 30 years there has been a move in the Western world to domesticate the hospital labour rooms so that they are less clinical in appearance. Fannon (2003), in a wide-ranging sociological critique of this trend, argues that we are left with hybrid spaces that are faking domesticity and homeliness when beneath the surface technology and professional hegemony are lurking with intent. She urges all stakeholders to own up to this hybrid compromise and not pretend that it mimics home birth. Surprisingly, there has not been much research into these softer aspects of hospital birth provision, though there has been substantial investigation into what could be called the relational aspects of labour care. It is to this heavily researched area that this chapter will turn first in exploring the many factors that shape birth environments.

Labour and interpersonal relationships

Over the years, a significant amount of research into different organisational models of midwifery care including teams, caseloads and midwifery group practices has been done. All of these schemes are premised on the principle that women benefit from establishing an ongoing relationship with their carers rather than being cared for by strangers within a fragmented model. Common sense tells us that journeying through such a significant rites of passage experience as childbirth is best done in the company of known carers. How many times do we have to repeat studies that keep telling us that these characteristics of a service are highly valued by women and consistently reduce birth interventions? It was therefore refreshing and challenging to hear a story coming out of South America that a country there has recognised that continuous support in labour was now a fundamental human right. They may legislate to make it illegal for maternity services not to provide this dimension to care. After all, they argued, the benefits have been proven again and again, across different countries and different decades. Even without the studies, it could be argued that indigenous birth practices have much to teach childbirth in the west about this aspect of labour care. Traditional birth attendants working with local women have for thousands of years harnessed the power of known birth companions in facilitating birth for the uninitiated woman. Western-style birth lost this crucial dimension when birth was hospitalised and done in the company of professionals who, mainly, were unknown to labouring women. It was not until the advent of doulas in US hospitals in the late 1970s that recognition was given to such a fundamental aspect of labour care.

The doula studies also examined the value of being supported throughout the entire labour and this aspect of care has now been extensively researched. Nine randomised controlled trials (RCTs) in Hodnett *et al.*'s (2007) systematic review concluded that continuous support during labour reduced Caesarean sections, pharmacological analgesia, assisted vaginal birth, low Apgar scores and labour length while women experienced more positive births. In addition, the authors make two telling points:

1. The most effective support may come from those not employed by the institution.
2. Continuous support will be less effective in a highly medicalised environment (Hodnett *et al.* 2002).

Rosen (2004) reviewed eight studies of labour support provided by five different categories of persons and concluded that care by known, untrained laywomen, starting in early labour was the most effective.

Taylor and colleagues (2000) explained this phenomenon by analysing stress responses in females. In a dramatic echo of childbirth physiology, they found that oxytocin was released in women exposed to stress and this triggered 'tending' and 'befriending' behaviours rather than the classical (male) response of 'fight and flight'. In a further mirroring of the hormonal cascade of labour, endogenous opiates, also released during the experience of stress, augment these effects.

Recently, the number of carers a woman has during her period of continuous support has been shown to be relevant to outcomes. The Caesarean section rate appears to increase in direct line with increasing number of carers. The researchers recommend keeping the number of changes of labour support persons to a minimum (Gagnon *et al.* 2007).

One could tease out some interesting implications from these findings, including a questioning of the common expectation that the male partner should be the principal birth companion. Midwives have long questioned the wisdom of this practice for some labours where a frightened, non-engaged male presence has had a negative impact. Equally challenging is the finding that non-medically trained carers and external to the institution are more effective at labour support. Research suggests that these individuals are more likely to have built a rapport prior to admission to hospital, are committed to staying with the woman throughout the labour (cannot be called away to help elsewhere on the delivery suite) and are not institutionally programmed to 'the way things are done here'. Midwives need to explore with women antenatally the selection of their birth companion, taking into account these findings. It challenges all parties to explore the doula option as the most appropriate person to fulfill this remit.

Aside from the consideration of best birth companion, midwives have argued for decades for providing continuous support in labour so that they can genuinely be 'with the woman'. It is likely that this organisational aspect alone would increase normal birth rates substantially. Yet achieving this goal remains an objective rather than an imperative for most services. That is a scandal in Western countries where investment can be found for many other expensive childbirth technologies and for extra posts for obstetric and anaesthetic subspecialisation. If there is a shortage of midwives, then consideration should be given to moving monies from obstetric and anaesthetic budgets.

Continuous support in labour is the priority as it potentially impacts on many more women than those who might benefit from highly specialised obstetric or anaesthetic services. At the same time, shift patterns should be reviewed in an effort to limit the number of carers a woman sees through her labour.

Continuity has been the subject of research and debate in midwifery for over 20 years now. One would be forgiven for concluding: is there any more we can learn? A cursory examination of the wider literature in health reveals there is because, of course, continuity has been of interest for many other areas of the health spectrum. Haggerty *et al.* (2005) summarise the literature this way:

- Informational continuity (patient story available to all relevant agencies)
- Management continuity (consistent, coherent care)
- Relational continuity (known carers)

All three contribute to a better patient experience and, arguably, better care. Midwifery care has focused more on relational continuity, possibly believing that the other two will follow, though this may not be the case. Nevertheless, a case can be made for this focus because of the unique features of midwife–woman relationship: its biologically determined longevity, its journey through a major rites of passage experience and the intimate nature of its focus. There are many organisational variants of relational continuity in midwifery services as already mentioned: teams, caseloads, group practices, named midwife. There has been enough research done around these options to glean some important lessons:

- Teams should number no more than six because, as numbers increase, 'a known midwife' becomes 'someone met once or twice' to eventually 'someone spoken of by a colleague' and continuity becomes meaningless (Flint 1993).
- Continuity needs differ depending on the phases of care. Keeping the number of carers to a minimum may be more important for labour and the post-natal period than antenatally (Green *et al.* 1998).
- Continuity between phases, especially having a known midwife for labour, is highly valued by women (Walsh 1999) and reduces labour interventions (Page *et al.* 1999; North Staffordshire Changing Childbirth Research Team 2000).

In relation to clinical outcomes and satisfaction with care, team and continuity variants generally reduce labour interventions, including epidural, induction of labour, episiotomy, neonatal resuscitation rates, and improve satisfaction.

Some of these benefits are linked to the role of the midwife as the lead carer because a number of other studies in various countries conclude that midwifery-led services are superior to obstetric-led models when caring for a low-risk group (Harvey *et al.* 1996; Homer *et al.* 2001), summarised now in a systematic review by Hatem *et al.* (2008). In addition, Tracy and Tracy (2003) showed that low technology, midwife-mediated services are cheaper, challenging the notion that closing free-standing birth centres (FSBCs) or under-investing in midwives will save money. The economic arguments around models of care are complex but services that choose to centralise provision, in part based on the economies of scale argument, should pay heed to Posnett's (1999) conclusion that there is a limit to what economies of scale can achieve. A point can be reached where large hospitals become more expensive per unit cost to run than small ones.

Attitudes and beliefs

It seems reasonable to assume that midwives choosing to work in home-birth and birth centre settings would be a self-selecting group and that they would exhibit beliefs and practices that are congruent with these environments. However qualitative research has painted a more complicated picture. Edwards (2000) discovered that some women in her Scottish home-birth study experienced a 'hospital birth at home' and Annandale (1988) coined the phrase 'ironic intervention' to represent the action of midwives routinely rupturing membranes in mid labour to avoid transfer out of a birth centre to a consultant unit for prolonged labour. Machin and Scamell (1997) described the 'irresistible nature of the biomedical metaphor' in explaining how women orientated to normal birth bought into medical interventions once they entered the hospital. It is becoming clear that assumptions cannot be made about the attitudes of midwives or women who choose birth centre options.

Coyle *et al.'s* (2001a, b) papers remind us that women who opt for birth centres expect to be cared for by midwives who share the same values around birth. Downe and McCourt (2008) espouse the importance of a focus on positive outcomes of birth, rather than on morbidity, captured in the term, 'salutogenesis' or well-being. Such a focus is imperative for birth centre staff as is a fundamental trust in the physiological processes of labour. This is where an explicit promotion of a philosophy of active birth and of the values behind a social model of care are so important for birth centre work. These approaches explicitly affirm birth physiology, and their impact on women antenatally has been demonstrated by Foster's (2005) audit of an antenatal education package based on these beliefs. Women who went through this programme had half the epidural rate of women who did not, confirming for the first time that preparation for childbirth classes can impact on the labour interventions.

It is therefore good practice to explore the motivation of midwives who apply for birth centre posts to gain insights into their beliefs and values. But prior to this, the philosophy and strategic direction of the birth centre needs articulating in information leaflets for women and in policy documents. Operationally, the opportunity should be provided antenatally for midwives to meet women who will access the centre for birth, ideally through repeat antenatal clinics or through childbirth education classes.

Facilitating midwifery contact with women reminds us once again of the importance of relational components to care and, as already outlined, there is a wealth of research confirming its significance for normal labour and birth (Hunter *et al*. 2008).

Redefining safety – human nesting

Providers' focus on birth environment has tended to be on safety for mother and baby. This is reflected in information leaflets on place of birth choices. However, recent birth centre research has illuminated an alternative 'take' on safety that links to the human expression of nesting (Walsh 2006a). The behaviour, values and beliefs of women and midwives in a FSBC strongly suggests this. Women chose the birth centre based on the homeliness of its décor and the nurturing ambience it projected. Midwifery activity also reflected these priorities. The adoption of nesting theory to explain these aspects of birth centre activity recalls its prominence in older textbooks of maternity care.

Nesting was mentioned in midwifery textbooks up to the mid-1980s where it was used to explain maternal behaviours during pregnancy (Myles 1981). During the first 12 weeks of gestation, nesting was said to cause tiredness and lethargy that slowed women's activity during the critical embryonic phase of fetal development. Nesting behaviours returned in the weeks preceding the birth and were marked by a drive to prepare the baby's immediate environment. Decorating the nursery, purchasing the layette, cleaning and tidying the home surrounds were said to be manifestations of nesting. For reasons that are not immediately apparent, references to nesting disappeared from midwifery textbooks around this time and only rarely appear in midwifery books today (England & Horowitz 1996). They survive in populist magazines on new motherhood (parents.com) and in the self-help literature around childbirth (Robertson 1997).

Nesting links humans to the large mammalian species where these behaviours are usually understood to be grounded in instinct – a much more problematic notion for humans because of the layers of socialisation and learned behaviours that suffuse human learning and development. In reference to human behaviour, Davis-Floyd and Arvidson (1997) prefer the term intuition to instinct as it encompasses emotional and thinking components. Using the characteristics of an intuitive response as identified by Bastick (1982), the women's focus on birth environment appears strongly intuitive in nature. Bastick named these characteristics of intuition as follows:

- Sudden, immediacy of awareness
- Association of affect with insight
- Non-analytical, non-rational, non-logical, gestalt nature of experience
- Empathic, preverbal
- Sense of certainty of the truth of insights

The women's comments were suggestive of some or all of these features:

> '... as soon as we walked in we thought - yep! This is the sort of place'
> 'I got stuck on it.'
> 'I could picture myself there'.
> It's a feeling rather than an empirical value system. A woman knows immediately when it's the right atmosphere.'
>
> (Walsh 2004, p. 145)

The sense of immediacy and certainty about the birth centre being an appropriate site for birth comes through here. The final comments articulate clearly the difficulty of explaining exactly why that certainty is felt and the visualisation confirms the involvement of the non-rational, emotionally mediated brain functions. The staff's comments reinforced this reading of the women's experience.

The dominance of feeling seems to win out over a more cerebral consideration of other factors and midwives explicitly linked what they observed in women to their understanding of animal behaviour:

> In relation to women feeling intuitively that it is right to give birth here, I think it is similar to animals finding the right spot to give birth and I just think – Yes it feels right, then they will do it.
>
> (Walsh 2004, p. 153)

Components of nesting

The intuitive 'feel' of this data reinforces the notion of nesting as an appropriate explanatory framework. Nesting activity is about preparing a safe place for offspring where, once born, they can be protected from harm. Animals and mammals, in particular, will go to extraordinary lengths to prepare such a place, and will guard it fiercely once birth has occurred (Attenborough 1990; Cronin *et al.* 1996). Protection and safety may be driving women's decisions here but applied in an alternative way that explores notions of safety beyond mortality and morbidity statistics. The possibility of seeing safety more broadly has been raised by Hirst (2005) in her review of maternity services in Australia. In part, she was responding to a 'cultural safety' agenda regarding maternity care and indigenous groups which Ramsden (2003) had first brought to public consciousness in New Zealand. But equally, one could speak of social and psychological safety and these dimensions to safety are strongly hinted at in the women's accounts. Being greeted by a staff member holding a baby impressed one woman, though at one level it appears a very normal occurrence in a maternity unit. Yet, due to institutional constraints related to health and safety, this would be an unlikely occurrence in a larger hospital. In this case the woman concluded that the birth centre was clearly a baby-friendly place where, by inference, their emotional and nurturing needs would be met. There is a sense of social safety in the request by a woman to have her teenage children present in the centre during her labour and women's direct communication with their babies *in utero* as they walk around the centre suggests strong connections to an emotional comfort zone or psychological safety.

Women's nesting response appears to be unrelated to the risk discourse of childbirth safety. Their thinking inverts the risk discourse's logic of protection and safety by deliberately choosing a non-medical environment for birth. Many redefined the birth centre as a hotel, 'like home', or a health farm, to disconnect it from a hospital ambience. For these women, protection and safety appeared to mean reducing the risk of iatrogenesis associated in their minds with hospital birth.

Nesting as protection and safety could also be linked to the friendliness, peace and relaxation that they experienced on visiting the centre. These qualities point to the balancing of the stress of labour experienced internally with peaceful surrounds externally.

Women were seeking a birth ambience characterised by compassion, warmth, nurture and love. This was not just in evidence at the birth centre by the welcome, hospitality and the care they received, but by the attention to detail that the staff had put into preparing the birth space. There is a sense in which the staff spend their working lives 'preparing for a baby'. At any moment, women may come through the door in labour and the staff's raison d'etre is providing for that eventuality. Their preparing is not an idle pastime but a sustained, continuous activity as they are constantly adapting, making-over and maintaining the birth space. It is environmental nurture. There was also a spatial dimension to honing environmental ambience – an absence of no 'no go' geographical locations within the centre. Both the women and staff interviews and the field notes recorded incidents of women, particularly during the evening and night, sitting down in the staff room and chatting with midwives and maternity care assistants (MCAs). The room was where staff went for their breaks and had a number of comfortable chairs, magazines and a television. Women and their relatives also entered the office where all the computing, telephone activity and shift handovers occurred. These actions break a strong taboo in institutions where space is used to distribute power and to construct identities (Halford & Leonard 2003). It contrasts with ethnographies of consultant delivery suites where there were not only prohibitions to some areas for patients, but also for some ranks of staff (Hunt & Symonds 1995; Yearley 1999).

Human nesting instinct appears to seek out the right emotional ambience for childbearing, which is as integral to establishing a protective, safe place for birth as are the immediate physical surrounds. This marks them out as different from other mammals who primarily seek solitude (Rosenberg & Trevathan 2003). Demere and colleagues (2002) observe that in the animal kingdom, the complexity of nesting increases as the need for parental care increases. A suitable nest is needed to continue the rearing of a newborn until it is mature enough to fend for itself. Therefore I would argue that because human offspring are developmentally very immature at birth in comparison to many other mammals (Allport 1997), women seek out this broader range of factors when selecting an appropriate place to birth. Part of this may be making an intuitive and rapid appraisal of emotional and environmental ambience.

These findings from researching care in birth centre suggest that both women and staff may manifest nesting-like behaviours when 'freed' from the culture of hospital birth. These behaviours conceptualise safety across several domains – physical, psychological and social, emphasising their mediation via relationships and the birth environment. The relationship focus involves hitherto an unrecognised dynamic in women's assessment of the suitability of the place of birth – its emotional ambience. Their interest in a suitable physical environment has been known about and responded to by services across the western world as Fannon (2003) elaborates on. What had not been recognised so far is the potential of staff to hone environmental ambience if given the remit and freedom to pursue this.

Reprising nesting as central to decision-making around the place of birth and to the preparations of maternity care staff for receiving a baby throws up distinctive challenges to current service provision. Three issues are worth considering for further research and practice:

- How women construct the notions of protection and safety in relation to the birth space when birth is within a hospital setting

- How staff would choose to construct environmental ambience if encouraged and enabled to do so
- What qualities in a hospital setting would women prioritise for optimum emotional ambience

If nesting helps explain women's and staff's emphasis on the birth environment's physical and emotional ambience, then how might some of the care interactions be conceptualised?

'Mother-like' care

A narrative of a young girl becoming very distressed during a long latent phase of labour and how the attending midwife responded to her is intriguing. The midwife got down on a mattress on the floor with her and held her in an embrace lasting two hours as the girl wept. It appeared to be a cathartic experience of emotional release such that the girl subsequently stood up and said she was ready. She went on to labour and birth within a few hours without any pain relief. In this situation, the midwife could be said to have intuited an appropriate response to the girl's distress that would not be found in textbooks or within the paradigm of a biomedical model. Leap and Anderson (2004) have written that a common response of midwives to the distress of labour is treating it with a variety of pharmacological pain-relieving agents. They argue for an alternative approach which they call 'working with pain'. This recognises that labour pain has a physiological purpose related to promoting the optimum hormonal response but that it can also indicate emotional distress. The midwifery skill is in discerning these differences. Simkin and Ancheta (2005), in their book on labour progress, explore the cause of labour delay from a holistic perspective, suggesting that simply diagnosing uterine inertia is too reductionist as an explanation. In many cases of delay, a psychological component is likely to be a contributory factor and they urge childbirth attendants to be sensitive to this possibility.

For the teenager, the 'becoming mother' journey had been a traumatic one and the midwife's empathic care for her in labour, had smoothed her path.

Another episode of care illustrated a similar dynamic. An hour after giving birth, Sarah called the midwife, complaining of abdominal pain. It was so severe she felt cold, clammy and faint. The midwife examined her but did not feel that there was any serious clinical reason for her pain. She then proceeded to cradle the woman in her arms, resting her head on her lap and holding it gently and massaging her hair and scalp in a very motherly, maternal way for the next 20 to 30 minutes.

During the post-natal interview, the woman reflected on the experience:

> She (midwife) was great afterwards because it was like having my Mum there. I remember having my head on her lap and she was just stroking the back of my head saying you will be all right. Just kind of nursing you which was invaluable. It was like you were her daughter.
>
> (Walsh 2004, p. 233)

Comfort and protection emanate from this incident.

Mothering manifested in another guise post-natally. Unlike post-natal stay times throughout the Western world, women at the birth centre frequently stayed for more than three days following a normal birth. During this time they were pampered and made to feel special. Birth centre staff seemed aware of the stresses of post-natal adjustment at home as another woman commented on:

> They said 'if you're happy to stay for the week and have that rest, then do it' ... And they said, 'you're just as important as what he is and if you don't feel well enough to go home, you just stay with us and let us look after him a bit longer. Be spoilt for a couple of days more because when you go home, it's a twenty four-hour job and there's no switch off'.
>
> (Walsh 2004, p. 237)

Women really appreciated the little treats they received from the staff which included ice drinks while in the jacuzzi, tea and biscuits for afternoon tea, and caring for their babies at night so the women could sleep. A staff member hand washed a nightdress for one woman who had very few items of clothes with her.

One of the birth centre staff who worked permanent nights, told a story of being asked to have a sleep when she came on duty because she was so exhausted from looking after terminally ill parents, illustrating a mothering response to the plight of a colleague. This anecdote borders on the subversive as sleeping on duty could be perceived as irresponsible. But here, it is an extension of the empathy shown to women and a poignant example of compassion to fellow colleagues.

In these accounts, the midwives express a 'mothering' dimension to care.

Sketching matrescence

In the stories of the young girl, held in an embrace and consoled by the midwife as she experienced early labour and of the woman comforted when in pain post-natally, the midwives respond intuitively. These were non-verbal, empathic actions that sprung from fairly immediate insight and awareness. There was no obvious logical or rational analysis guiding them to embrace the women in the way they did. Their actions may have been preceded by a biophysical assessment which eliminated pathology in their minds but then the midwives appeared to tap into a protective, nurturing reservoir that could be understood as 'matrescent' or 'of matrescence' (Thomas 2001) – becoming mother. Matrescence was first coined by Raphael (1973) to emphasise that birth often 'becomes' a new mother as well as a new baby, an idea that has been echoed since by Wickham (2002) and Thomas (2001). Thomas writes of matrescence as spiritual formation drawing analogies with the Judaeo-Christian tradition. Using neglected Old Testament imagery of the fecundity of God in giving birth to creation, of nurturing the people of Israel as a mother suckles her child at the breast, and of protecting the nation from harm as a hen protects its chickens, she argues for a new spiritual examination of birth as a rite of passage experience. It is these images of nurture and protection that can be applied to the caring by the birth attendants here.

Thomas (2001) explored another, more clearly ethical dimension to matrescence in her reflections on the physicality of pregnancy (two in one), and of childbirth (one becoming two). Cosslett (1994) commenting on this, notes that the concept can radically challenge the idea of the autonomous, individual subject. This connection between mother and child, though severed physically by the cutting of the cord, remains intact as the child grows, drawing selflessness and agape (Christian notion of disinterested love as opposed to erotic love) from her. It is a kind of unconditional love that finds meaning in giving.

Matrescent care, understood in this way, incorporates an ethical disposition. If authentic, it would manifest more broadly than in just relationships with the birth centre women. One would expect to witness its effect among staff. The night staff's experience when she was asked to have a sleep is one poignant example.

This action can all be seen as matrescent in the sense of 'mothering', nurturing and protecting work colleagues. Cosslett's idea of connection to 'other' overriding the needs of the autonomous self is demonstrated by these actions.

It parallels to the metaphor of 'home' regularly spoken of by the women, so the staff used the analogy of 'family'. However caution is required. Notions of home and family, idealised here as a site and environment of nurture and belonging, can be problematised. For some women and their children, home and family are places of abuse, rejection and deprivation (Mooney 1994; Barlow & Birch 2004). Easy elision of an optimum birth environment with the domestic setting is misleading, unless contextual meanings are made explicit. It was clear from the data that the use of this language here was intended to convey positive interpretations of home and family.

In the same way, feminist critiques of the social construction of motherhood problematises essentialist characteristics ascribed to the role (Oakley 1993). These roles have stereotyped women as instinctive carers and homemakers, masking women's disadvantage in the private domestic sphere compared with men's position and power in the public sphere (Bordo 1993; Upton & Han 2003). For this reason, 'matrescence' is a better term than 'maternalism' as the latter is laden with this gender baggage. I understand matrescence as a skill in facilitating becoming a mother, which has generic application to either gender.

Underlying the women's gratitude for their experience of post-natal care in the birth centre may be the reality that, although becoming a mother is a major rites-of-passage event, western cultures have all but lost its ritual marking. Kitzinger (2000) writes regarding indigenous cultures, of the 'sacred lying-in periods', often up to 40 days, when the woman and her baby are in a transitional, liminal stage. Other women nurture the woman into motherhood so that the mother is freed of her usual responsibilities and can 'grow with' her baby. The activity and focus of carers is to protect, to nurture and to cherish the new mother and baby.

Qualitative research into consultant delivery suites tends to reveal them as hierarchical in structure and bureaucratic in processes (Hunt & Symonds 1995; Hunter 2004) in contrast to birth centres where structures are flatter and processes more pragmatic with considerable autonomy residing with birth centre staff (Walsh 2004). Compromised autonomy was a recurrent theme in midwives' accounts of working on labour wards (Ball *et al.* 2003; Pollard 2003) and activity in consultant units tend to be more task-driven and regulated (Lankshear *et al.* 2005) which differs from birth centres where tasks are more relationally mediated (Walsh 2006b). There are two studies of the labour ward environments where findings were largely positive. Berg (2005) and Price and Johnson (2006) conclude that midwives were able to practice using a combination of affective/intuitive skills and rational/scientific skills without hierarchical and institutional pressures impinging on them.

Conclusion

The birth environment powerfully shapes and impacts on the birth experience of women and carers. There is nothing neutral in this context with environment, attitudes and relationships all contributing in an enabling or disabling way. It may be that birth centres and home birth have something significant to teach us about the use of intuition and instinct in correcting a clinical bias that has arisen around institutional birth over the past 40 years. When allowed to be expressed, these behaviours appear to link humans to their mammal heritage of nesting but also facilitate a psychosocial dimension to safety, mediated profoundly through matrescent care. The challenge for institutional birth settings is to harness this largely untapped source of nurture and encourage its expression for the vast majority of women who birth in this context.

References

Allport S (1997) *A Natural History of Parenting*. New York, Harmony.

Annandale E (1988) How midwives accomplish natural birth: managing risk and balancing expectation. *Social Problems* 35(2): 95–110.

Attenborough D (1990) *The Trials of Life*. London, Collins.

Ball L, Curtis P, Kirkham M (2003) *Why do Midwives Leave?* London, Royal College of Midwives.

Barlow J, Birch L (2004) Midwifery practice and sexual abuse. *British Journal of Midwifery* 12(2): 72–5.

Bastick T (1982) *Intuition: How we Think and Act*. New York, John Willey & Sons, Inc.

Berg MA (2005) Midwifery model of care for childbearing women at high risk: genuine caring in caring for the genuine. *Journal of Perinatal Education* 14(1): 9–21.

Bordo S (1993) *Unbearable Weight: Feminism, Western Culture and the Body*. London, University of California Press.

Cosslett T (1994) *Women Writing Childbirth: Modern Discourses on Motherhood*. Manchester, Manchester University Press.

Coyle K, Hauck Y, Percival P, Kristjanson L (2001a) Ongoing relationships with a personal focus: mother's perceptions of birth centre versus hospital care. *Midwifery* 17: 171–81.

Coyle K, Hauck Y, Percival P, Kristjanson L (2001b) Ongoing relationships with a personal focus: mother's perceptions of birth centre versus hospital care. *Midwifery* 17: 182–93.

Cronin G, Simpson G, Hemsworth P (1996) The effects of gestation and farrowing environments on saw and piglet behaviour and piglet survival and growth in early lactation. *Applied Animal Behaviour Science* 46: 175–92.

Davis-Floyd R, Arvidson P (1997) *Intuition: The Inside Story. Interdisciplinary Perspectives*. New York, Routledge.

Demere T, Hollingsworth B, Unitt P (2002) Nests and nest-building animals. *Field Notes* Spring 3: 13–5.

Downe S, McCourt C (2008) From being to becoming: reconstructing childbirth knowledges. In Downe S (ed) *Normal Childbirth; Evidence and Debate*, 2nd edition. London, Churchill Livingstone.

Edwards N (2000) Woman planning homebirths: their own views on their relationships with midwives. In Kirkham M (ed) *The Midwife-Woman Relationship*. London, MacMillan, 55–91.

England P, Horowitz R (1996) *Birthing from Within*. Albuquerque, Partera Press.

Fannon M (2003) Domesticating birth in the hospital: "Family-centred" birth and the emergence of "homelike" birthing rooms. *Antipode* 35(3): 513–35.

Flint C (1993) *Midwifery Teams and Caseloads*. London, Butterworth Heinemann.

Foster J (2005) Innovative practice in birth education. In Nolan M, Foster J (eds) *Birth and Parenting Skills: New Directions in Antenatal Education*. London, Elsevier Science.

Gagnon A, Meier K, Waghorn K (2007) Continuity of nursing care and its link to caesarean birth rate. *Birth* 34(1): 26–31.

Green J, Coupland B, Kitzinger J (1998) *Great Expectations: A Prospective Study of Women's Expectations and Experiences of Childbirth*. Cambridge, Child Care and Development Group.

Haggerty J, Reid R, Freeman G, Starfield B, Adair C, McKendry R (2005) Continuity of care: a multidisciplinary review. *British Medical Journal* 327: 1219–21.

Halford S, Leonard P (2003) Space and place in the construction and performance of gendered nursing identities. *Journal of Advanced Nursing* 42(2): 201–8.

Harvey S, Jarrell J, Brant R, Stainton C, Rach D (1996) A randomised controlled trial of nurse/midwifery care. *Birth* 23: 128–35.

Hatem M, Sandall J, Devane D, Soltani H, Gates S (2008) Midwife-led versus other models of care for childbearing women. *Cochrane Database of Systematic Reviews* (4).

Hirst C (2005) *Rebirthing: Report of the Review of the Maternity Services in Qld*. Brisbane.

Hodnett ED, Gates S, Hofmeyr GJ, Sakala C (2007) Continuous support for women during childbirth. In *The Cochrane Library (Cochrane Review)*, Issue 1. Chichester, John Wiley & Sons, Ltd.

Hodnett E, Lowe N, Hannah M, Willan A (2002) Effectiveness of nurses as providers of birth labour support in North American Hospitals. *Journal of the American Medical Association* 288: 1373–81.

Homer C, Davis G, Brodie P, *et al.* (2001) Collaboration in maternity care: a randomised trial comparing community-based continuity of care with standard hospital care. *British Journal of Obstetrics and Gynaecology* 108: 16–22.

Hunt S, Symonds A (1995) *The Social Meaning of Midwifery*. Basingstoke, MacMillan.

Hunter B (2004) Conflicting ideologies as a source of emotion work in midwifery. *Midwifery* 20(3): 261–72.

Hunter B, Berg M, Lundgren I, O'lafsdo'ttir O, Kirkham M (2008) Relationships: the hidden threads in the tapestry of maternity care. *Midwifery* 24: 132–7.

Kitzinger S (2000) *Rediscovering Birth*. London, Little Brown & Company.

Lankshear G, Ettorre E, Mason D (2005) Decision-making, uncertainty and risk: exploring the complexity of work processes on NHD delivery suites. *Health, Risk and Society* 7(4): 361–77.

Leap N, Anderson P (2004) The role of pain in normal birth and the empowerment of women. In Downe S (ed) *Normal Childbirth; Evidence and Debate.* London, Churchill Livingstone.

Machin D, Scamell M (1997) The experience of labour: using ethnography to explore the irresistible nature of the bio-medical metaphor during labour. *Midwifery* 13: 78–84.

Mooney J (1994) *The Hidden Figure: Domestic Violence in North London.* Islington, Islington Police and Crime Prevention Unit.

Myles M (1981) *Myles Textbook for Midwives.* Edinburgh, Churchill Livingstone.

North Staffordshire Changing Childbirth Research Team (2000) A randomised study of midwifery caseload care and traditional 'shared-care'. *Midwifery* 16(4): 295–302.

Oakley A (1993) *Essays on Women, Medicine and Health.* Edinburgh, Edinburgh University Press.

Page L, McCourt C, Beake S, Hewison J (1999) Clinical interventions and outcomes of One-to-One midwifery practice. *Journal of Public Health Medicine* 21(3): 243–8.

Pollard K (2003) Searching for autonomy. *Midwifery* 19: 113–24.

Posnett J (1999) Is bigger better? Concentration in the provision of secondary care. *British Medical Journal* 319: 1063–65.

Price M, Johnson M (2006) An ethnography of experienced midwives caring for women in labour. *Evidence-Based Midwifery* 4(3): 101–6.

Ramsden I (2003) *Cultural Safety and Nursing Education in Aotearoa and Te Waipounamu,* available from: http://culturalsafety.masey.ac.nz/RAMSDEN%20 THESIS.pdf (accessed December 2008).

Raphael D (1973) *Tender Gift: Breast Feeding.* London, Prentice Hall.

Robertson A (1997) *The Midwife Companion.* Sydney, Ace Graphics.

Rosen P (2004) Supporting women in labour: analysis of different types of caregivers. *Journal of Midwifery and Women's Health* 49: 24–31.

Rosenberg K, Trevathan W (2003) Birth, obstetrics and human evolution. *British Journal of Obstetrics and Gynaecology* 109(11): 1199–206.

Simkin P, Ancheta R (2005) *The Labour Progress Handbook.* Oxford, Blackwell Science.

Taylor S, Klein L, Lewis B *et al.* (2000) Biobehavioural responses to stress in females. *Psychological Review* 107(3): 411–29.

Thomas T (2001) Becoming a mother: matrescence as spiritual formation. *Religious Education* 96(1): 88–105.

Tracy S, Tracy M (2003) Costing the cascade: estimating the cost of increased obstetric intervention in childbirth using population data. *BJOG: An International Journal of Obstetrics and Gynaecology* 110(8): 717–24.

Upton R., Han S (2003) Maternity and its discontents. *Journal of Contemporary Ethnography* 32(6): 670–92.

Walsh D (1999) An ethnographic study of women's experience of partnership caseload midwifery practice: the professional as friend. *Midwifery* 15(3): 165–76.

Walsh D (2004) *Becoming mother: an ethnography of a free-standing birth centre.* PhD Thesis, University of Central Lancashire.

Walsh D (2006a) 'Nesting' and 'Matrescence': distinctive features of a free-standing birth centre. *Midwifery* 22(3): 228–39.

Walsh D (2006b) Subverting assembly-line birth: childbirth in a free-standing birth centre. *Social Science and Medicine* 62(6): 1330–40.

Wickham S (2002) *Reclaiming Spirituality in Birth*. [On-line]. available from: http://www.withwoman.co.uk/contents/info/spiritualbirth.html (accessed 2003).

Yearley C (1999) Pre-registration student midwives: fitting in. *British Journal of Midwifery* 7(10): 627–31.

Chapter 5
Labour Rhythms

Denis Walsh

Introduction

This chapter reviews the latest developments in normal labour, especially in relation to the emerging critique of the labour progress paradigm. The requirement to vigilantly monitor labour progress is a recent development in labour care, with its main exponents writing about this imperative from the 1950s onwards. An alternative paradigm of labour rhythms will also be explored, and its understanding extended to the second stage of labour.

Once the flexibility of the labour rhythms paradigm is adopted, practitioners are released from the bondage of repeated vaginal examinations (VE) as the marker of normal labour pattern. A variety of other skills can come into play that arguably had been lost from earlier birth attendants as the VE became the monitor of progress par excellence. These will be reviewed, though their evidence base, at least in relation to research, is paltry.

Labour progression has been the focus of extensive research over the past 40 years but virtually all of it suffers from contextual narrowness, having been exclusively carried out in large maternity hospitals. When writing about intrapartum skills the paucity of any studies outside of these environments limits not only the ability to premise writing on conventional evidence sources but also undermines attempts to explain the rich variety of personal anecdote around individual women's labours. Research into out-of-hospital birth settings is imperative in the urgent quest to explore and explain labour patterns.

Origins of the progress paradigm

Emanuel Friedman was the first to graphically record cervical dilatation over time and measure this in a cohort of women. His work in the mid-1950s became seminal in influencing our understanding of average lengths of labour for primigravid and multigravid women and the sigmoid-shaped Friedman curve was incorporated into obstetric and midwifery textbooks for the next 50 years (Friedman 1954). The curve represented early, middle and later phases of the first stage of labour.

In the early 1970s, Phillpott and Castle (1972) added the partogram to labour records and amplified the cervicograph to give guidance for what to do if labours were slow. Using just the active phase of the first stage of labour, they drew an alert line at the 1 cm/hour rate, a transfer line at 2 hours behind the alert line and an action line 2 hours behind that. The alert line was a signal to the clinician to monitor closely, the transfer line to literally transfer physically to a major hospital and the action line to rupture membranes and administer syntocinon. Philpott and Castle were working in remote area of Rhodesia and were concerned about the disastrous consequences of obstructed labours.

Studd (1973) measured cohorts of women admitted to UK hospitals at differing stages of cervical dilatation and plotted their dilatation over time, raising the interesting possibility that British women might labour at different rates to African or North American women.

All three of these cervicograph variations were adapted and added to by O'Driscoll in his protocol of 'active management of labour' (O'Driscoll & Meagher 1986). This interventionist approach had strict criteria for labour diagnosis and aggressive management of slow progress with early recourse to artificial rupture of membranes and intravenous syntocinon if labour did not progress at 1 cm/hour. The active management of labour protocol was responsible for the convention that labours should adhere to the 1 cm/hour template which is much stricter than Philpott's guideline of the early 1970s. Though the active management of labour went out of fashion during the 1990s when it was realised that the only effective component of the package was continuous support during labour (Frigoletto *et al.* 1995), its championing of syntocinon for the augmentation of labour continues to be popular today. UK studies show that up to 57% of low-risk primigravid women are prescribed it (Mead 2004), with similar rates in Australia (Tracey *et al.* 2007), suggestive of a collapse in the belief that nulliparous women can labour physiologically.

Organisational factors

This clinical imperative that long labours could indicate pathology may not have gained credence without the changes in organisational structures in how maternity care was delivered, in particular, the centralising movement of the second half of the 20th century. With more and more women giving birth in larger and larger hospitals, there was organisational pressure to process women through delivery suites and post-natal wards. Martin (1987) had railed against assembly-line childbirth in the 1980s but it was not until Perkins's (2004) comprehensive and considered critique of USA maternity care policy that the adoption of an essentially business/industrial model by maternity hospitals has been made so explicit. Perkins cited Henry Ford car assembly line as the template for the organisation of USA maternity hospital activity.

One of us (DW) elaborated on this critique in a study of childbirth at a free-standing birth centre (FSBC) in the United Kingdom (Walsh 2006a). Temporal differences were among the most striking between this setting and maternity hospitals. Women's labours were not on a time line and there was no pressure to free up rooms for new occupants. The corollary of hospitals with time restrictions on labour length is that more women can labour and birth within their space. It comes as little surprise to find that the hospitals still practising active management of labour are among the largest in Europe with over 8000 births/year (Murphy-Lawless 1998). Midwives' anecdotes and ethnographic research point to the pressures that exist in big units to 'get through the work' and deal with the labour 'nigglers' (Hunt & Symonds 1995).

The time pressures that are applied to women's labours in hospital therefore have their origins in both a clinical and organisational imperative. These pressures will not be addressed simply by revising clinical parameters around labour length, important though that endeavour is, but by simultaneously challenging the centralising tendency of maternity care provision.

An emergent critique

A backlash against the clinical imperative of labour progress was beginning to appear in the late 1990s when Albers (1999) concluded from her research that nulliparous women's labours were longer than what Friedman said. She found that in a low-risk population of women cared for by midwives in nine different centres in the USA, some active phases of labour were twice the length of Freidman's cohort (17.5 hours vs. 8.5 hours for nulliparas and 13.8 hours vs. 7 hours for multiparas) without any consequent morbidity. Cesario's (2004) later study found a similar average length of labour to Friedman but a wider range of normal. Primiparous women remained in the first stage for up to 26 hours and multiparous women for 23 hours without adverse effects. A more recent randomised controlled trial (RCT) showed that if prescriptive action lines that limit labour length are used with primigravid women, over 50% will require intervention with the authors calling for a review of labour length orthodoxies (Lavender *et al.* 2006).

Obstetric journals were also beginning to question Friedman's curve. Zhang and colleagues (2002) examined the patterns of cervical dilatation in 1329 nulliparous women and found slower dilatation rates in the active phase, especially before 7 cm, where the slowest group were all below Friedman's 1 cm/hour threshold. They concluded that current diagnostic criteria for protracted or arrested labour may be too stringent, citing important contextual differences in current practice to Friedman's day. Among these are the medical advances for managing longer labours like syntocinon, epidural anaesthesia and fetal monitoring and the mean increase in maternal body mass and fetal weight with the latter probably contributing to slower labours. We would add to this the increase in general health of the current generation of women compared with 50 years ago, making them less vulnerable to the effects of long labours.

Gurewitsch *et al.*'s (2002) interesting paper contributed newer data on labour rhythms at the other end of parity – grand multiparous women. They found that the latent phase of labour could last till up to 6 cm and that progression after that mimics lower order parity women, challenging the convention that grand multiparous women labour more quickly.

What these papers suggest to us is that there is more physiological variation between women than previously thought. Recent criticisms of quantitative evidence sources support this. The limitations of methods based on homogenising women statistically towards an average have already been questioned in Chapter 1 but here is a good example. Midwives have always known that many women do not fit the average of a 1 cm/hour dilatation rate and even more fundamentally, may not physiologically mimic the parameters of the average cervix. Their cervix may be fully dilated at 9 or 11 cm! Given the infinite variety in women's physical appearance and psychosocial characteristics, it seems entirely reasonable to expect subtle differences in their birth physiology.

In recent years a better understanding of the hormones regulating labour contributes to this more complex picture of physiological varia-tion. Odent (2001) and Buckley (2004) have shown us that the hormonal cocktail influencing these processes is appropriately called the 'dance of labour'. These hormones' delicate interactions mediated by environ-mental and relational factors resemble the rhythm, beauty and harmony of skilled dancers. Sarah Buckley elaborates on these in Chapter 12.

Finally, a somewhat muted backlash against the organisational im-perative of processing women has appeared since 2003 (Perkins 2004; Walsh 2006a). The advent of organisational models like birth centres, both free-standing and alongside, has provided an alternative to the centralised delivery suite model. Birth centres rarely birth more than 1500 women/year and do not therefore feel the temporal pressures of busy labour wards. The backlash is muted though by the con-tinued centralising tendency. Consultant maternity units of less than 3000 birth/year, at least in the United Kingdom, are under pressure to close or merge on a tertiary centre site. Already we have maternity hospitals with an excess of 8000 births/year.

Rhythms in early labour

The division of the first stage of labour into latent and active is clinician-based and not necessarily resonant with the lived experience of labour as women with long latent phases have been trying to tell us for ages. The progress template has led us down a distinctly non-woman centred cul-de-sac here. We cannot, when a woman comes into hospital, validate her description of labour pains for 7 days because we dare not record a length of labour greater than 24 hours. We therefore invent euphemisms for her experience that allows us to classify her story as not being genuine labour – spurious labour, false labour or simply and starkly 'you're not in labour'. Gross and colleagues (2003) have illuminated our understanding of the phenomena of early labour by revealing how eclectically it presents in different women and how women vary in their self-diagnosis. Less than 60% of woman experienced contractions as the starting point of their labours. The remainder described fluid loss (28%), constant pain (24%), blood-stained loss (16%), gastrointestinal symptoms (6%), emotional upheaval (6%), and sleep alterations (4%) as heralding the start of labour, none of which fit the classic textbook definition. Gross suggests we change the direction of our questioning from eliciting the pattern of contractions to simply enquiring 'how did you recognise the start of labour'?

Burvill (2002) and Cheyne *et al.* (2006) point out that the midwifery diagnosis of labour in hospital is not simply a unilateral clinical judgement but a complex blend of balancing the totality of the woman's situation with institutional constraints like workloads, guidelines, continuity concerns, justifying decisions to senior staff and risk management. Contrast this with care at a home birth or free-standing birth centre (FSBC) where the organisational and clinical parameters are secondary to women's lived experience and care is driven by the latter (Walsh 2006a).

Twenty years ago, Flint (1986) counselled that early labour was best experienced at home with access to a midwife and this remains the ideal for low-risk women. Maternity services have realised since that time that the worst place to be is on a delivery suite because, as early and recent research shows, women just end up having more labour interventions (Hemminki & Simukka 1986; Rahnama *et al.* 2006). This is because of the organisational imperative of processing women through the system. The last thing a busy labour ward needs is the 'nigglers' (Hunt & Symonds 1995) 'clogging up the place' and taking rooms from the genuine labourers. Recent studies have showed the value of triage facilities or early labour assessment centres if home assessment in early labour is not an option. Women who attend them have less labour interventions (Lauzon & Hodnett 2004). Jackson *et al.* (2003) counselled the value of attending a FSBC and Turnbull *et al.* (1996) of seeing a midwife and not an obstetrician. Individualising care, ongoing informational and relational continuity are all important elements of best practice for the latent phase of labour. Lindgren and colleagues (2008) recent study of home-birth transfers in Sweden highlighted a hitherto unknown effect of relational continuity – the fact that when women were not attended by their known primary care midwife, they had more intrapartum transfers. This stands in stark contrast to caseload schemes where home-birth rates went up when early labour support at home led to the choice of a home birth in women who where undecided (Benjamin *et al.* 2001).

Rhythms in mid labour

What clinicians understand as the active phase of the first stage of labour has been the main focus of partogram recordings over the past 50 years. We have discussed the relaxation in times lines around this issue in recent years and now want to explore the decoupling of the phenomena of labour slowing or stopping from the presumption that this represents pathology. Apart from strong anecdotal evidence that some women experience a latent period in advanced labour, it was not until Davis *et al.*'s (2002) paper on labour 'plateaus' that statistical data was available. Their retrospective examination of thousands of records of home-birth women discovered that some had periods when the cervix stopped dilating temporarily in active labour. This was not interpreted as pathology by their birth attendants, and after variable periods of time, cervical progression began again. Some women even had two 'plateaus' in their labours. Gaskin's (2003) description of 'pasmo' indicated that physiological delays were known about in 19th century. If we then engage with the individuality of the labour experience for different women, the subtlety of hormonal interactions and the mediating effects of environment and companions, it is entirely feasible that actually labour could be understood as a 'unique normality', varying from woman to woman (Downe & McCourt 2008). Midwifery skill is in facilitating its individual expression in women in our care.

Recent research into the use of differing action lines (2 hours and 4 hours behind the 1 cm/hour line) in the active phase of labour has shown that the allowing for a slower rate of cervical dilatation does not result in more Caesarean sections and, importantly, women were just as satisfied with longer labours (Lavender *et al.* 2006). The *Guide to Effective*

Care in Pregnancy and Childbirth (Enkin *et al.* 2000) now recommends a cervical dilatation rate of 0.5 cm/hour in nulliparous women. One large UK consultant unit has recommended a minimum VE interval of 12 hours for nulliparous to reflect a loosening in attitude towards labour progression (Thorton 2006, Personal communication).

The ubiquity of VE as a practice in labour is inextricably linked to the progress paradigm. It deserves some appraisal as a common childbirth intervention to see if its widespread use is justifiable. It does not pass Chalmers *et al.*'s (1989) first test that it is necessary to enhance normal physiological processes. Devane's (1996) systematic literature review failed to identify the research basis for this procedure which reveals the power of the labour progress paradigm, effectively driving the adoption of the procedure on the basis of custom and practice. It also fails the second test of minimal untoward side effects that do not undermine its original intent. The literature around sexual abuse (Robohm & Buttenheim 1996) and post-traumatic stress disorder (Menage 1996) indicate that women who have experienced these find VE very problematic. Then there is the enlightening paper by Bergstrom *et al.* (1992), still a classic of phenomenological method and of the value of qualitative research. Her video taping of VE in US labour wards revealed the ritual that has evolved around the practice to legitimise such an intrusion into the private space. In essence, she shows the surgical construction of a practice, undertaken by strangers that would be totally unacceptable in any other circumstance except in an intimate sexual context between consenting adults. The adoption of a passive patient role and the marked power differential between them and the clinician were other taken-for-granted behaviours. More recently Stewart (2005) came to similar conclusions in a UK-based study. Warren (1999) reminds us that two important questions need asking before any VE is carried out:

- Why do I need to know this information now?
- Is there any other way I can obtain it?

Alternative skills for assessing labour

It is interesting to speculate how other skills would emerge if delivery suites and labour wards, for the period of a week, placed a moratorium on VE in low-risk women. Would it throw midwives and obstetricians into a panic, knowing that they could not monitor labour events by VE?

There is a surprising dearth of any research examining alternatives to VE for labour care, given the rich anecdotes that surround this area. Midwives have always taken into account the character of contractions, a woman's response to them and the findings from abdominal palpation.

Stuart (2000) is possibly unique in relying on abdominal palpation instead of VE to ascertain progress and most midwives weigh the results of VE above contractions and behaviour. It is the practices that are substitutional for vaginal exams that are the most interesting. Hobbs (1998) advocated the 'purple line' method, a line that runs from the distal margin of the anus up between the buttocks said to indicate full dilatation when it reaches the natal cleft. Byrne and Edmonds (1990) reported that 89% of women developed the line. Frye (2004), in her extremely comprehensive manual of care during normal birth, writes of monitoring temperature change in the lower leg. As labour progresses a coldness on touch is noted to move from the ankle up the leg to the knee. Over recent years I have heard from a number of sources of the marker on the forehead of a woman. Possibly originating from traditional birth attendant practices in Peru, this involved feeling for the appearance of a ridge running from between the eyes up to the hairline as labour progresses.

More knowledge comes from intuitive perceptions that many midwives may recognise but find hard to articulate, and even harder to write down as illustrated by the following story. An experience of intuition was related by home-birth midwives who noted in their own bodies the desire to defecate when women they were caring for were approaching full dilatation. A midwife in Australia's tropical north, told me how she used the ebb and flow of the tide to gauge how indigenous island women laboured. They tended to birth at high tide so, as the birthing suite overlooked a tidal bay, she knew they were approaching second stage of labour when the tide was high. Dutch midwives speak of observing the behaviour of the domestic cat who leaves the birth room as full dilatation is reached. The transitional phase between first and second stages has been studied by Baker and Kenner (1993) who noted the common vocalisations that mark it.

These are just a few examples of anecdotes that abound in this area. It is an area ripe for observational research but also for articles mapping the richness of midwives' experience. The intuitive hunches of midwives are in danger of being lost as they exist largely as oral stories, not written accounts, possibly because they might be discredited by an evidence orthodoxy that rates empirical verifiability as the standard.

Finally, there is the domain of emotional nuance reading that may impact hugely on how labour unfolds. (Kennedy *et al.* 2004). One of us (DW) recalled one such episode in the birth centre study (Walsh 2006b) when a teenage girl arrives in early labour, very distressed. The midwife asked her mother and sister to leave the room and gently enquired as to how she was. She burst into tears and over the next 2 hours, the midwife held her in an embrace on a mattress on the floor as the girl sobbed and sobbed. Then she said she was ready and went on to have a normal, rather peaceful birth. In other settings the girl may have been offered an epidural but this was not pain distress but emotional distress and the skill of the midwife was in her intuitive emotional nuance reading of that and how to bring comfort and support.

'Being with', not 'doing to' labouring women

The quest to dismantle assembly-line birth, removing women from the intrapartum timeline and rehabilitating belief in 'unique normality' of labour for individual women challenges us to radically rethink our focus and orientation to normal labour care. Hints of a different way of situating ourselves with women are in the writings of midwives and they speak in paradox and metaphor. Leap (2000a) tells of 'the less we do, the more we give' and Kennedy (2000) of 'doing nothing well' in her insightful study of expert US midwives. Fahy (1998) conceptualises the work of the midwife as 'being with' women, not 'doing to' them and Anderson (2004) quips that good labour care requires the midwife 'to drink tea intelligently'. All these writers are alluding not to a temporally regulated activity marked by task completions but to a disposition towards compassionate companionship with women that is a 'masterly inactivity' (RCM 2006). As a birth centre midwife offered during an interview: 'it's about being comfortable when there is nothing to do'.

These ideas are countercultural in an environment heavily inscribed with a 'doing' ethos as maternity hospitals are and also an anathema for the medical model where there is a 'compulsion to act' (Grol & Grimshaw 2003). It is challenging in a resource-tight health service where time and motion analysis are skewed to activity measurement. Yet Chalmers *et al.* (1989), as already mentioned in Chapter 1, the doyen of evidence-based maternity care, understood the truism that sometimes 'what really counts, cannot be counted' and I suggest that supportive labour care fits precisely into this category.

Definition of second stage

The reductionist nature of the biomedical definition of the second stage of labour has generated more than its fair share of 'doing good by stealth' behaviours by midwives (Kirkham 1999), particularly regarding its length. It is an especially brave midwife who will record the 6-hour second stage that included several hours of latency. It is far more comfortable to retrospectively assign the start so that the time comes in under whatever the guideline locally requires. Most of us have 'been there' and adopted the visualisation of the presenting part as our reference marker for the start of second stage.

Midwives know that women's bodies simply do not fit the template of the biomedical definition, either because they have a 'rest and be thankful' phase after full dilation or they involuntarily push before. Both of these fall outside of the normative physiology. Ascertaining the start of the second stage even with a confirmatory VE was always problematic anyway. As a midwifery mentor pointed out to a student during her training, if there is no cervix palpable on examination, then you are already too late – full dilatation occurred sometime before. Or the midwives who deliberately record full dilation at 9 cm or 11 cm because they argue the improbability that every women in the world has a cervix that dilates to 10 cm exactly. Of course they are facetiously commenting on the nonsense that birth anatomy and physiology is uniform across all women.

The artificial imposition of labour stages is classically challenged here because of the first to second stage transition: that mysterious phenomena, virtually ignored by childbirth textbooks except by one of us (SD) in the most recent edition of Myles (Downe 2003). Yet transition is one of the earliest observed labour behaviours by students on birth suites and its recognition and care is a key practical skill for the midwife to acquire. Writing about transition more often appears in lay childbirth literature, in books on natural birth and the occasional midwifery journal. This highlights the fact that transition is a 'lived phenomena', not easily reducible to scientific measurement and not held to be of clinical interest to obstetric researchers.

Woods (2006) gives an excellent summary of what is known about transition to date and it remains a priority for midwifery research. She describes a spectrum of experiences and emotions (from inner calm to acute distress) that occur in many women in the latter half of labour just prior to the pushing phase. Mander (2002), in an important paper, focuses on labour pain in transition and the challenge this poses for the midwife. It is a stern test of a 'working with pain' approach but wise midwives develop strategies to support women through (Flint 1986), discerning the difference between this and pain indicative of pathology (Leap 2000b).

The biomedical model's delineation of the stages of labour seems to primarily serve the purpose of establishing time frames for each. If time frames take on less significance, then midwives will be freer to work with the lived experience of transition and second stage and arguably offer better individualised care. The assembly-line imperative is as much in evidence in second stage as in first, even more so because birth suite staff seem to believe that they can directly rescue a protracted second stage – hence the cheerleading scenario or rugby scrum analogy that is sometimes observed here. In an overdue contribution on the experiential and psychological aspects of second stage,

Anderson's (2000) interviews with women were very revealing. They spoke of

- the paradox of being in control and 'letting go';
- their altered states of consciousness;
- experiencing a sense of timelessness;
- wanting the midwife to be a safe anchor, someone to put trust in and a calm, quiet, unobtrusive presence;
- unhelpful aspects of care were being treated as a 'naughty schoolgirl', being told off, intrusive interventions e.g. fetal monitoring, requiring to be on bed, interruptions and being undermined.

Most of their comments relate to aspects of care deleteriously affected by time constraints. One way out of this temporality bind is to adjust the definition of the start of second stage. Long (2006) makes an important contribution to redefining this by changing the criteria of full dilatation of the cervix to 'when the presenting part has passed through the cervix and is below the ischial spines'. This alteration, she argues, would allow for the physiological variations observed in practice of latent episodes after reaching full dilatation. Once the presenting part has passed through the cervix and has descended beyond the ischial spines, then bearing down will occur as the fetus enters the perineal phase (Roberts 2003) or encounters the 'fetal ejection reflex' (Sutton 2001).

An acknowledgement of a latent element to the second stage of labour and a subsequent lengthening of the time frame has appeared in obstetric journals in recent years (Fraser *et al.* 2000). Its curious and ironic source is epidural anaesthesia. Anaesthetists and obstetricians became alarmed at the assisted vaginal birth rates with epidurals and at the fetal distress associated with prolonged instructed pushing. They began researching passive descent, in some studies up to 5 hours (Hansen *et al.* 2002), before active pushing was commenced. Now it is common practice to wait at least 2 hours in many consultant units. A blatant double standard exists in these very same units where women without epidurals are only 'allowed' 1 hour. The perverse thinking here defies any logic. It is safe to permit a woman to languish on a bed, immobile, probably with syntocinon augmenting her expulsive contractions, for several hours if she has an epidural but not if she is labouring physiologically without drugs, probably upright and free to move at will?

Time and fetal health

Many obstetricians and paediatricians appear to believe there is direct link between the length of second stage and fetal health and this primarily drives times restrictions on second stage. A examination of the evidence, all of it from obstetric journals, does not support this conclusion.

Four large retrospective observational studies have been conducted over the past 15 years. Saunders *et al.* (1992) examined 25 000 women and found the length of second stage was not associated with low Apgar scores or neonatal unit admissions. Menticoglou *et al.* (1995) looked at 6000 nulliparous women, some of whom had second stages lasting longer than 5 hours, concluding that there was no increase in low 5 min Apgar scores, neonatal seizures, and neonatal unit admissions in those women. Janni *et al.* (2002) oft quoted study also concluded that there was no association between the length of second stage and neonatal morbidity. Finally, Myles and Santolaya (2003) confirmed all previous findings in their study of 4700 women whose second stages lasted up to 4 hours. Some of these studies found links to maternal morbidity such as infection and bleeding but these were explained by labour practices or first stage factors.

These studies refute the assumed link between time in second stage and fetal compromise and support a recommendation to abandon arbitrary time constraints in normal labours. This recommendation needs to be combined with ensuring best practice in encouraging upright posture and spontaneous pushing, both of which will optimise fetal health. The only qualifying factor is that there is some evidence that when the presenting part is on the pelvic floor, fetal lactic acid begins to accumulate and this may be reflected in a deterioration in fetal heart patterns (Nordstrom *et al.* 2001).

Early pushing

We are indebted to Bergstrom and colleagues (1997) for vividly capturing women's distress with the phenomena of early bearing down, which was not because of the physiological experience but because of their carers' responses. 'I've gotta push. Please let me push' is a lesson in choosing a paper's title to catch the reader's attention. For a topic where there is such ingrained custom and practice, one would expect there to be a substantial research base. Not only has it not been researched, like transition, little has been written about it. This makes it all the more remarkable that even Enkin *et al.* (2000) describe early pushing as a form of care unlikely to be beneficial. In the absence of research, this key evidence source felt able to comment on it.

Like spontaneous rupture of membranes at term (VE is required to exclude cord prolapse), so early bearing down has spawned practices based, at best, on worse case scenario thinking and, at worst, on myth. Student midwives have been told that it will lead to an oedematous lip of cervix which, if left untreated, will slough off leading to haemorrhage. That tends to focus the mind of the midwife: to get the woman lying on her side breathing on entonox or, if that fails, siting an epidural. For midwives committed to physiological birth, it is the dissonance generated by this that is so difficult. On the one hand we are encouraging women to trust their instinctual urges except in this case.

One of us (SD) has scoped this issue comprehensively and surveyed midwives' approaches to it. Using midwives' responses to a variety of vignettes, she categorised the midwives' actions under technologic, equivocal or physiologic. She repeated the survey 7 years later and found a trend towards more physiologic actions, reflecting a stronger normal discourse abroad in midwifery culture (Downe 2008). Thematic analysis revealed that organisational factors like time constraints and custom and practice 'rules', place of birth and how midwives integrated their experiences over time regardless of years qualified were all influential in dealing with dissonance. Downe argues for a paradigm of 'unique normality' that incorporates a spread of physiology still within the orbit of normal to address the early pushing phenomena, as well as calling for more research.

Attitudes and philosophy

How we integrate experiences that 'catch us out' e.g. when we encourage instinctive pushing behaviours and later discover a stalled labour at 5 cm, is formational to our practice journey. Recent writing has stressed the notion of being comfortable with uncertainty in normal childbirth care (Sookhoo & Biott 2002; Winter & Cameron 2006; Downe & McCourt 2008). The ability to not necessarily adjust one's care because of a suboptimal outcome e.g. to resist the temptation after the experience above to always do a confirmatory VE when signs of second stage appear, takes experience and a supportive environment. You have to be able to say: 'That was the exception and I know the vast majority of the time I can trust the physiology'. It is even harder to hold this position in a birth suite where intervention is common and regular exposure to non-medicated, physiological labours is the exception.

In the second stage of labour as Anderson (2000) demonstrated, attitudinal change to enhance women's autonomy is imperative because of the history of disempowerment over recent centuries. How often do women ask about breathing and pushing as though they have little confidence that these behaviours will manifest instinctively?

Conclusion

An attempt has been made in this chapter to challenge the labour progress paradigm and, in relation to normal labour, suggest the rhythms alternative. This is not to say that a woman whose uterus is working powerfully but whose labour is stalled does not require appropriate intervention. However, even here, as Simkin and Ancheta (2005) counsel, physiological interventions like posture and mobility should be tried prior to invoking the traditional medical interventions like rupturing of membranes and syntocinon augmentation.

This is to say that women can labour at different rates and that progressive rhythms can be interspersed with resting, quiescent periods. It is unlikely though that the labour progress mentality can be fully addressed without challenging the organisational imperative found in very large hospitals. This requires a whole systems rethink that predicates care on the simple principle that 'small is beautiful'.

References

Albers L (1999) The duration of labour in healthy women. *Journal of Perinatology* 19(2): 114–9.

Anderson T (2000) Feeling safe enough to let go: the relationship between the woman and her midwife in the second stage of labour. In Kirkham M (ed) *The Midwife-Woman Relationship*. London, Routledge.

Anderson T (2004) Conference presentation. The impact of the age of risk for antenatal education. NCT Conference, Coventry, 13th March 2004.

Baker A, Kenner A (1993) Communication of pain: vocalisation as an indicator of the stage of labour. *Australian and New Zealand Journal of Obstetrics and Gynaecology* 33(4): 384–5.

Benjamin Y, Walsh D, Taub N (2001) A comparison of partnership caseload midwifery care with conventional team midwifery care: labour and birth outcomes. *Midwifery* 17(3): 234–40.

Bergstrom L, Roberts J, Skillman L, Seidel J (1992) 'You'll feel me touching you, sweetie'. Vaginal Examinations during the Second Stage of Labour. *Birth* 19(l): 10–8.

Bergstrom L, Seedily J, Schulman-Hull L, Roberts J (1997) 'I gotta push. Please let me push!' Social interactions during the change from first to second stage labour. *Birth* 24(3): 173–80.

Buckley S (2004) Undisturbed birth – nature's hormonal blueprint for safety, ease and ecstasy. *Midirs* 14(2): 203–9.

Burvill S (2002) Midwifery diagnosis of labour onset. *British Journal of Midwifery* 10(10): 600–5.

Byrne D, Edmonds D (1990) Clinical methods for evaluating progress in first stage of labour. *Lancet* 335(1681): 122.

Cesario S (2004) Re-evaluation of Freidman's labour curve: a pilot study. *Journal of Obstetrics, Gynaecology and Neonatal Nursing* 33: 713–22.

Chalmers I, Kierse M, Neilson J *et al.* (1989) *A Guide to Effective Care in Pregnancy and Childbirth.* Oxford, Oxford University Press.

Cheyne H, Dowding D, Hundley V (2006) Making the diagnosis of labour: midwives' diagnostic judgement and management decisions. *Journal of Advanced Nursing* 53(6): 625–35.

Davis B, Johnson K, Gaskin I (2002) The MANA Curve – Describing plateaus in labour using the MANA database. 26th Triennial Congress, ICM, Vienna, Abstract No 30.

Devane D (1996) Sexuality and midwifery. *British Journal of Midwifery* 4(8): 413–20.

Downe S (2003) Transition and the second stage of labour. In Fraser D, Cooper A (eds) *Myles Textbook for Midwives*, 14th edition. Edinburgh, Churchill Livingstone, 487–505.

Downe S (2008) The early pushing urge: practice and discourse. In Downe S (ed) *Normal Birth – Evidence and Debate.* London, Churchill Livingstone.

Downe S, McCourt C (2008) From being to becoming: reconstructing childbirth knowledges. In Downe S (ed) *Normal Childbirth; Evidence and Debate.* London, Churchill Livingstone.

Enkin M, Kierse M, Neilson J *et al.* (2000) *A Guide to Effective Care in Pregnancy and Childbirth.* Oxford, Oxford University Press.

Fahy K (1998) Being a midwife or doing midwifery. *Australian Midwives College Journal* 11(2): 11–6.

Flint C (1986) *Sensitive Midwifery.* London, Heinemann.

Fraser W, Marcoux S, Krauss I *et al.* (2000) Multi-centre, randomised controlled trial of delayed pushing for nulliparous women in the second stage of labour with continuous epidural analgesia. *American Journal of Obstetrics and Gynaecology* 182: 1165–72.

Friedman E (1954) The graphic analysis of labour. *American Journal of Obstetrics and Gynaecology* 68: 1568–75.

Frigoletto F, Lieberman E, Lang J *et al.* (1995) A clinical trial active management of labour. *New England Journal of Medicine* 333: 745–50.

Frye A (2004) *Holistic Midwifery, Care of the Mother and Baby from Onset of Labour Through the First Hours After Birth*, Vol. 11. Portland, Labry's Press.

Gaskin IM (2003) Going backwards: the concept of 'pasmo'. *The Practising Midwife* 6(8): 34–6.

Grol R, Grimshaw (2003) From best evidence to best practice: effective implementation of change in patient's care. *Lancet* 362: 1225–30.

Gross M, Haunschild T, Stoexen T, Methner V, Guenter H (2003) Women's recognition of the spontaneous onset of labour. *Birth* 30(4): 267–71.

Gurewitsch E, Diament P, Fong J *et al.* (2002) The labour curve of the grand multipara: does progress of labour continue to improve with additional childbearing? *American Journal of Obstetrics and Gynaecology* 186: 1331–8.

Hansen S, Clark S, Foster J (2002) Active pushing versus passive fetal descent in the second stage of labour: a randomised controlled trial. *Obstetrics and Gynaecology* 99: 29–34.

Hemminki E, Simukka R (1986) The timing of hospital admission and progress of labour. *European Journal of Obstetrics, Gynaecology and Reproductive Biology* 22: 85–94.

Hobbs L (1998) Assessing cervical dilatation without VEs. *The Practising Midwife* 1(11): 34–5.

Hunt S, Symonds A (1995) *The Social Meaning of Midwifery*. Basingstoke, MacMillan.

Kennedy H, (2000) A model of exemplary midwifery practice: results of a Delphi study including commentary by Ernst K. *Journal of Midwifery and Women's Health* 45 (1): 4–19.

Kennedy H, Shannon M, Chuahorm U, Kravetz M, (2004) The landscape of caring for women: a narrative study of midwifery practice. *Journal of Midwifery and Women's Health* 49: 14–23.

Jackson D, Lang J, Ecker J, Swartz W, Heeren T (2003) Impact of collaborative management and early labour admission in labour on method of delivery. *Journal of Obstetrics, Gynaecology and Neonatal Nursing* 32(2): 147–57.

Janni W, Schiessl B, Peschers U *et al.* (2002) The prognostic impact of a prolonged second stage of labour on maternal and fetal outcome. *Acta Obstetrica Gynaecologica Scandinavia* 81: 214–21.

Kirkham M, (1999) The culture of midwifery in the National Health Service in England. *Journal of Advanced Nursing* 30: 732–9.

Lauzon L, Hodnett E (2004) Labour assessment programs to delay admission to labour wards (Cochrane Review). *The Cochrane Library*, Issue 1. Chichester, John Wiley & Sons, Ltd.

Lavender T, Alfirevic Z, Walkinshaw S (2006) Effect of different partogram action lines on birth outcomes. *Obstetrics and Gynaecology* 108: 295–302.

Leap N, (2000a) The less we do, the more we give. In Kirkham M (ed) *The Midwife-mother Relationship*. London, MacMillan, 1–18.

Leap N (2000b) Pain in labour towards a midwifery perspective. *Midirs Midwifery Digest* 10(1): 49–53.

Lindgren H, Hildingsson I, Christensson K (2008) Transfers in planned homebirths related to midwife availability and continuity: a nationwide population-based study. *Birth* 25(1): 9–15.

Long L (2006) Redefining the second stage of labour could help to promote normal birth. *British Journal of Midwifery* 14(2): 104–6.

Mander R (2002) The transitional stage. *The Practising Midwife* 5(1): 10–2.

Martin E, (1987) *The Woman in the Body: A Cultural Analysis of Reproduction*. Milton Keynes, Open University Press.

Mead M (2004) Midwives' perspectives in a 11 UK maternity units. In Downe S (ed) *Normal Childbirth: Evidence and Debate*. London, Churchill Livingstone.

Menage J (1996) Post-traumatic stress disorder following obstetric/gynaecological procedures. *British Journal of Midwifery* 4(10): 532–3.

Menticoglou S, Manning F, Harman C *et al.* (1995) perinatal outcome in relation to second stage duration. *American Journal of Obstetrics and Gynaecology* 173(3): 906–12.

Murphy-Lawless J, (1998) *Reading Birth and Death: A History of Obstetric Thinking*. Cork, Cork University Press.

Myles T, Santolaya J (2003) Maternal and neonatal outcomes in patients with a prolonged second stage of labour. *Obstetrics and Gynaecology*, 102: 52–8.

Nordstrom L, Achanna S, Naka K, Arulkumaran S (2001) Fetal and maternal lactate increase during active second stage of labour. *British Journal of Obstetrics and Gynaecology* 108: 263–8.

Odent M (2001) New reasons and new ways to study birth physiology. *International Journal of Gynaecology and Obstetrics* 75: S39–S45.

O'Driscoll K, Meager D (1986) *Active Management of Labour.* London, W.B. Saunders.

Perkins B (2004) *The Medical Delivery Business: Health Reform, Childbirth and the Economic Order.* London, Rutgers University Press.

Phillpott R, Castle W (1972) Cervicographs in the management of labour on primigravidae 1. The alert line for detecting abnormal labour. *Journal of Obstetrics and Gynaecology of the British Commonwealth* 79: 592–8.

Rahnama P, Ziaei S, Faghihzadeh S (2006) Impact of early admission in labour on method of delivery. *International Journal of Gynaecology and Obstetrics* 92(3): 217–20.

Roberts J (2003) A new understanding of the second stage of labour: implications for nursing care. *Journal of Obstetric, Gynaecological and Neonatal Nursing* 32(6): 794–801.

Robohm J, Buttenheim M (1996) The gynaecological care experience of adult survivors of childhood sexual abuse: a preliminary investigation. *Women and Health* 24(3): 59–75.

Royal College of Midwives (2006) *Campaign for Normal Birth.* http://www. rcmnormalbirth.org.uk/default.asp?sID=1099658666156 (accessed December 2008).

Saunders N, Paterson C, Wadsworth J (1992) Neonatal and maternal morbidity in relation to the length of the second stage of labour. *British Journal of Obstetrics and Gynaecology* 99(5): 381–5.

Simkin P, Ancheta R (2005) *The Labour Progress Handbook Oxford.* Oxford, Blackwell Science.

Sookhoo M, Biott C (2002) Learning at work: midwives judging progress in labour. *Learning in Health and Social Care* 1(2): 75–85.

Stewart M (2005) 'I'm just going to wash you down': sanitizing the vaginal examination. *Journal of Advanced Nursing* 51(6): 587–94.

Stuart C (2000) Invasive actions in labour: where have all the old trick gone? *The Practising Midwife* 3(8): 30–3.

Studd J (1973) Partograms and nomograms of cervical dilatation in management of primigravid labour. *British Medical Journal* 4: 451–5.

Sutton J (2001) *Let Birth be Born Again.* Auckland, Birth Concepts UK.

Tracey S, Sullivan E, Wang Y (2007) Birth outcomes associated with intervention in labour amongst low risk women: a population-based study. *Women and Birth* 20(2): 41–8.

Turnbull D, Holmes S, Cheyne H *et al.* (1996) Randomised controlled trial of efficacy of midwifery-managed care. *Lancet* 348: 213–8.

Walsh D (2006a) Subverting assembly-line birth: childbirth in a free-standing birth centre. *Social Science and Medicine* 62(6): 1330–40.

Walsh D (2006b) 'Nesting' and 'Matrescence': distinctive features of a free-standing birth centre. *Midwifery* 22(3): 228–39.

Warren C (1999) Invaders of privacy. *Midwifery Matters* 81: 8–9.

Winter C, Cameron J (2006) The 'stages' model of labour: deconstructing the myth. *British Journal of Midwifery* 14(8): 454–7.

Woods T (2006) The transitional stage of labour. *Midirs* 16(2): 225–8.

Zhang J, Troendle J, Yancey M (2002) Reassessing the labour curve. *American Journal Of Obstetrics and Gynaecology* 187: 824–8.

Chapter 6
Evidence for Neonatal Transition and the First Hour of Life

Judith Mercer and Debra Erikson-Owens

Introduction

Birth is perhaps the most dramatic physiologic event any human will experience. How it is conducted may have effects that last a lifetime. New information shatters our complacency and increases fear about the damage done to infants by some of the birth and newborn practices we hold as routine and insignificant. For instance, evidence is building that immediate cord clamping may create harm such as iron deficiency anaemia in term infants and intraventricular haemorrhage (IVH), sepsis, and the need for more transfusions in preterm infants (Mercer *et al.* 2006; Hutton & Hassan 2007; Rabe *et al.* 2008). Iron deficiency anaemia can affect a child's ability to develop normally and achieve his or her full potential (Lozoff & Georgieff 2006; Lozoff *et al.* 2006a, 2006b; Lozoff 2007) and IVH and sepsis in preterm infants often results in later developmental delay (Vohr *et al.* 2003; Stoll *et al.* 2004).

Previously, we focused our concerns on the amount of iron and blood volume lost with immediate cord clamping (Yao *et al.* 1969; Cernadas *et al.* 2006) but recent information about stem cells has added another dimension for consideration and research. Stem cells have a miraculous ability to heal. In animal models, they have been found to repair heart, brain, liver, lung and muscle tissue as well as endothelial cells lining blood vessels. Immediate cord clamping robs a term infant of almost one billion of these miracle cells at birth (Haneline *et al.* 1996). Blood banks designed to save the baby's stem cells for the future have been established without any longitudinal research on the safety or impact of immediate cord clamping and the interference with the infant receiving his or her full allotment of stem cells at birth. Yet, in rat studies, injection of human cord blood stem cells within 24 hours after injury can prevent cerebral palsy (Meier *et al.* 2006). This animal study, along with other studies on the healing power of stem cells, demands that the safety of ICC at birth be studied with inclusion of long-term follow-up of children.

In the first minutes after birth, the infant spans two worlds – the world of the fetus and the world of the newborn. When oxygen-rich blood is allowed to course through the intact cord, the newly born infant is afforded a protected time of adjustment and discovery. Handling the infant slowly, gently and lovingly and placing him or her on the mother's abdomen allows for a gentle transition between these life stages. This precious time of taking in between mother and baby is like no other. There are emotional, physiologic, bacteriologic, hormonal and spiritual exchanges between the mother and the infant during this special time. Yet, in a busy hospital environment, the magnitude of this human achievement is likely to be overlooked. Immediate cord clamping, separation of the infant from its mother, suctioning and other 'pressing' newborn tasks often take precedence over the mother and infant's time of intimacy and connectedness. This important period of dual transition from fetus to newborn and from pregnancy to motherhood, inadequately referred to as the fourth stage of labour, is ripe for examination.

A critical goal of pregnancy, labour and birth, is to have a healthy vigorous newborn. A strong, alert newborn is ready to be a fully functioning partner for the mother during the initial bonding time. The practices and interventions used during birth and the immediate post-partum period can either support or disrupt the newborn's adjustment during this important first hour. Many of these practices are not based on evidence. For instance, recent literature suggests supportive birth practices should encourage at least 1 hour of uninterrupted contact between the healthy newborn and its mother (and father) (Varney *et al.* 2004; AAP 2005). This chapter will look at the time of immediate neonatal transition and review birth and early post-partum practices that are influential in the support or disruption of the first hour of life. Evidence-based approaches will be offered, when available, to support best practice during the time of normal immediate newborn transition.

Birth practices

During the birth process, allowing time for restitution of the shoulders and delaying cord clamping reduces physiologic stress that the infant will experience. Birth interventions such as the somersault manoeuvre for a tight nuchal cord, milking the cord if one must 'cut and run' or performing resuscitation at the perineum offer alternative ways to ensure that an infant will get an adequate blood volume. Clearing the nose, mouth or stomach is not necessary and can interfere with early initiation

Table 6.1 Supportive and disruptive birth practices in healthy newborns: birth.

Birth practices	Supportive birth practices	Disruptive birth practices
Restitution (Varney *et al.* 2004)	Wait for restitution (one to two contractions) before delivering shoulders	Rapid delivery of shoulders and excessive traction on the neck
Timing of cord clamping (Gupta & Ramji 2002; Emhamed *et al.* 2004; Cernadas *et al.* 2006; Chaparro *et al.* 2006; Hutton & Hassan 2007)	Delayed for at least 2 minutes but left intact until pulsations stop is preferable	Immediate or early (within 20 seconds) cord clamping
Nuchal cord (If tight and will not slip over head) (Varney *et al.* 2004; Mercer *et al.* 2005)	Somersault manoeuvre	Double clamp and then cut immediately
Suction (Cordero & Hon 1971; Widstrom *et al.* 1987; Estol *et al.* 1992; Carrasco *et al.* 1997; Waltman *et al.* 2004)	Not necessary	Routine-nasal, oral and/or gastric suctioning
Resuscitation (Mercer *et al.* 2000; Tan *et al.* 2005; Kattwinkel 2006)	At the perineum with an intact cord; room air first (for 90 seconds) and follow NRP guidelines	Cut cord immediately, bring infant to Resuscitair and resuscitate following NRP guidelines
Cord milking (McCausland *et al.* 1949; Colozzi 1954; Whipple *et al.* 1957)	Quickly milk the umbilical cord two to four times if must 'cut and run'	Not considered
Quieting the infant (Leboyer 1975, 2002)	If breathing and colour are good, support quieting	Methods to stimulate to make infant cry

of breastfeeding. Table 6.1 presents an overview of the interventions and practices used at birth that can either support or disrupt the infant's transition. Each practice is discussed in the following sections.

Restitution

Restitution occurs after the head of the infant is born and the shoulders rotate from a transverse position to an anterior-posterior position in order to facilitate easier birthing (Varney *et al.* 2004). The restitution contraction is a 'catch-up' contraction. The body of the uterus is practically empty – probably hips and feet of the fetus only remain – and this very powerful contraction pushes the infant down the birth canal and squeezes blood from the placenta into the infant in preparation for the first breath. This contraction occurs 1–3 minutes after delivery of the head. The clinical 'management' of the time of restitution varies throughout the world. Some providers wait patiently after delivery of the head, allowing the shoulders to restitute and assist birth with the next contraction while others immediately begin downward traction on the head and neck and deliver the infant in less than 30 seconds. The combination of rushing and manipulation often begins the disruption of the normal physiologic transition of birth and is unnecessary, with potential to harm the infant and the mother.

Active management of the third stage of labour

Active management of the third stage of labour (AMTSL) is practised by many providers worldwide as a strategy to reduce the incidence of postpartum haemorrhage (WHO 2007). The three components of AMTSL include the prophylactic administration of a uterotonic drug to the mother either at the birth of the shoulders or within 1 minute after birth, cord clamping and cutting (timing varies among practitioners) and the use of controlled cord traction after cord clamping to facilitate the delivery of the placenta (Prendiville *et al.* 2000; McDonald & Middleton 2008). In some parts of the world, AMTSL includes fundal massage after delivery of the placenta to prevent atony (WHO 2003). The conduct of AMTSL can be supportive, rather than disruptive, during the first few minutes after birth. A simple delay in the timing of cord clamping, before the delivery of the placenta, can ensure that the infant receives adequate blood and red cell volume without any additional haemorrhage risk for the mother (Chaparro *et al.* 2008; McDonald & Middleton 2008). (See Appendix A)

Umbilical cord clamping

Delaying the time of cord clamping at birth is a vital part of a normal, gentle transition and creates a continuation of the peace and harmony that should accompany every birth. It is extremely important for the infant's well-being as it allows the newly born infant to straddle the world of the fetus and the neonate, pausing for a few moments and allowing time to fill its capillary beds (especially the lungs) with oxygen-rich blood (Mercer & Skovgaard 2002). With delayed cord clamping (DCC), the infant receives more blood volume, red blood cells (RBCs) and haematopoietic stem cells (HSC) than when the cord is cut immediately. The blood volume received with DCC is not just an 'extra' 30% of volume. Rather, it is the transfer of blood volume that was originally in the placenta fulfilling respiratory and other functions. At birth, this blood moves into the infant's lung. The cardiac output to the lung changes from 8–10% in utero to 45% in the immediate newborn period and demands an increased blood volume. For a term 3.5-kg infant, this represents about 70 mL of blood which is available to the infant if the cord is left intact (Yao *et al.* 1969). With ICC, blood must be borrowed from the capillary beds of the newborn's other organs in order to fill the expanding lung. This 'borrowing' of blood volume creates a deficit in other organs, which also require adequate blood volume to fulfill their specified functions for the first time independent from the placenta.

Studies on DCC in term infants since 1980 include two systematic reviews (van Rheenen & Brabin 2004; Hutton & Hassan 2007), eight randomised controlled trials (RCTs) (Nelson *et al.* 1980; Oxford Midwives Research Group 1991; Geethanath *et al.* 1997; Grajeda *et al.* 1997; Gupta and Ramji 2002; Emhamed *et al.* 2004; Cernadas *et al.* 2006; Chaparro *et al.* 2006) and five well-designed controlled trials (Kliot & Silverstein 1984; Linderkamp *et al.* 1992; Nelle *et al.* 1993, 1995, 1996). All show absence of harm with DCC. In the latest systematic review, Hutton and Hassan (2007) examined 15 trials that included 1912 newborns. Delayed clamping occurred in 1001 infants while 901 infants received ICC. Results favoured DCC at 5 days with higher haematocrit levels (RR 12, 95% CI 8.5–15, $p < .001$); at 2–3 months with higher mean ferritin concentrations (WMD 17.89 µg/L, 95% CI 16.6–19, $p < .001$) and less anaemia (RR 0.53, CI 0.4–0.7, $p < .001$); and at 6 months of age with higher levels of stored iron in a subgroup of infants (Hutton & Hassan 2007).

Studies on DCC in preterm infants (since 1980) include two systematic reviews (Rabe *et al.* 2004, 2008) which include 13 RCTs (one with milking the cord). Cord clamping in preterm infants is usually delayed between 30 and 60 seconds. The studies on DCC in preterm infants showed absence of harm with delay and benefits such as less respiratory distress (Kinmond *et al.* 1993), less need for blood transfusion (McDonnell & Henderson-Smart 1997; Rabe *et al.* 2000; Hosono *et al.* 2008), less IVH (Hofmeyr *et al.* 1988, 1993; Mercer *et al.* 2006) and less late-onset sepsis (Mercer *et al.* 2006). In the latest meta-analysis of 10 studies, Rabe *et al.* (2008) found reduced rates of neonatal transfusion for hypotension or anaemia ($p < .005$), and IVH ($p < .002$). No long-term outcomes could be adequately examined (Rabe *et al.* 2008).

Red cell volume

An adequate red cell volume (RCV) is essential for oxygen delivery, effective tissue functioning, normal pH, and circulatory integrity.

Infants with DCC obtain about 50% more RBC (Yao *et al.* 1969). RBC are the only cells in the body that carry oxygen and carbon dioxide to and from the cells and lungs. Jones *et al.* (1990) estimate that infants need about 45 mg/kg of RBC for adequate oxygen carrying capacity. Many studies provide evidence for the physiologic benefit of increased red cell and blood volume due to DCC. These include higher haematocrit levels (Oh & Lind 1966; Nelle *et al.* 1998), better skin perfusion and higher temperature (Oh & Lind 1967; Pietra *et al.* 1968), less hypovolaemia (Yao *et al.* 1969; Nelle *et al.* 1998), and a 12–20% increased RBC flow to the brain and gut (Nelle *et al.* 1995). Infants with an adequate blood volume are warmer (Oh & Lind 1967), better perfused (Pietra *et al.* 1968; Nelle *et al.* 1995, 1998), show increased renal blood flow, higher urine output, and greater ability to concentrate urine and retain sodium (Oh *et al.* 1966).

Stem cells

When an infant receives more blood volume, he or she should also receive a greater allotment of HSC. HSC found in human cord blood have incredible potential for healing (Meier *et al.* 2006). They have been used successfully to treat a wide variety of metabolic and haematologic disorders, immune deficiencies, and cancers (Moise 2005). In animal models, they have been found to repair heart, brain, liver, lung, muscle, and endothelial cells lining blood vessels. A unique property of stem cells is that they can self-renew and have the ability to differentiate into more mature cell types (Wobus & Boheler 2006). Stem cells have a remarkable ability to migrate to damaged areas within the body and can differentiate into such cells as glia, oligodendrocytes and cardiomyocytes. This is regulated by an array of signaling proteins or cytokines (Lapidot *et al.* 2005). Evidence suggests that HSC and leukocytes can migrate to and help repair damaged tissue during times of inflammation (Rojas *et al.* 2005). When cord clamping is delayed, the 3.5-kg infant will obtain more than one billion of these highly activated cells. Male infants have a higher content of stem cells collected even when corrected for birthweight (Cairo *et al.* 2005; George *et al.* 2006).

Overtransfusion

Neonatologists and paediatricians often raise concerns about over-transfusion. They fear that the infant will get too much blood leading to circulatory overload, polycythaemia and hyperviscosity, hyperbilirubinaemia and respiratory distress. We have been able to find little research evidence to support this concern. New available evidence suggests that these fears are unfounded. In a recent meta-analysis of term infants with DCC, the haematologic benefits far outweighed any concerns

(Hutton & Hassan 2007). Hutton and Hassan (2007) found no increase in hyperbilirubinaemia and no increase in symptomatic polycythaemia. More infants in the DCC group had a haematocrit value greater than 65% but were asymptomatic and did not require any treatment. Fear of overtransfusion appears to result from older studies that used radioactively tagged albumin to measure blood volume in some sick infants (Linderkamp *et al.* 1977; Saigal & Usher 1977). Albumin readily crosses the capillary membranes and will falsely elevate the blood volume measurement.

Immediate cord clamping and iron deficiency and anemia

Iron deficiency is the most common nutrient deficiency in the world (Hutton & Hassan 2007) and poses a significant public health problem worldwide for infants and toddlers (Eden 2003). Infants have high iron requirements needed to support normal growth thus leaving them at risk for iron deficiency after the first 4–6 months of life (Hutton & Hassan 2007). Poor iron stores in the first year of life can lead to iron deficiency anaemia which has the potential to cause harm to the developing brain (Lozoff *et al.* 2006a). Lozoff and colleagues (2006b) have demonstrated that adolescents, in their late teens, who had anaemia as infants experienced higher rates of behavioural and developmental impairment even when the anaemia had been successfully treated in infancy (Lozoff & Georgieff 2006). This suggests anaemia in early life, even when adequately treated, may have long-term effects. Recently, Shafir *et al.* (2008) reported the association of poorer motor function in 9–10 month old children with iron deficiency with or without anaemia (Shafir *et al.* 2008). This small study suggests that iron deficiency is not necessarily benign. New evidence supports DCC as a low-tech, low-cost birth practice intervention which can improve infant iron stores. Immediate clamping of the umbilical cord can deprive the term infant of approximately 60–100 mL of whole blood or 50 mg/kg of iron (Wardrop & Holland 1995; Mercer 2001; Chaparro *et al.* 2006). Dewey and Chaparro (2007) suggest that DCC can provide adequate iron stores for the first 6–8 months of age.

Tight nuchal cord

A nuchal cord occurs in up to 30% of all births. A tight nuchal cord occurs less often. The management of a tight nuchal cord can vary among obstetrical providers and very little evidence has been found to support cord management practices other than what was found in case reports and a survey of American midwifery practices (Mercer 2001).

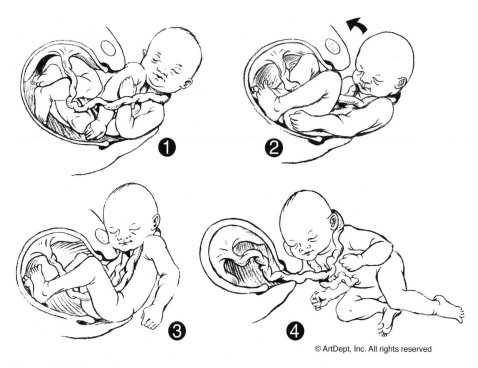

Figure 6.1 Somersault manoeuvre.

Schorn and Blanco (1991) first introduced a technique known as the somersault manoeuvre as an alternative to the usual practice of ICC of the cord when a tight nuchal cord is encountered at birth (see Figure 6.1). Mercer *et al.* (2005) recommends using the somersault manoeuvre followed by DCC when a tight nuchal cord is present. The somersault manoeuvre not only preserves the integrity of the cord but facilitates the practice of DCC which is particularly important as many infants with a tight nuchal cord experience some degree of hypovolaemia (Cashore & Usher 1973; Vanhaesebrouck *et al.* 1987; Iffy *et al.* 2001; Mercer *et al.* 2005).

Resuscitation

Most midwives who practice in out-of-hospital settings, especially at home, resuscitate infants at the perineum with the cord intact. This procedure allows the infant to be physiologically supported via continued placental respiration while resuscitation is underway. It does not seem logical to cut the cord immediately and remove a non-breathing infant from his only source of support. We challenge and question the wisdom of severing the cord immediately at birth when an infant is depressed and then moving the infant to the Resuscitair. This practice is especially to be avoided in an out-of-hospital setting where other support is not available (Mercer & Skovgaard 2004).

Developing evidence points at perfusion as the key factor in adult resuscitation, such as in the case of cardiac arrest. The 2005 American Heart Association guidelines for cardiopulmonary resuscitation (CPR) places increasing importance on chest compressions (AHA 2005). Ewy (2005) advocates reconceptualising CPR as 'cardiocerebral' resuscitation (CCR) and recommends continuous chest compressions (CCC-CPR), without interruption for ventilations (Ewy 2005). This recommendation is based on animal models in which cardiac arrest survival increased to 80% when CCC-CPR was applied, compared to 13% with standard CPR (Ewy *et al.* 2006). Maintenance of perfusion to the heart and brain is the critical factor in protecting function and impacting survival. Hypovolaemic infants, such as those with ICC, may lack the crucial blood volume needed to adequately perfuse the heart and brain. Resuscitating an infant at the perineum, with an intact umbilical cord, allows the infant access to its placental blood – a step that may be essential for recovery. We caution against ICC to obtain a cord blood gas. A limp, pale, non-breathing infant benefits from placental transfusion while resuscitation is underway.

Cord milking

In situations when the infant is slow to start or the clinician believes they must 'cut and run', milking the umbilical cord can facilitate the movement of blood from the placenta to the infant quickly. The clinician supports the umbilical cord in one hand and grasps the cord between the thumb and index finger of the other. The cord is milked the entire length two to four times, vigorously, from the perineum (or the cord insertion site on placenta, if Caesarean) towards the infant's umbilicus. In nine clinical trials involving 746 term babies, cord milking was shown to accelerate the transfer of blood and red cells while causing no harm (McCausland *et al.* 1949; Siddall *et al.* 1952; Siddall & Richardson 1953; Colozzi 1954; Whipple *et al.* 1957; Lanzkowsky 1960; Usher *et al.* 1963; Walsh 1969; Hosono *et al.* 2007). Infants who received cord milking had significantly higher haematocrit and haemoglobin levels compared to infants with ICC. Colozzi (1954) recommended cord milking as a valuable technique which can provide rapid volume expansion especially in those infants who appear hypovolaemic-pale, limp and languid at birth (Colozzi 1954).

In preterm infants, Hosono and colleagues (2008) have documented the cardiovascular benefit of increased BP (from increasing circulatory volume) in 24- to 28-week preterm infants with cord milking. The mean initial BP was higher in the cord milking group (28 vs. 34, $p = .03$) suggesting that cord milking was an important technique to improve organ perfusion. Infants also needed fewer transfusions (Hosono *et al.* 2008). Hosono *et al.* also found that preterm infants who received cord milking at birth had significantly less total number of blood transfusions (1.7 vs. 4.0, $p = .02$) (Hosono *et al.* 2008).

Suctioning

Suctioning is a common practice after birth with no true benefit demonstrated for the neonate. The clearing of the infant's nose and mouth at birth with a bulb syringe is often routine practice recommended in most obstetrical texts. However, four small controlled trials conducted on a total of 177 vigorous, healthy term infants suggest that there is no benefit from routine suctioning. The evidence suggests the practice should be abandoned (Cordero & Hon 1971; Estol *et al.* 1992; Carrasco *et al.* 1997; Waltman *et al.* 2004).

Another common practice – suctioning the infant's gastric contents in order to prevent aspiration or regurgitation – should also be abandoned. Widstrom *et al.* (1987) studied the effect of gastric suction on circulation and the subsequent breastfeeding behaviours of 21 infants. He found that infants who were suctioned had more episodes of bradycardia and higher blood pressures and breastfeeding initiation was delayed. This small study found harm and no benefit from gastric suctioning. When meconium was present, suctioning the infant prior to the birth or suctioning vigorous infants after birth showed no benefit and did not prevent meconium aspiration syndrome (Wiswell *et al.* 2000; Vain *et al.* 2004). The American Academy of Pediatrics (AAP 2005) strongly urges avoiding the overly aggressive suctioning of the oropharynx, oesophagus or trachea as it potentially can interfere with breastfeeding (AAP 2005).

Early post-partum practices

The ultimate goal of presenting this information is to attempt to identify practices that will contribute to the well-being of the newborn infant and thus his or her ability to fully participate with the mother during the initial period of maternal–infant bonding. Initial bonding is dependent on mother and infant both being well and intact and is facilitated by the use of skin-to-skin (STS) care and early breast stimulation and feeding. All of the practices discussed here support infant wellness and are outlined in Table 6.2.

Table 6.2 Supportive and disruptive birth practices in healthy newborns: first hour after birth.

Birth practices	Supportive birth practices	Disruptive birth practices
Initial bonding (Leboyer 1975, 2002; Kennell & Klaus 1998a, 1998b; Klaus & Kennell 2001; Odent 2002; AAP 2005)	Prevent separation at birth; foster closeness and interaction; delay tasks	Interrupted; infant and mother separated in order to complete tasks
Skin to skin (Fardig 1980; van den Bosch & Bullough 1990; Kennell & Klaus 1998a, 1998b; Klaus and Kennell 2001; Odent 2002; Anderson *et al.* 2003; Ferber & Makhoul 2004; AAP 2005; Carfoot *et al.* 2005; Fransson *et al.* 2005; Vaidya *et al.* 2005; Moore *et al.* 2007)	After drying, place newborn directly on maternal bare skin (abdomen)	Infant placed under radiant heater shortly after birth
Breastfeeding (Kennell & Klaus 1998a, 1998b; Klaus & Kennell 2001; Odent 2002; AAP 2005)	Encourage early initiation STS, infant kept with mother until at least first feed accomplished	Delayed; separates infant and mother to complete tasks

Initial bonding

The first hour of life is a time for the miracle of birth to unfold – a time for the mother and infant to become attuned to one another. During this interlude of attunement, the mother and infant are unusually open to the discovery of one another. Therefore, it is a period when the mother and infant need to be free from interference (Simonds *et al.* 2007). During this first hour of life, healthy mothers and infants should remain together. Care providers should practice the 'art of cautious intervention', remaining unobtrusive but paying close attention (Odent 1984). We believe that the midwife has a special role in overseeing the fourth stage of labour, serving as the infant's advocate. The midwife's role must include informing and preparing parents about how fourth stage is optimally conducted, carrying out a gentle labour and birth, and especially serving as a guardian of 'normality' during the immediate post-partum period.

Hormonal releases play an important part in mother–infant bonding and necessitate physical contact between the mother and infant. Peak releases of maternal oxytocin have been documented as a response to the neonate's movements and actions (i.e. touching and licking) as well as early breastfeeding (Nissen *et al.* 1995; Matthiesen *et al.* 2001). Fuchs *et al.* (1991) demonstrated that these peak releases of oxytocin occur during the second stage of labour. High levels of oxytocin (natural) activate the olfactory bulb which may increase the ability of both mother and infant to bond to each other's smells (Gimpl & Fahrenholz 2001). The sweet smell of a baby's breath is noted in the naming of a fragrant flower in its honour. Bonding is also enhanced and supported by STS care and early breastfeeding.

Skin-to-skin care

STS care at birth is the placement of the naked infant prone on the mother's abdomen, directly on her skin (see Appendix A). The infant (and mother) is covered with a blanket and a cap may be placed on the infant's head. STS care is known to have benefit in term and preterm infants. Not only does it enhance thermoregulation (keeps infants warmer) and breastfeeding success but it assists in metabolic and bacteriological adaptation and newborn behavioural states (Anderson *et al.* 2003; Ferber & Makhoul 2004; Carfoot *et al.* 2005; Fransson *et al.* 2005; Vaidya *et al.* 2005). Keeping an infant warm after birth is an important part of the first hour of newborn transition. Infants are vulnerable to heat loss because of their large surface area, lack of subcutaneous tissue and skin permeability to water but placing the dried infant STS on the bare maternal abdomen can prevent heat loss through convection and evaporation (Mercer *et al.* 2007).

For the mother, STS care provides the gentle touch of her newborn as he or she squirms and pushes in the attempt to find the breast. This early contact causes the mother's pituitary to release additional oxytocin. This oxytocin helps to contract the uterus and expel the placenta but also engenders appropriate maternal caring and protective responses found in most mammalian species (Gimpl & Fahrenholz 2001).

Klaus *et al.* (1995) reported that infants seldom cry during the first 90 minutes after birth when placed STS with their mothers. In contrast, he found that infants placed in a bassinet cry 30 to 40 seconds every 5 minutes. STS is a natural precursor to early breastfeeding. The cord can be left intact during STS care until the placenta is ready to deliver (see Appendix A).

Early initiation of breastfeeding

There is no doubt that human milk is uniquely superior to all substitute feeding preparations for human infants. There is evidence of reduced rates of sudden infant death syndrome (SIDS) and Type I and II diabetes, and improved cognitive development in breastfed infants. Benefits to the mother include quicker involution and return to prepregnancy weight, but also decreased bleeding, and, later in life, lower rates of breast and ovarian cancer and less osteoporosis (AAP 2005). Community benefits include lower annual health care costs for mothers and infants, lower parental absenteeism, and reducing the environmental burden of the large volume of disposable waste associated with formula containers (AAP 2005).

Care practices do affect initiation of breastfeeding. Forster and McLachlan (2007) recommend that continuous support for women during labour, continuous STS care and early initiation of breastfeeding (in the first hour) are three important factors that enhance breastfeeding success.

All tasks, such as weighing, injections and eye prophylaxis, can wait until after this first breastfeed is accomplished. In 2005, AAP published a policy statement on breastfeeding and the use of human milk. This document lists 15 recommendations for healthy term infants to support early initiation of breastfeeding and suggests that 'healthy infants should be placed and remain in direct STS contact with their mothers immediately after delivery until the first feeding is accomplished . . . dry the infant, assign Apgar scores, and perform the initial physical assessment while the infant is with the mother' (p. 498–9) (AAP 2005). The tasks of newborn care such as measuring and weighing, eye care and injections of vitamin K, vaccines, etc. can be safely deferred until the completion of the infant's first breastfeed.

Conclusions

Care practices and how they are conducted at birth and during the fourth stage of labour may have effects that will last a lifetime. Immediate cord clamping, separation of the infant from his mother, suctioning and other 'pressing' newborn tasks can be disruptive and need to be avoided so as not to take precedence over the mother and infant's time of intimacy and connectedness. Recent literature encourages at least 1 hour of uninterrupted contact between the healthy newborn and its mother (and father) including direct skin contact with the mother immediately after delivery lasting until the first feeding is accomplished (AAP 2005). This important period of time of transitioning, both for the neonate and mother, requires supportive and thoughtful care underpinned by a philosophy of patience, peacefulness and personal interest while using the 'art of cautious intervention' (Dick Read 1944; Odent 1984, 2002).

References

AAP (2005) Breastfeeding and the use of human milk. *Pediatrics* 115(2): 496–506.

AHA (2005) American Heart Association guidelines for cardiopulmonary resuscitation and emergency cardiovascular care. *Circulation* 112(IV): 1–203.

Anderson G, Moore E, Hepworth J *et al*. (2003) Early skin-to-skin contact for mothers and their healthy newborn infants. *Cochrane Database of Systematic Reviews* (2).

van den Bosch C, Bullough C (1990) Effect of early suckling on term neonate's core body temperature. *Annals of Tropical Paediatrics* 10(4): 347–53.

Cairo MS, Wagner EL, Fraser J *et al*. (2005) Characterization of banked umbilical cord blood hematopoietic progenitor cells and lymphocyte subsets and correlation with ethnicity, birth weight, sex, and type of delivery: a Cord Blood Transplantation (COBLT) Study report. *Transfusion* 45(6): 856–66.

Carfoot S, Williamson P, Dickson R *et al*. (2005) A randomised controlled trial in the north of England examining the effects of skin-to-skin care on breast feeding. *Midwifery* 21(1): 71–9.

Carrasco M, Martell M, EStol PC *et al*. (1997) Oronasopharyngeal suction at birth: effects on arterial oxygen saturation. *The Journal of Pediatrics* 130(5): 832–4.

Cashore WJ, Usher R (1973) Hypovolemia resulting from a tight nuchal cord at birth. *Pediatric Research* 7: 399.

Cernadas J, Carroli G, Pellegrini L *et al*. (2006) The effect of timing of cord clamping on neonatal venous hematocrit values and clinical outcome at term: a randomized controlled trial. *Obstetrical and Gynecological Survey* 61(9): 564–5.

Chaparro CM, Lutter C, Camacho-Hubner AV *et al*. (2008) *Essential Delivery Care Practices for Maternal and Newborn Health and Nutrition*. Washington DC, PAHO & USAID.

Chaparro CM, Neufeld LM, Alavez TG *et al*. (2006) Effect of timing of umbilical cord clamping on iron status in Mexican infants: a randomised controlled trial *Lancet* 367(9527): 1997–2004.

Colozzi A (1954) Clamping of the umbilical cord: its effect on the placental transfusion. *The New England Journal of Medicine* 250(15): 629–32.

Cordero L Jr, Hon EH (1971) Neonatal bradycardia following nasopharyngeal stimulation. *The Journal of Pediatrics* 78(3): 441–7.

Dewey KG, Chaparro CM (2007) Session 4: mineral metabolism and body composition iron status of breast-fed infants. *The Proceedings of the Nutrition Society* 66(3): 412–22.

Dick Read G (1944) *Childbirth Without Fear. The Principles and Practice of Natural Childbirth*. London, Pinter & Martin Ltd.

Eden AN (2003) Preventing iron deficiency in toddlers: a major public health problem. *Contemporary Pediatrics* 20(2): 57–67.

Emhamed MO, van Rheenen P, Brabin BJ *et al*. (2004) The early effects of delayed cord clamping in term infants born to Libyan mothers. *Tropical Doctor* 34(4): 218–22.

Estol PC, Piriz H, Basalo S *et al.* (1992) Oro-naso-pharyngeal suction at birth: effects on respiratory adaptation of normal term vaginally born infants. *Journal of Perinatal Medicine* 20(4): 297–305.

Ewy GA (2005) Cardiocerebral resuscitation: the new cardiopulmonary resuscitation. *Circulation* 111(16): 2134–42.

Ewy GA, Kern KB, Sanders AB *et al.* (2006) Cardiocerebral resuscitation for cardiac arrest. *The American Journal of Medicine* 119(1): 6–9.

Fardig J (1980) A comparison of skin-to-skin contact and radiant heaters in promoting neonatal thermoregulation. *The Journal of Nuclear Medicine* 25(1).

Ferber SG, Makhoul IR (2004) The effect of skin-to-skin contact (kangaroo care) shortly after birth on the neurobehavioral responses of the term newborn: a randomized, controlled trial. *Pediatrics* 113(4): 858–65.

Forster DA, McLachlan HL (2007) Breastfeeding initiation and birth setting practices: a review of the literature. *Journal of Midwifery and Women's Health* 52(3): 273–80.

Fransson AL, Karlsson H, Nilsson K *et al.* (2005) Temperature variation in newborn babies: importance of physical contact with the mother. *Archives of Disease in Childhood: Fetal and Neonatal Edition* 90(6): F500–4.

Fuchs AR, Romero R, Keefe D *et al.* (1991) Oxytocin secretion and human parturition: pulse frequency and duration increase during spontaneous labor in women. *American Journal of Obstetrics and Gynecology* 165(5 Pt 1): 1515–23.

Geethanath RM, Ramji S, Thirupuram S *et al.* (1997) Effect of timing of cord clamping on the iron status of infants at 3 months. *Indian Pediatrics* 34: 103–6.

George TJ, Sugrue MW, George SN *et al.* (2006) Factors associated with parameters of engraftment potential of umbilical cord blood. *Transfusion* 46(10): 1803–12.

Gimpl G, Fahrenholz F (2001) The oxytocin receptor system: structure, function, and regulation. *Physiological Reviews* 81(2): 629–83.

Grajeda R, Perez-Escamilla R, Dewey KG *et al.* (1997) Delayed clamping of the umbilical cord improves hematologic status of Guatemalan infants at 2 mo of age. *The American Journal of Clinical Nutrition* 65(2): 425–31.

Gupta R, Ramji S (2002) Effect of delayed cord clamping on iron stores in infants born to anemic mothers: a randomized controlled trial. *Indian Pediatrics* 39(2): 130–5.

Haneline LS, Marshall KP, Clapp DW *et al.* (1996) The highest concentration of primitive hematopoietic progenitor cells in cord blood is found in extremely premature infants. *Pediatric Research* 39(5): 820–5.

Hofmeyr GJ, Bolton KD, Bowen DC *et al.* (1988) Periventricular/intraventricular haemorrhage and umbilical cord clamping. Findings and hypothesis. *South African Medical Journal* 73(2): 104–6.

Hofmeyr GJ, Gobetz L, Bex PJ *et al.* (1993) Periventricular/intraventricular hemorrhage following early and delayed umbilical cord clamping. A randomized controlled trial. *The Journal of Current Clinical Trials Curr Clin Trials* [Online] Doc No 110.

Hosono S, Mugishima H, Fujita H *et al.* (2007) Umbilical cord milking reduces the need for red cell transfusions and improves neonatal adaptation in infants born less than 29 weeks' gestation: a randomized controlled trial. *Archives of Disease in Childhood: Fetal and Neonatal Edition* 93(1): F14–9.

Hosono S, Mugishima H, Fujita H *et al.* (2008) Umbilical cord milking reduces the need for red cell transfusions and improves neonatal adaptation in infants born less than 29 weeks' gestation: a randomized controlled trial. *Archives of Disease in Childhood: Fetal and Neonatal Edition* 93(1): F14–9.

Hutton EK, Hassan ES (2007) Late vs early clamping of the umbilical cord in full-term neonates: systematic review and meta-analysis of controlled trials. *The Journal of the American Medical Association* 297(11): 1241–52.

Iffy L, Varadi V, Papp E *et al.* (2001) Untoward neonatal sequelae deriving from cutting of the umbilical cord before delivery. *Medicine and Law* 20(4): 627–34.

Jones JG, Holland BM, Holland BM *et al.* (1990) Total circulating red cells versus haematocrit as the primary descriptor of oxygen transport by the blood. *British Journal of Haematology* 76: 288–94.

Kattwinkel J (ed) (2006) *Textbook of Neonatal Resuscitation.* Washington DC, American Academy of Pediatrics and American Heart Association.

Kennell J, Klaus M (1998a) Bonding by Kennell and Klaus. *Pediatrics in Review* 19(12): 433.

Kennell JH, Klaus MH (1998b) Bonding: recent observations that alter perinatal care. *Pediatrics in Review* 19(1): 4–12.

Kinmond S, Aitchison TC, Holland BM *et al.* (1993) Umbilical cord clamping and preterm infants: a randomized trial. *British Medical Journal* 306: 172–5.

Klaus M, Kennell J (2001) Commentary: routines in maternity units: are they still appropriate for 2002? *Birth* 28(4): 274–5.

Klaus MH, Kennell JH, Klaus PH *et al.* (1995) *Bonding: Building the Foundations of a Secure Attachment and Independence.* Cambridge, Perseus.

Kliot D, Silverstein L (1984) Changing maternal and newborn care: a study of the Leboyer approach to childbirth management. *New York State Journal of Medicine* 84: 169–84.

Lanzkowsky P (1960) Effects of early and late clamping of umbilical cord on infant's haemoglobin level. *British Medical Journal* 5215: 1777–82.

Lapidot T, Dar A, Kollet O *et al.* (2005) How do stem cells find their way home? *Blood* 106(6): 1901–10.

Leboyer F (1975) *Birth without Violence.* New York, Knopf.

Leboyer F (2002) *Birth without Violence. Revised Edition of the Classic.* Rochester, Healing Arts Press.

Linderkamp O, Holthausen H, Seifert J *et al.* (1977) Accuracy of blood volume estimations in critically ill children using 125I-labelled albumin and 51Cr-labelled red cells. *European Journal of Pediatrics* 125(2): 143–51.

Linderkamp O, Nelle M, Zilow EP *et al.* (1992) The effect of early and late cord-clamping on blood viscosity and other hemorheological parameters in full-term neonates. *Acta Paediatrica* 81(10): 745–50.

Lozoff B (2007) Iron deficiency and child development. *Food and Nutrition Bulletin* 28(Suppl 4): S560–71.

Lozoff B, Beard J, Connor J *et al.* (2006a) Long-lasting neural and behavioral effects of iron deficiency in infancy. *Nutrition Reviews* 64(5 Pt 2): S34–43; discussion S72-91.

Lozoff B, Georgieff MK (2006) Iron deficiency and brain development. *Seminars in Pediatric Neurology* 13(3): 158–65.

Lozoff B, Jimenez E, Smith JB *et al.* (2006b) Double burden of iron deficiency in infancy and low socioeconomic status: a longitudinal analysis of cognitive test scores to age 19 years. *Archives of Pediatrics and Adolescent Medicine* 160(11): 1108–13.

Matthiesen AS, Ransjo-Arvidson AB, Nissen E *et al.* (2001) Postpartum maternal oxytocin release by newborns: effects of infant hand massage and sucking. *Birth* 28(1): 13–9.

McCausland A, Holmes F, Schumann W *et al.* (1949) Management of cord and placental blood and its effect upon the newborn: part 1. *California Medicine* 71(3): 190–6.

McDonald SJ, Middleton P (2008) Effect of timing of umbilical cord clamping of term infants on maternal and neonatal outcomes. *Cochrane Database of Systematic Reviews* (2): CD004074.

McDonnell M, Henderson-Smart DJ (1997) Delayed umbilical cord clamping in preterm infants: a feasibility study. *Journal of Paediatrics and Child Health* 33: 308–10.

Meier C, Middelanis J, Wasielewski B *et al.* (2006) Spastic paresis after perinatal brain damage in rats is reduced by human cord blood mononuclear cells. *Pediatric Research* 59(2): 244–9.

Mercer J (2001) Best evidence: a review of the literature on umbilical cord clamping. *Journal of Midwifery and Women's Health* 46(6): 402–14.

Mercer J, Erickson-Owens D, Graves B *et al.* (2007) Evidence-based practices for the fetal to newborn transition. *Journal of Midwifery and Women's Health* 52(3): 262–72.

Mercer J, Nelson C, Skovgaard R *et al.* (2000) Umbilical cord clamping: beliefs and practices of American nurse-midwives. *Journal of Midwifery and Women's Health* 45(1): 58–66.

Mercer J, Skovgaard R (2002) Neonatal transitional physiology: a new paradigm. *The Journal of Perinatal and Neonatal Nursing* 15(4): 56–75.

Mercer J, Skovgaard R (2004) Fetal to neonatal transition: first, do no harm. In Downe S (ed) *Normal Childbirth: Evidence and Debate.* Edinburgh, Elsevier Science.

Mercer JS, Skovgaard RL, Peareara-Eaves J *et al.* (2005) Nuchal cord management and nurse-midwifery practice. *Journal of Midwifery and Women's Health* 50(5): 373–9.

Mercer JS, Vohr BR, Mcgrath MM *et al.* (2006) Delayed cord clamping in very preterm infants reduces the incidence of intraventricular hemorrhage and late-onset sepsis: a randomized, controlled trial. *Pediatrics* 117(4): 1235–42.

Moise KJ Jr (2005) Umbilical cord stem cells. *Obstetrics and Gynecology* 106(6): 1393–407.

Moore ER, Anderson GC, Bergman N *et al.* (2007) Early skin-to-skin contact for mothers and their healthy newborn infants. *Cochrane Database of Systematic Reviews* (3): CD003519.

Nelle M, Fischer S, Conze S *et al.* (1998) Effects of later cord clamping on circulation in prematures (Abstract). *Pediatric Research* 44: 420.

Nelle M, Kraus M, Bastert G *et al.* (1996) Effects of Leboyer childbirth on left- and right systolic time intervals in healthy term neonates. *Journal of Perinatal Medicine* 24(5): 513–20.

Nelle M, Zilow EP, Bastert G *et al.* (1993) The effect of Leboyer delivery on blood viscosity and other hemorheologic parameters in term neonates. *American Journal of Obstetrics and Gynecology* 169(1): 189–93.

Nelle M, Zilow EP, Bastert G *et al.* (1995) Effect of Leboyer childbirth on cardiac output, cerebral and gastrointestinal blood flow velocities in full-term neonates. *American Journal of Perinatology* 12(3): 212–6.

Nelson N, Enkin MW, Saigal S *et al.* (1980) A randomized trial of the Leboyer approach to childbirth. *New England Journal on Medicine* 302: 655–60.

Nissen E, Lilja G, Widstrom AM *et al.* (1995) Elevation of oxytocin levels early post partum in women. *Acta Obstetricia et Gynecologica Scandinavica* 74(7): 530–3.

Odent M (1984) *Birth Reborn*. New York, Pantheon Books.

Odent M. (2002) The first hour following birth: don't wake the mother! *Midwifery Today International Midwifery* 61 (Spring 2002): 9–12.

Oh W, Lind J (1966) Venous and capillary hematocrit in newborn infants and placental transfusion. *Acta Paediatrica Scandinavica* 55(1): 38–48.

Oh W, Lind J (1967) Body temperature of the newborn infant in relation to placental transfusion. *Acta Paediatrica Scandinavica* 172S: 137–45.

Oh W, Oh MA, Lind J *et al.* (1966) Renal function and blood volume in newborn infant related to placental transfusion. *Acta Paediatrica Scandinavica* 55: 197–210.

Oxford Midwives Research Group (1991) A study of the relationship between the delivery to cord clamping interval and the time of cord separation. *Midwifery* 7(4): 167–76.

Pietra GG, D'Amodio MD, Leventhal MM *et al.* (1968) Electron microscopy of cutaneous capillaries of newborn infants: effects of placental transfusion. *Pediatrics* 42(4): 678–83.

Prendiville WJ, Elbourne D, McDonald S *et al.* (2000) Active versus expectant management in the third stage of labour. *Cochrane Database of Systematic Reviews* (3): CD000007.

Rabe H, Reynolds G, Diaz-Rossello J *et al.* (2004) Early versus delayed umbilical cord clamping in preterm infants. *Cochrane Database of Systematic Reviews* (4): CD003248.

Rabe H, Reynolds G, Diaz-Rossello J *et al.* (2008) A systematic review and meta-analysis of a brief delay in clamping the umbilical cord of preterm infants. *Neonatology* 93(2): 138–44.

Rabe H, Wacker A., Hulskamp G *et al.* (2000) A randomised controlled trial of delayed cord clamping in very low birth weight preterm infants. *European Journal of Pediatrics* 159(10): 775–7.

van Rheenen P, Brabin BJ (2004) Late umbilical cord-clamping as an intervention for reducing iron deficiency anaemia in term infants in developing and industrialised countries: a systematic review. *Annals of Tropical Paediatrics* 24(1): 3–16.

Rojas M, Xu J, Mora AL *et al.* (2005) Bone marrow-derived mesenchymal stem cells in repair of the injured lung. *American Journal of Respiratory Cell and Molecular Biology* 33(2): 145–52.

Saigal S, Usher RH (1977) Symptomatic neonatal plethora. *Biology of the Neonate* 32(1–2): 62–72.

Schorn MN, Blanco JD (1991) Management of the nuchal cord. *Journal of Nurse-Midwifery* 36: 131–2.

Shafir T, Angulo-Barroso R, Jing Y *et al.* (2008) Iron deficiency and infant motor development. *Early Human Development.*

Siddall R, Crissey R, Knapp W *et al.* (1952) Effects of cesarean section babies of stripping or milking of the umbilical cord. *American Journal of Obstetrics and Gynecology* 63(5): 1059–64.

Siddall RS, Richardson RP (1953) Milking or stripping the umbilical cord; effect on vaginally delivered babies. *Obstetrics and Gynecology* 1(2): 230–3.

Simonds W, Katz Rothman B, Norman B *et al.* (2007) *Laboring On. Birth in Transition in the United States.* New York, Routledge.

Stoll BJ, Hansen NI, DAdams-Chapman I *et al.* (2004) Neurodevelopmental and growth impairment among extremely low-birth-weight infants with neonatal infection. *The Journal of the American Medical Association* 292(19): 2357–65.

Tan A, Schulze A, O'Donnell C *et al.* (2005) Air versus oxygen for resuscitation of infants at birth. *Cochrane Database of Systematic Reviews* (2).

Usher R, Shephard M, Lind J *et al.* (1963) The blood volume of the newborn infant and placental transfusion. *Acta Paediatrica* 52: 497–512.

Vaidya K, Sharma A, Dhungel S *et al.* (2005) Effect of early mother-baby close contact over the duration of exclusive breastfeeding. *Nepal Medical College Journal* 7(2): 138–40.

Vain NE, Szyld EG, Prudent LM *et al.* (2004) Oropharyngeal and nasopharyngeal suctioning of meconium-stained neonates before delivery of their shoulders: multicentre, randomised controlled trial. *Lancet* 364(9434): 597–602.

Vanhaesebrouck P, Vanneste K, de-Praeter C *et al.* (1987) Tight nuchal cord and neonatal hypovolaemic shock. *Archives of Disease in Childhood* 62(12): 1276–7.

Varney H, Kriebs J, Gegor C *et al.* (2004) *Varney's Midwifery.* Boston, Jones and Bartlett Publishers.

Vohr BR, Allan WC, Westerveld M *et al.* (2003) School-age outcomes of very low birth weight infants in the indomethacin intraventricular hemorrhage prevention trial. *Pediatrics* 111(4 Pt 1): e340–6.

Walsh SZ (1969) Early clamping versus stripping of card: comparative study of electrocardiogram in neonatal period. *British Heart Journal* 31(1): 122–6.

Waltman PA, Brewer JM, Rogers BP *et al.* (2004) Building evidence for practice: a pilot study of newborn bulb suctioning at birth. *Journal of Midwifery and Women's Health* 49(1): 32–8.

Wardrop CAJ, Holland BM (1995) The roles and vital importance of placental blood to the newborn infant. *Journal of Perinatal Medicine* 23: 139–43.

Whipple GA, Sisson TR, Lund CJ *et al.* (1957) Delayed ligation of the umbilical cord; its influence on the blood volume of the newborn. *Obstetrics and Gynecology* 10(6): 603–10.

WHO (2003) *Managing Complications for Pregnancy and Childbearing. A Guide for Midwives and Doctors*. Geneva, WHO.

WHO (2007) *Recommendations for the Prevention of Postpartum Haemorrhage. Making Pregnancy Safer*. Geneva, WHO.

Widstrom AM, Ransjo-Arvidson AB, Christensson K *et al.* (1987) Gastric suction in healthy newborn infants. Effects on circulation and developing feeding behaviour. *Acta Paediatrica Scandinavica* 76(4): 566–72.

Wiswell TE, Gannon CM, Jacob J *et al.* (2000) Delivery room management of the apparently vigorous meconium-stained neonate: results of the multicenter, international collaborative trial. *Pediatrics* 105(1 Pt 1): 1–7.

Wobus A, Boheler K (eds) (2006) Stem cells. *Handbook of Experimental Pharmacology*. Berlin, Heidelberg, Springer-Verlag.

Yao AC, Moinian M, Lind J *et al.* (1969) Distribution of blood between infant and placenta after birth. *Lancet* 2(7626): 871–3.

Appendix A

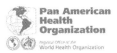

Essential delivery care practices for maternal and newborn health and nutrition

The first minutes after birth are a very vulnerable period for both mother and newborn. The care that is provided during this time is critical to ensure not only their immediate survival but also to improve their longer-term health and nutrition. Active management of the third stage of labor (AMTSL), the optimal timing of umbilical cord clamping, early skin-to-skin contact between mother and newborn, and early breastfeeding initiation are safe, effective, feasible and evidence-based care practices that should be offered by a skilled birth attendant to all mothers and their infants in the continuum of maternal-neonatal care.

What are the recommended practices and why are they essential for maternal and infant health and survival?

1. Active management of the third stage of labor (AMTSL)

What is it?

■ AMTSL includes three steps:[1,2]

1) Administration of an uterotonic drug (e.g. 10 IU of oxytocin intramuscularly) soon after delivery of the infant to avoid uterine atony. If oxytocin is not available, 400-600 μg of misoprostol can be given orally.

2) Delayed clamping and cutting of the umbilical cord followed by delivery of the placenta by controlled cord traction: After clamping and cutting the cord, keep slight tension on the cord and await a strong uterine contraction. Very gently pull downwards on the cord while stabilizing the uterus by applying counter traction with the other hand placed just above the mother's pubic bone.

3) Uterine massage immediately following delivery of the placenta, and every 15 minutes for the first two hours.

Why is it important?

■ Fourteen million cases of postpartum hemorrhage (PPH) are estimated to occur annually on a global level.[3] PPH is the leading cause of maternal mortality worldwide, contributing to 25% of all maternal deaths,[3] and uterine atony is the most common cause of PPH.

■ AMTSL has been shown to significantly reduce the incidence of PPH from uterine atony by 60%,[4] the incidence of postpartum blood loss of 1 L or more and the need for costly and risky blood transfusions,[1] and prevent complications related to PPH. **AMTSL can not only help prevent the disability and death of a mother at delivery but also ensure a better chance at survival for her infant, as maternal and neonatal survival are inextricably linked.**

2. Optimal timing of umbilical cord clamping

What is it?

■ The optimal time to clamp the umbilical cord for all infants regardless of gestational age or fetal weight is when the circulation in the cord has ceased, and the cord is flat and pulseless (approximately 3 minutes or more after birth).[5] After the infant is delivered and dried with a clean dry cloth, a fully reactive infant may be placed prone on the maternal abdomen and covered with a warm dry blanket until cord pulsations cease and the cord is clamped and cut.

Why is it important?

■ For the first minutes after birth, there is still circulation from the placenta to the infant, the majority of which occurs within three minutes,[5] generally coinciding with the end of cord pulsations.

■ Clamping the umbilical cord immediately (within the first 10 to 15 seconds after delivery) prevents the newborn from receiving adequate blood volume and consequently sufficient iron stores. **Immediate cord clamping has been shown to increase the incidence of iron deficiency and anemia during the first half of infancy,[6] with lower birth weight infants and infants born to iron deficient mothers being at particular risk.[7] Up to 50% of infants in developing countries become anemic by 1 year of life,[8] a condition which can negatively and perhaps irreversibly affect mental and motor development.[9] According to one longitudinal study, Costa Rican children with chronic iron deficiency in infancy had 10 to 25 point lower cognitive test scores at 19 years of age, when compared to similar children with adequate iron status.[10]** Waiting to clamp the umbilical cord allows a physiological transfer of placental blood to the infant which provides sufficient iron reserves for the first 6 to 8 months of life,[11] preventing or delaying the development of iron deficiency until other interventions—such as the use of iron-fortified foods—can be implemented.

■ **For premature and low birth weight infants, immediate cord clamping can also increase the risk of intraventricular hemorrhage,[12,13] and late-onset sepsis.[13] In addition, immediate cord clamping in these infants increases the need for blood transfusions for anemia and low blood pressure.[12]**

3. Early initiation of breastfeeding and mother-to-infant skin-to-skin contact

What is it?

■ As soon as the newborn is stable and breathing, he/she may be placed on the mother's chest, prone, in skin-to-skin contact, with a warm, dry cloth covering the infant's back and the mother's chest. Routine delivery room procedures (such as cleaning and weighing) should be delayed for at least the first hour.[14]

Why is it important?

■ In addition to regulating infant temperature[15] and enhancing maternal-infant bonding[16]–essential for neonatal survival–immediate and uninterrupted skin-to-skin contact between the mother and infant promotes early initiation of breastfeeding[17] and is associated with a longer duration of exclusive breastfeeding in infancy.[16] **Beginning breastfeeding immediately and exclusively (i.e. within the first hour) is fundamental to survival in the neonatal period[18] and beyond: in Latin America and the Caribbean, it is estimated that 66% of infant deaths due to diarrheal disease and acute respiratory infection occurring between 0 to 3 months of age could be prevented by exclusive breastfeeding.[19]** Early breastfeeding also may benefit the mother, as suckling stimulates maternal oxytocin secretion,[20] promoting uterine contractions[21] and possibly reducing maternal bleeding. Routine delivery room practices that separate the mother and infant (such as cleaning and weighing the infant) have been shown to negatively impact early initiation of breastfeeding,[22] as continuous, uninterrupted skin-to-skin contact may optimize the baby's success at the first breastfeed.[17] During this period together, health care staff should monitor the condition of both mother and newborn, and provide unobtrusive breastfeeding assistance if necessary, using an approach that takes into account maternal comfort and her desire for modesty.

In summary

These are *evidence-based, cost-effective, safe and simple* practices to reduce maternal morbidity and mortality and improve newborn and infant survival, health and nutrition.

To whom should these practices be offered?

All mothers should be offered AMTSL and immediate skin-to-skin contact with their infant after delivery and delayed cord clamping should be considered for every infant except in the case of asphyxiation where early cord clamping may be necessary in order to provide immediate resuscitative measures.

How can these practices be implemented together?

There are still remaining questions as to how to implement AMTSL with optimal cord clamping, in combination with early skin-to-skin contact and initiation of breastfeeding. A proposed sequence of steps based on potential feasibility and the available evidence supporting each practice is presented below. †

1. After delivery, immediately dry the infant. Then place the reactive infant, prone, on the mother's abdomen.* Keep the infant covered with a dry cloth or towel to prevent heat loss.

*If the infant is pale, limp, or not breathing, it is best to keep the infant at the level of the perineum to allow optimal blood flow and oxygenation while resuscitative measures are performed. Early cord clamping may be necessary if immediate attention cannot be provided without clamping and cutting the cord.

2. Give oxytocin (10 IU, intramuscularly) soon after delivery.

3. **After cord pulsations have ceased (approximately 3 minutes after delivery),** clamp and cut the cord following strict hygienic techniques.

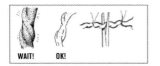

WAIT!   OK!

4. Place the infant directly on the mother's chest, prone, with the newborn's skin touching the mother's skin. While the mother's skin will help regulate the infant's temperature, cover both the mother and infant with a dry, warm cloth or towel to prevent heat loss. Cover the baby's head with a cap or cloth.

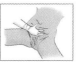

5. Deliver the placenta by controlled cord traction on the umbilical cord and counter-pressure to the uterus.

6. Massage the uterus through the abdomen after delivery of the placenta.

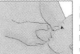

7. During recovery, palpate the uterus through the abdomen every 15 minutes for two hours to make sure it is firm and monitor the amount of vaginal bleeding.

8. Aim to delay routine procedures (e.g. weighing, bathing) for at least the first hour so that mother and baby can be together in uninterrupted skin-to-skin contact and begin breastfeeding. If necessary, offer to assist the mother with the first breastfeed, being sensitive to her need for modesty.

---

†Figures adapted by Martha Cifuentes from "Active management of the third stage of labor (AMSTL)" POPPHI, (available at http://www.pphprevention.org/job_aids.php) and "A Book for Midwives", Hesperian Foundation (available at http://www.hesperian.org/publications_download_midwives.php).

References

1. World Health Organization (WHO). WHO Recommendations for the Prevention of Postpartum Haemorrhage. Geneva: World Health Organization: Department of Making Pregnancy Safer, 2007.

2. World Health Organization (WHO). MPS Technical Update: Prevention of postpartum haemorrhage by active management of the third stage of labour. Geneva: World Health Organization, 2006.

3. World Health Organization (WHO) Department of Reproductive Health and Research. Maternal mortality in 2000: Estimates developed by WHO, UNICEF, and UNFPA. Geneva, 2004.

4. Prendiville WJ, Harding JE, Elbourne DR, Stirrat GM. The Bristol third stage trial: active versus physiological management of the third stage of labour. *BMJ* 1988;297:1295-1300.

5. van Rheenen P, Brabin BJ. A practical approach to timing cord clamping in resource poor settings. *BMJ* 2007;333:954-958.

6. Hutton EK, Hassan ES. Late vs. early clamping of the umbilical cord in full-term neonates: systematic review and meta-analysis of controlled trials. *JAMA* 2007;297(11):1241-52.

7. Chaparro CM, Neufeld LM, Tena Alavez G, Eguia-Liz Cedillo R, Dewey KG. Effect of timing of umbilical cord clamping on iron status in Mexican infants: a randomised controlled trial. *Lancet* 2006;367:1997-2004.

8. Gillespie S, Johnston JL. Expert Consultation on Anemia: Determinants and Interventions. Ottawa: The Micronutrient Initiative, 1998.

9. Lozoff B, Georgieff MK. Iron deficiency and brain development. *Semin Pediatr Neurol* 2006;13:158-165.

10. Lozoff B, Jimenez E, Smith JB. Double burden of iron deficiency in infancy and low socioeconomic status: a longitudinal analysis of cognitive test scores to age 19 years. *Arch Pediatr Adolesc Med* 2006;160(11):1108-1113.

11. Dewey KG, Chaparro CM. Session 4: Mineral metabolism and body composition Iron status of breast-fed infants. *Proc Nutr Soc* 2007;66(3):412-422.

12. Rabe H, Reynolds G, Diaz-Rossello J. Early versus delayed umbilical cord clamping in preterm infants. *Cochrane Database Systematic Reviews* 2004;Issue 4. Art. No.: CD003248. DOI: 10.1002/14651858.CD003248.pub2.

13. Mercer JS, Vohr BR, McGrath MM, Padbury JF, Wallach M, Oh W. Delayed cord clamping in very preterm infants reduces the incidence of intraventricular hemorrhage and late-onset sepsis: A randomized controlled trial. *Pediatrics* 2006;117:1235-1242.

14. American Academy of Pediatrics (AAP). Policy Statement: Breastfeeding and the use of human milk. *Pediatrics* 2005;115(2):496-506.

15. Christensson K, Siles C, Moreno L, et al. Temperature, metabolic adaptation and crying in healthy full-term newborns cared for skin-to-skin or in a cot. *Acta Paediatr* 1992;81(607):488-493.

16. Moore ER, Anderson GC, Bergman N. Early skin-to-skin contact for mothers and their healthy newborn infants. *Cochrane Database of Systematic Reviews* 2007;Issue 3.:Art.No.: CD003519. DOI: 10.1002/14651858.CD003519.pub2.

17. Righard L, Alade MO. Effect of delivery room routines on success of first breast-feed. *Lancet* 1990;336:1105-1107.

18. Edmond KM, Zandoh C, Quigley MA, Amenga-Etego S, Owusu-Agyei S, Kirkwood BR. Delayed breastfeeding initiation increases risk of neonatal mortality. *Pediatrics* 2006;117:380-386.

19. Betran AP, de Onis M, Lauer JA, Villar J. Ecological study of effect of breast feeding on infant mortality in Latin America. *BMJ* 2001;323(7308):303-306.

20. Matthiesen AS, Ransjö-Arvidson AB, Nissen E, Uvnäs-Moberg K. Postpartum maternal oxytocin release by newborns: effects of infant hand massage and sucking. *Birth* 2001;28(1):13-19.

21. Chua S, Arulkumaran S, Lim I, Selamat N, Ratnam SS. Influence of breastfeeding and nipple stimulation on postpartum uterine activity. *BJOG* 1994;101(9):804-805.

22. Awi DD, Alikor EA. Barriers to timely initiation of breastfeeding among mothers of healthy full-term babies who deliver at the University of Port Harcourt Teaching Hospital. *Niger J Clin Pract* 2006;8(1):57-64.

Acknowledgments

This document was written by Camila Chaparro. Chessa Lutter and A. Virginia Camacho Hubner were the responsible technical officers and provided comments and technical oversight. An earlier draft was circulated at the Regional Technical Consultation for the Regional Action Plan on Neonatal Health, August 28-30, 2007. We would like to thank and acknowledge the following individuals for their valuable comments: Fernando Arango Gómez, Guillermo Carroli, Kathryn Dewey, José Luis Díaz Rossello, Joaquín Guillermo Gómez Dávila, Ornella Lincetto, Matthews Mathai, Judith Mercer, Hedwig van Asten and Patrick van Rheenen. We would also like to recognize Yehuda Benguigui and Ricardo Fescina for their support in the development of this document.

This publication has been made possible thanks to support from the Regional Office of Sustainable Development, Office for Latin America and the Caribbean, United Statues Agency for International Development, under the terms of Grant No. LAC-G-00-04-00002-00. The ideas and opinions expressed do not necessarily reflect the point of view of the United Statues Agency for International Development, USAID.

For more information, please contact:

Unit on Child and Adolescent Health
Pan American Health Organization
525 23rd Street, NW, Washington D.C. 20037
Website: http://www.paho.org • Telephone: (202) 974-3519

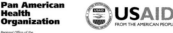

Chapter 7
Midwifery Presence: Philosophy, Science and Art

Holly Powell Kennedy, Tricia Anderson and Nicky Leap

> Always, I think, impressing upon families that you are there for them while they're in labor. I think that's so essential because if you set someone up to believe that this is possible and there's no one there who can carry that out, they're left in the hands of unskilled professionals who don't know how to facilitate normal birth and that's not fair.
>
> (Kennedy & Shannon 2004)

Introduction

The Oxford English Dictionary (2007) defines *presence* as a verb, noun, characteristic or influence. As a verb, presence is 'the state of being with or in the same place.' As a noun, it is 'the place or space in front of or around a person; the immediate vicinity of a person'. This use can refer to ceremonial or formal attendance, such as with royalty. A person can be described to 'have' presence, such as a characteristic or demeanour (stateliness, bearing). This can project an influence upon others, suggesting inner strength or force of personality merely by being present. As such, embodiment is implied in the definition. Finally, presence of mind is 'the ability to remain calm and take quick, sensible action.' We believe that all of these definitions have meaning in the care of childbearing women. How a midwife[1] defines and uses presence is likely to vary depending on philosophical beliefs and exposure to those who actively use it as part of their repertoire. In an increasingly technical world of childbirth, it is a skill that either may be undeveloped or unable to be implemented effectively.

The American College of Nurse-Midwives (ACNM) (2004) specifically identifies the value of presence in their philosophy of midwifery. In similar vein, the Australian College of Midwives' *Philosophy Statement for Midwifery* (ACM 2004) identifies that the original meaning of the word 'midwife' means 'with woman' and that 'this meaning shapes midwifery's philosophy, work and relationships'. The Royal College of Midwives (RCM 2007) describes this to aspiring midwives as, 'A midwife does more than just deliver babies. Because she is *present* at every birth, whether at home or in hospital, she touches everyone's life'. We assert that presence is a multifaceted, complex concept, essential to working with women and their families during childbirth. Teaching novice midwives or sceptical administrators and managers the value of presence remains a continuing challenge. The purpose of this chapter is to explore the use and meaning of presence in midwifery practice, with a particular focus on the dynamics of how this relates to being with women during labour and birth. We will argue that presence is both process and outcome, with evidence supporting its clinical value. We also passionately believe that presence is a midwifery art. At its pinnacle it is beautiful to behold, but often invisible to the unschooled eye that does not notice or value the quiet midwife in the corner of the room, watching and listening, but letting the woman 'get on with it' in her own way. We have chosen favourite songs as metaphorical examples to illustrate the 'art of midwifery presence.'[2]

A philosophical view of midwifery presence

Childbirth is a significant junction in a woman's life as she brings forth a new person into the world. Her beliefs, values, relationships and knowledge will influence how she sees and experiences pregnancy and birth, including how she interacts with the midwife, and perhaps other practitioners, during the childbearing year. Practitioners' beliefs, values, relationships and knowledge will also influence how they work with the woman as their worlds intimately unite during the labour and birth. Understanding women's needs in childbirth must integrate these dimensions to provide optimal care. Midwifery presence can be a powerful instrument and the act of being present or 'with woman' can have multiple facets, from gathering data to establishing and developing a mutually trusting relationship.

We have chosen the philosophical lens of interpretive phenomenology to explore the meaning of midwifery presence. Heideggerian phenomenology rejects Cartesian duality (separation of mind and body) in traditional science because it hinders our understanding of what it is to be a person. Leonard (1994) describes this perspective as a filter that 'constrains our ability to understand human agency' (p. 45). Hermeneutics is the 'science of interpretation' – the goals of humanities and social science are the understanding of our world and that of others, in contrast to the natural sciences which more often seek explanation (Benner 1994). Heiddeger believed it was essential to understand the existential structures of living and what it means to live in the world, particularly around our relationship with time. It is in this discovery that we move closer to understanding human life through the lived experience (Benner 1994). This requires recognition of the complexity of human life and a willingness to acknowledge that all phenomena can never be fully known or proven. It requires an ability to be open to a more fluid and encompassing worldview that may be very different from your own. Neither is right or wrong, but all can exist in a situated, temporal world. In other words, knowledge is always situated in the world at hand, relative and dynamic. We have used five dimensions of phenomenology described by Benner and Wrubel (1989) to frame our exploration of midwifery presence through four clinical stories.

Situation: The ability to understand the person's circumstances and history, both current and past is an important aspect of care. Each midwife is taught to 'take' a history in order to understand the woman's background and how that might influence the current pregnancy and birth. However, there is far more about a woman's situation that can influence how childbirth unfolds than is often on the clinical data collection form. Although we might never truly know or completely understand another person's situation, a relationship built on trust and continuity is likely to give us deeper understandings of a woman's circumstances. The ability to be present allows the midwife to use all of her senses to gather clues on the woman's situation.

> She knew me, she knew my family, she knew my profession, it was wonderful. It was like going to visit a friend every single time.
>
> (Kennedy & Shannon 2004, p. 18)

Embodiment: The responses of the body are often taken for granted, yet they enable us to recognise and react quickly. Benner (1994) calls this 'skilful comportment and perceptual emotional responses' (p. 104). This is similar to 'presence of mind' and can be reflected in the midwife's embodied hand skills that act almost without thought or actions, sometimes appearing to be based on intuition rather than based on rational reasoning. Presence is the powerful embodiment of 'being with woman' as the midwife sits quietly at hand, steps away to let the woman be on her own, or actively works with her hand-in-hand during a trying moment. This can also reflect the midwife's or woman's demeanour. A calm, unruffled presence and quiet words of encouragement, sometimes called *midwifery muttering* (Leap 2000), can create a relaxed environment just as panic can induce chaos.

> I could hear them talking, I wasn't really aware of my surroundings too much, I was just concentrating on my contractions, but I could hear just nice, comforting words coming from behind me.

Temporality: The experience of lived time incorporates understanding the present from knowledge of the past. A midwife will practise based on her past experiences, just as women will react to the challenges of childbirth based on their experiences. The intersections of each person's temporality with others can influence how the process unfolds. It also accounts for understandings of present time and associated meanings. This is particularly significant since experience of time is altered for many women in labour and birth (Beck 1994). Anderson (2000) suggested that temporal distortion for labouring women may produce altered states of consciousness similar to those produced by meditation and losing track of time becomes a coping strategy. How the midwife attends a woman in labour may be dictated by rules about time allowed for the process to happen. All of these temporal aspects converge and can affect the childbirth experience. We believe the important meaning of temporality is that although childbirth occurs in the present, it is influenced by the past and will shape the future.

> It wasn't a particular long labor, so they tell me. To me it seemed like a while.
>
> (Kennedy 2001, unpublished data)

Concerns: Knowledge of what is meaningful to each person or what really matters will affect the provision and experience of childbirth care (Carolan & Hodnett 2007). Beliefs and values intensely shade each person's view of the world. What is critically important to the woman may be vastly different from what is important to the midwife – it represents another intersection for connection or separation. Each woman comes to birth desiring different things shaped by culture, experience and situation. Sometimes these are consciously known to her and communicated to her care providers. At other times they become apparent in the labour if you are open to observing for their clues.

> It was all about me and what I needed. She was there. She was with us the whole time. She wasn't the ring leader, I was.
>
> (Kennedy 2001, unpublished data)

Common meanings: There are cultural and/or linguistic meanings or assumptions common to each individual, but which may differ among individuals and can give rise to misunderstandings. Meaning in each person's world is shaped through these perspectives. Understanding definitions of events and acts is crucial to construct care that meets the woman's needs as an individual. For example, 'safety' as it applies to birth may be defined differently by the woman, the midwife, the obstetrician and the risk management team – each of their definitions have potential to shape the processes of care.

I kept the door closed, but somehow or other though the information just sort of goes out to the hospital floor that she's been pushing for two hours and what was I going to do about it?

(Kennedy 2001, unpublished data)

The goal of interpretive phenomenology is to understand everyday experiences and for this chapter, we will use it as the lens to understand the use of midwifery presence as an embodied part of our practice. What does it mean to say there is value in 'presence'? What does it mean to 'be present' or to be 'with woman'? The first step in our exploration will be to present the science that best describes this phenomenon.

The scientific evidence for midwifery presence

The act of presence: Exploring the concept of midwifery presence requires a willingness to realise that there can never be one formula that can describe causation with certainty. Our work is rife with uncertainty. For example, merely placing a midwife with the woman during her labour does not guarantee improved outcomes. Rather, presence is likely to be one of many factors in providing care. Downe and McCourt (2008) described this from the perspective of complexity theory that accounts for the interconnection of events and rejects the idea that there is one 'right' way to accomplish an end. Most of the literature has examined presence in nursing care, with a smaller group of studies focused on midwifery practice and even less in medicine. A related concept is that of continuous support during childbirth. The latter is likely a broader concept and less specific definition of presence, but is important to explore and is addressed later in this chapter.

Presence was specifically discussed by Lehrman (1988) and Kennedy (1995, 2000) in their early theory development in midwifery. Lehrman (1988) defined it as 'one on one personal attention and constant availability of the nurse-midwife in labor' and this was positively associated with the woman's self-esteem and satisfaction with care (p. 44). Kennedy's (1995, 2000) and Kennedy and Shannon (2004) research has revealed presence as a process that incorporated intimacy, respect, patience and creating physical and emotional space conducive to birth. 'She sits down, she asks you questions about the past year ... things that are really related to your passion, what you are doing' (2004, p. 17). Hunter (2002) conducted a comprehensive review of the literature to understand the concept of 'being with woman' and described midwifery philosophy and physiological arguments for the practice. She reviewed 13 qualitative studies on midwifery care (from both midwives' and women's experiences) and identified women's value of midwifery support, sensitivity to women's needs, clinical expertise, control in decision-making, and advice/information provided by the midwife. She argued that there is empirical evidence for the value of 'being with' women in labour and the two representative attributes of this concept are (1) providing available human presence and (2) social support as indicated by the woman's emotional, physical, spiritual and psychological needs. However, the literature lacked clarity about the embodiment of presence – what it really looks like in action and what it means for the midwife, woman and/or her family.

Kennedy (2000) described the 'art of doing nothing well' in her Delphi study of exemplary US midwives and women for whom they cared. This meant vigilant attendance, but not necessarily intervening in the process. Much of this work was invisible to others who were unaware of the 'actions' of presence during which mutual trust was established.

> Much of what midwives do during early labor doesn't even look like 'doing' ... I speak for myself and the long honorable tradition of midwifery when I describe this 'work' as mastery in doing 'nothing.' It is a specific skill that must be learned and developed, no less so than any of those busy medical skills associated with the 'doing-ness' of hospital-based obstetrics. As a community midwife, I sit for many long hours doing this 'nothing' silently observing while listening to the parents talk about their hopes and dreams, fears and frustrations.
>
> (Kennedy 2000, p. 12)

Leap (2000) explored the notion of 'the less we do, the more we give' in relation to empowerment and suggested that, by minimising disturbance, direction, intervention and authority, the potential for physiology, common sense and instinctive behaviour is maximised. In doing so, trust is placed with the childbearing woman and power is shifted toward the woman. She described how she learned from watching midwives sitting quietly in the corner of the room where the woman was labouring, in watchful anticipation, being very quiet and non-directive:

> Our expertise as midwives rests in our ability to watch, to listen and to respond to any given situation with all of our senses. This will include the conscious and subconscious 'knowing' that has been generated from our experience and learning. It also involves a 'cluefullness' as we respond to the overt and covert clues from women and their worlds. The skill lies in knowing when to inform, suggest, act, seek help and, most importantly, when to be still or when to withdraw and remove ourselves (p. 5–6).

In a similar vein, Anderson (2002) discussed the midwife as a significant intervention and the importance of deconstructing routine procedures that may interfere with the normal processes of labour. She also described this as part of our 'invisible' work because when we do not 'do' – our work cannot always be seen, and hence valued. Berg (2005) describes this as 'enduring presence', linked to the requirement to provide care with dignity. It includes nearness and availability; 'I give her my time, show her that I have time for her. I stop and I sit down' (p. 13).

There is abundant literature on the concept of presence as provided by nurses. In the United States, as well as some other countries, nurses provide the front line of care during parturition, thus the research on their use of presence is relevant. Explorations of the concept cover all types of nursing practice, including perinatal care. Tavernier (2006) conducted a concept analysis from the scientific evidence on presence and defined it as the 'mutual act of intentionally focusing on the patient through attentiveness to their needs by offering of one's whole self to be with the patient for the purpose of healing' (p. 154). Sandelowski (2002) examined the visible nature of nursing and how nurses define themselves. Part of how they saw their work was expressed as 'being there and available, which goes beyond spectatorship' and 'emotional, personal, and existential availability' (p. 64). However, she noted that nurses can be physically in place, but not fully present to the person. This is often complicated by multiple aspects of the health care arena, including technological interventions that remove the nurse from the bedside or draw her gaze to the machine rather than the person.

Covington (2005) noted that presence creates a 'safe space' for patients built upon trust and connection. Using presence is something that is learned and comes with experience. Arbon (2004) believes that less experienced nurses focus more on safety and technological aspects of care. 'With time and experience nurses become more adept at these fundamental nursing activities, more comfortable and confident . . . and can focus more attention of the caring, interpersonal and connecting side of practice' (p. 154). When patients are asked what they wish from nurses they describe the desire to be heard, to be respected for their decisions, and to be treated with compassion and understanding (Aquino-Russell 2005). Women's experiences with those providing care in childbirth reflect the importance of building relationship and a safe place to birth, especially when it is absent. 'Nobody came over and stroked my hair or just held my hand and said, you know we're coming right with you' (Mackinnon *et al.* 2005, p. 32). Too often, modern maternity care is beset with technological complexities which create structural practices that disrupt this relationship. Malone (2003) calls this 'distal nursing'. One example is the evolution of central fetal monitoring which removes the clinician from the bedside to watch the fetal response to labour at a distal location; thus the woman's response and the use of presence to create a safe space is lost.

The physiology of presence: Quantifying the association of midwifery presence with clinical outcomes is challenging. Theoretically, presence (or the absence of it) may be most closely related to stress theory in which the experience of stress activates physiological mechanisms (catecholamines) for fight or flight (Shannon *et al.* 2007). The ability of the body to manage this physiologically is called *allostasis*. As stressors persist, there is allostatic overload and diminishment of the body's ability to balance stress. In an illness situation, this can result in increased pathology or altered healing. In childbirth it can result in decreased ability to cope with the rigours of labour. Hunter's (2002) review of the physiological literature suggested that a sustaining presence enhances women's ability to cope with the stress of fear, pain and anxiety of childbirth. Touch helped women cope, feel comforted, and decreased systolic blood pressure and pulse rates. Buckley (2004) noted that women as human beings have varying needs for privacy, some preferring more personal support, and others prefer complete privacy. Creating the ability for a woman to birth in a situation that feels safe and supported through midwifery presence is more likely to help her achieve a birth with minimal intervention. Each intervention holds potential for a cascade of further interventions and long-term effects for the mother and infant (Kitzinger 2005).

Drawing on the significant research of Kerstin Uvnas-Moberg (2003) at the Karolinska institute in Stockholm, Sweden, Tricia Anderson (2006) described an inverse relationship between trust and oxytocin. When a woman is stressed, anxious or on her guard, oxytocin levels will drop. Conversely, if oxytocin levels rise there is an activation of the parasympathetic nervous system, lowering of blood pressure and pulse rates, increased circulation to skin and mucous membranes, lowered levels of stress hormones, and more effective digestion and nutrition uptake.

Tricia called this the *calm and connect* response that improves breastfeeding, infant digestion, and stimulation of growth and healing. When a woman is threatened, trust flees, but when she feels safe her body's physiology works in synchrony to permit her to open to the sensations needed to give birth. Presence, when used skilfully can be the bridge to trust. 'I kept looking up and you were there and calm; you said I could do it and so I knew I could' (Anderson 2006). Tricia's work on 'calm and connect' also draws on theory proposed initially by psychologists from the University of California, Los Angeles (Taylor *et al.* 2002). Their model, called *tend and befriend* adds another dimension to the 'fight-or-flight' response to stress. Taylor and colleagues suggested that the research describing 'flight and fight' responses was carried out on male animals and men. They propose that females are more likely to respond to stressful situations by protecting themselves and their young through nurturing behaviours and forming alliances with a larger social group, predominantly with other females. These responses developed because females tend to be the primary caregivers of their young, with pregnancy, lactation and caring behaviours taking precedence over a readiness for flight and aggression. In evolutionary terms, it is argued, fleeing too readily in dangerous situations might put a female's offspring at risk. The argument for the 'tend and befriend' response to stress draws on evidence from research from animal and human studies, notably studies of neurohormonal activity and social psychology. The 'tend and befriend' – or 'calm and connect' – response is linked to the brain's attachment and nurturing systems, in particular the production of female reproductive hormones. These hormones, notably oxytocin and endogenous opioid peptide mechanisms counteract the metabolic activity of the traditional 'fight-or-flight' responses of increased heart rate, blood pressure and cortisol levels. Furthermore, these neurohormonal processes promote caregiving activities and attachment between mothers and their young (Taylor *et al.* 2002). The importance of oxytocin in the promotion of trust and social behaviour is increasingly being identified (Kosfeld *et al.* 2005). The continuing exploration of how all of this relates to the promotion of well-being for labouring women is the challenge that Tricia hands onto us as an important part of her legacy.

Linked to increasing understandings of neurohormonal processes and labour is the notion of non-disturbance, described initially by Michel Odent (1984). Reducing stimulation to the neuro-cortex facilitates the release and interplay of the neurohormonal processes of physiological labour, including the woman's own endogenous opioids. The sight of a woman who has entered her own 'zone' or altered state of consciousness during powerful labour is one which brings a quiet delight and sense of confidence in a midwife who is 'present' at a woman's labour. Midwives have probably always recognised this withdrawal that accompanies strong, uncomplicated labour. A retired midwife who practised in Battersea, London in the 1940s reflected on her experience:

> I think myself that the system has a certain amount of sedative in itself that it releases at a time like that. I'm sure it has, because I've seen people that just looked as if they were half sozzled – and they didn't have anything! Just looked like somebody 'gone' – and they hadn't had any dope!
>
> I think the body does release something into the system. If it's not interfered with by giving dope, it will work. But I think when you interfere, it won't work then.
>
> (Leap & Hunter 1993, p. 168–169)

Sometimes, this midwifery non-disturbance stretches to protecting the woman from the fears and anxieties of her labour supporters, explained by another retired midwife who worked in pre-NHS Devon:

I think she was a primip. All the house was very anxious and all the rest of it. So they said, 'What could they do?' So I said, 'Oh well, keep quiet and let her go. Sit down and have a game of cards, or do something.' When I went back and had a look in, there they all were most religiously playing cards! It worked!

(Leap & Hunter 1993, p. 169)

Continuous support in labour: A synonym for presence is 'being there.' A similar concept to presence in labour is that of continuous support. Hodnett and colleagues (2007) conducted a systematic review of continuous labour support in 16 trials across 11 countries with a sample of over 13 000 women birthing in a variety of settings. Continuous support, especially when it was provided early in labour, was associated with higher rates of spontaneous birth, less use of pain medications, somewhat shorter labours, and greater levels of satisfaction. Interestingly, continuous support was more effective when provided by women other than hospital staff. Drawing specific linkages for these findings is challenging. A systematic review of women's satisfaction in relationship to the pain of labour and birth found that pain was not the overriding factor (Hodnett 2002). Satisfaction was associated with (1) personal expectations, (2) amount of support from caregivers, (3) quality of the caregiver–patient relationship, and (4) involvement in decision-making. This suggests that it is not about *what is done* but about *how women felt* in terms of support and personal control. In other words, 'presence' may be the strongest contributory factor.

This review suggests there is a theoretical and scientific basis for the use of midwifery presence when caring for women during labour and birth. The next section will describe from a variety of studies what this looks like in action. Four vignettes will be presented and discussed using the dimensions of phenomenology discussed by Benner and Wrubel (1989).

The art of midwifery presence

Kennedy and Shannon (2004) found that midwives often describe their work using artistic terms, both in process and outcome. These include 'orchestration' and 'dancing' with women and within the health care setting. It is an 'art' to bring all of the players together to achieve the best production possible. The woman is the central actor and the midwife and others are supporting cast. The 'art' of practice is often mentioned as if it is oppositional to science. We believe that presence and continuous support are linked to clinical outcomes, thus they represent part of the science of our practice. However, *how* the midwife provides presence may clearly depict the art and embodiment of practice. It is a skill of knowing when to step in and when to step out – an intricate blend of listening, responding and acting only when required.

Exemplary midwives in Kennedy's (2000) study believed the most important outcome was 'optimal health of the mother and infant in the given situation' (p. 8). Most midwifery philosophies view health as holistic going beyond physical to emotional, psychological, social and spiritual dimensions. The vignettes chosen represent not only the woman's various dimensions of health, but also the midwives' experience, because in order to be fully present to others it is important to be present to oneself. In recognition of the artful side of practice, we have chosen favourite songs of ours to provide the backdrop for the stories. All names are pseudonyms.

The Long and Winding Road

The Beatles' lyrics for the *Long & Winding Road* (Lennon & McCartney 1970) tell a story of pain, tears and a difficult journey, and suggests an untold story. The following story evokes that metaphor as the midwife teases out the hidden story that is blocking the woman's way through her labour.

> Hard, hard, hard first labour ... I did know by this time that things were not going well ... So I had asked her a question about this or that and wasn't getting anywhere. Finally, leaning on the end of the bed I said, 'Tell me about your mother.' She was quiet for a moment and said, 'Which one?' I said, 'Well, anyone you want to talk about.' I didn't have a clue what she meant. So she began to talk and I remember it was three in the morning, between three and four. You know we talk about teasing out membranes so they won't break off. This felt like the hardest work I ever did because it was like teasing the story out. She didn't really want to go there and I couldn't push her to go there. But I could just tease it, I didn't want it to break you know ... It took an hour to get there ... In that hour with that story coming out agonizingly slow ... this poopy labour that was going nowhere, I became aware that the contractions were getting bigger and stronger. She was paying no attention to her contractions at this point. She'd had not anything for pain, but she just kept wanting to talk ... as she talked, the contractions kept getting stronger and stronger and closer together. I mean from an hour of the time she finished telling the story, she was overwhelmed with labour. Within an hour of that she had the baby.
>
> (Kennedy 2001, unpublished data)

This woman took an hour to tell a long and winding story of grief and mothering from her past in the middle of a labour that had stalled. Over the years we have heard many, many similar stories that told of hidden fears. Examining the meaning of this story, we see a woman who came to her birth with issues that may have held her labour up. Because the situation permitted the midwife to sit with her, probe, and listen to her concerns, she was able to tell her story. The temporality of the story was revealed in past events creating a barrier to how this woman saw herself as a current daughter and future mother. In the recounting of the story the midwife did not play the role of psychologist – she simply listened and let the woman get on with her labour.

A Hard Day's Night

The opening chord of the Beatles' *A Hard Day's Night* is universally recognised by anyone familiar with their music (Lennon & McCartney 1964). It portrays the desire to be nurtured after a hard day's work. Labour is hard, and often very long with day turning to night and then to day again – for both the woman and midwife.

We have chosen a poem to reflect the 24 × 7 days per week temporal nature of labour and birth when allowed to unfold on its own. Written by the baby's father and given to the midwife as a gesture of appreciation, the poem unfolds the call into night and shadows the midwife's presence against the woman's triumph.

Wise woman

So comes our time, the waiting done
No more hicks and cups of berry tea
Nor diary scan for due date be
Now clock hands mark the beat of nature's surge

Turn down the lights, let calm be here
With music make a gentle place
And to a sleepy voice the call
'Wise Woman. Come. Our dance begins'

And so we three a fourth entice
With whispers speak as though within a sacred place
Wise woman, me, our champion to support
Her corporeal triumph to embrace

Through timeless night wise woman gentle weaves
Her practised craft; her words and timely deeds
As guiding spirit, both there and not there
Her un-present presence our moments to allow

(Martin Vincent, with permission)

A sense of background presence, quiet strength, and expertise is communicated in these gentle words. The father's sense of timeless life cycles is echoed as the woman triumphs with the midwife in the background.

Let it Be

In the song *Let it Be*, Lennon and McCartney (1970) convey the power of a strong presence with whispered words of wisdom during the hour of darkness.

> At one point she went into the bathroom and shut the door. After a while, she let me come in. She had been in there crying, and she just said she didn't know whether she could do this. Then her labour began to just peter out ... she had stayed at 6–7 cm for a long time ... Then he [husband] starts to get tense and little bit anxious ... he was hovering. Not only was it bothering Cindy, I think that it was bothering me too. I set him some task to do; I don't remember what it was, go do something in the kitchen. But at this point Cindy didn't even seem to want me much. She just really wanted space. I left her alone and I saw her go into the bedroom. After a while, I followed her in there and she was standing with her head on her hands, just standing at the bed, just blocking everything out. She made no acknowledgment that I had come into the room. So I didn't say anything. I just watched her for a little while and I sort of went and stood somewhat near her but not right next to her. Then she simply fell to the floor. She didn't do over like a pole, like she had fainted. She just melted to the floor like someone who had utterly given up everything. Of course, I was startled. I looked down at her and her color looked OK. I reached down and her pulse was OK but she just lay on the floor. She didn't move a muscle. She had just melted onto the floor. I still hadn't said anything to her, and I really didn't know what to say or what to do. So I lay down on the floor beside her but I laid at her back side. She was sort of on her side and I laid where she didn't see me but she of course knew I was there. I just lay beside her ... After a while I became aware that she was having contractions. I just lay there and listened and those contractions just picked up and picked up. I still hadn't said a word to her. So I got up and said, 'Cindy, I've got to get the doppler and listen to the baby. I haven't listened to the baby in a while.' I said, 'I know that Adam is very anxious outside. Do you want him in here?' That's the first words she said to me in all that time and said, 'Not now.' I got up and went out and got the doppler. Of course, he

was frantic, 'I want to go in there, why can't I go in there?' All I could do is say, 'I know how much you love her Adam. She needs for you right now to give her this space. When it's time, I know she's going to want you to be with her.' I listened to the baby, the baby was fine. I think it was not an hour, or maybe an hour and a half and she was fully dilated and feeling pushy. 'Cindy you've got to be clear about what you do and don't want' ... So we came out to the place that she had chosen to give birth.

(Kennedy 2001, unpublished data)

Cindy went on to give birth in the room she had planned. She was able to give the midwife direction about what was helping her and what was not, particularly about the presence of others in the room. Her disappearance had been to move away from those she was not comfortable with at the birth. When she first attended the birth, the midwife had not been aware of Cindy's situation. As the labour evolved, she slowly was able to clue into the woman's concerns through presence, observation and gentle probing. She was able to assess her physical well-being as she fell to the ground and simply stayed with her. The common meanings were likely different for the husband (who was anxious and felt excluded), the woman (who needed space) and the midwife – who had the safety of the woman to consider and the role of mediator. She was able to bridge the two and create the space for the woman to choose to birth when she was ready. We tried to imagine this in a busy hospital labour ward where there is no place for a woman to escape and too often no midwife to provide the skilled presence to know when to 'let it be' by creating that safe place for the woman.

I Am Woman

Helen Reddy led the chorus of women's claiming of power in the 1970s with the song *I Am* Woman (Reddy & Burton 1972). The strength, wisdom and power of a woman was birthed through pain but was rewarded by her invincibility and realisation that she could do anything.

My midwife walked a fine line flawlessly. On the one hand, when I, sobbing, told her I didn't want to raise a retarded child, she sympathetically agreed, neither would she. She, thus, shared in our common humanity without making me feel less a person. On the other hand, she held and treated my baby as a precious, beautiful gift. That too, helped me overcome my own fears of being rejected and stigmatized since my baby was retarded. She helped me rise to the occasion

(Kennedy 2000, p. 11)

This minimalist quote presents the uncertainty of the situation – of childbirth. Even with all of the testing, monitoring and safety nets – the outcome of birth is not certain. But is not that life, where the only certain things are death and taxes? Midwifery presence – when skilled and imbued with acts of human kindness, can turn moments around. In the quote above, a woman was confronted with a child with Down's syndrome and was devastated as much by her reaction as she was by the child. Her midwife, by her presence and actions, showed her that her humanness was her strength – it turned the corner.

Conclusion

'I feel that good midwifery practice is essentially silent in that it helps a woman toward achievements which she rightly sees as hers and not as the midwife's' (Kirkham 2000, p. 197).

The cameos and songs above allow us to consider how situation, embodiment, temporality, concerns and common meanings play a role in midwifery presence. The midwife has engaged with each situation using all of her senses. As identified by Dreyfus and Dreyfus (2005) this emotional investment allows the practitioner to develop an embodied awareness that promotes intuitive responses and holistic approaches. The midwives draw on what Dreyfus and Dreyfus refer to as 'a vast repertoire of situational discriminations' (p. 787) in making embodied decisions about what needs to be done and how to do it. This includes picking up the clues from the past – the woman's and the midwife's past – that may be influencing the present. The significance of this and the meaning that each individual woman ascribes to her experience can have a profound effect on her life, particularly as most women describe an altered state of consciousness in straightforward labour. One woman articulated this in reflecting on her birth experience and the role the midwife played within that experience:

> To begin to understand the power of 'presence', in this context of the birthing process, is to be open to other realities. Phrases and words like: 'out-of-body experience'; 'visible/invisible'; aberration, are a real phenomenon in my birth experience. I believe it's related to the ability to appreciate and understand the cycle of life and death; the change of seasons – all things organic and inorganic. This 'way of being', was obvious at the first point of contact with my midwife. It has no decipherable language, and yet I felt 'trust' immediately. 'Presence' gave me the self-belief that I could do it – and give birth, knowing, whatever the outcome I would find my way.
>
> (Akosua Asante 2008, Personal communication)

As discussed earlier, the sense of trust described here may play a significant role in promoting oxytocin and physiological labour. As Hall and Taylor (2004) have pointed out, trust is a multifaceted process – the midwife needs to have an awareness of self and be able to trust her instincts as well as those of the woman she attends. This includes understandings of the potential role of fear in affecting outcomes and experiences. The development of trust is likely to be facilitated where the woman and her midwife have the opportunity to develop a relationship (Huber & Sandall 2006). However, debates continue about whether continuity of care in itself is more important than the philosophy of care in terms of women feeling well supported during labour (Carolan & Hodnett 2007). What is undeniable is that whether the labouring woman and her midwife have met before or not; the way in which the midwife enacts her 'presence' will be acutely remembered by the woman for the rest of her life (Leap & Hunter 1993; Simkin 1999).

Notes

1 We are using the term midwife consistently through this chapter. However, we recognise that other practitioners can provide similar care, including the use of 'presence' when caring for childbearing women. However, we believe the use of presence is a hallmark of exemplary midwifery care. Since most midwives (but not all) are women we will also use the pronoun 'she' for ease of reading.

2 This chapter was designed by Tricia Anderson and Holly Kennedy and hopes to convey the critical importance of presence in the midwife's repertoire of caring for women. They believed that conveying the artful nature of this skill required a creative approach, thus they designed a chapter using music, poetry and stories to illustrate their thoughts. Sadly, Tricia died in October 2007 before the chapter was completed. However, she remains an author because her artful creativity was at the heart of planning its presentation. Nicky Leap, a good friend and also a creative midwife, stepped in to help finish the chapter. Nicky and Holly thank Tricia for all she gave to women, midwifery and to us. Although we have lost her earthly company, her 'presence' will always be with us.

References

ACM (2004) *Australian College of Midwives Philosophy for Midwifery*. Canberra. http://www.acmi.org.au/AboutUs/ACMPhilosophyforMidwifery/tabid/256/Default.aspx (Retrieved 4/02/08).

ACNM (2004) *Philosophy of the American College of Nurse-Midwives*, MD. Silver Spring. http://www.midwife.org/philosophy.cfm. (Retrieved 29/01/08).

Anderson T (2000) Feeling safe enough to let go: the relationship between a woman and her midwife during the second stage of labour. In Kirkham M (ed) *The Midwife–Mother Relationship*, Chapter 1. New York, Palgrave, 92–119.

Anderson T (2002) Peeling back the layers: a new look at midwifery interventions. *MIDIRS, Midwifery Digest* 12(2): 208.

Anderson T (2006) Midwifery as alchemy. Is trust the key? 3rd International Research Conference on Normal Birth, Grange-Over-Sands, England, June 2006.

Aquino-Russell CE (2005) Practice possibilities for nurses choosing true presence with persons who live with a different sense of hearing. *Nursing Science Quarterly* 18(1): 32–6.

Arbon P (2004) Understanding experience in nursing. *Journal of Clinical Nursing* 13: 150–7.

Beck CT (1994) Women's temporal experiences during the delivery process. A phenomenological study. *International Journal of Nursing Studies* 31(3): 245–52.

Benner P (1994) The tradition and skill of interpretive phenomenology in studying health, illness, and caring practices. In Benner P. (ed) *Interpretive Phenomenology. Embodiment, Caring, and Ethics in Health and Illness*. Thousand Oaks, Sage Publications, 99–128.

Benner PE, Wrubel J (1989) *The Primacy of Caring: Stress and Coping in Health and Illness*. Menlo Park, Addison-Wesley Publishing Company.

Berg M (2005) A midwifery model of care for childbearing women at high risk: genuine caring in caring for the genuine. *Journal of Perinatal Education* 14(1): 9–21.

Buckley S (2004) Unlocking the potential for normality. *The Practising Midwife* 7(6): 15–7.

Carolan M, Hodnett E (2007) 'With woman' philosophy: examining the evidence, answering the questions. *Nursing Inquiry* 14(2): 140–52.

Covington H (2005) Providing a safe space for patients. *Holistic Nurse Practitioners* 19(4): 169–72.

Downe S, McCourt C (2008) From being to becoming: reconstructing childbirth knowledges. In Downe S (ed) *Normal Childbirth: Evidence and Debate*, 2nd edition. London, Churchill Livingstone.

Dreyfus HL, Dreyfus SE (2005) Peripheral vision: expertise in real world contexts. *Organization Studies* 26(5): 779–92.

Hall J, Taylor M (2004) Birth and spirituality. In Downe S (ed) *Normal Childbirth: Evidence and Debate*. Edinburgh, Churchill Livingstone.

Hodnett E (2002) Pain and women's satisfaction with the experience of childbirth: a systematic review. *American Journal of Obstetrics and Gynecology* 186: 160–72.

Hodnett ED, Gates S, Hofmeyr GJ, Sakala C (2007) Continuous support for women during childbirth. *Cochrane Database of Systematic Reviews*, (3), Art. No.: CD003766. DOI: 10.1002/14651858.CD003766.pub2.

Huber U, Sandall J (2006) Continuity of care, trust and breastfeeding. *MIDIRS Midwifery Digest* 16(4): 445–9.

Hunter LP (2002) Being with woman: a guiding concept for the care of labouring women. *Journal of Midwifery and Women's Health* 31(6): 650–7.

Kennedy H, (2001) *Exemplary Midwifery Practice Research Project*. San Francisco, Unpublished data.

Kennedy HP, Shannon MT (2004) Keeping birth normal: research findings on midwifery care during childbirth. *Journal of Obstetrical, Gynecologic, and Neonatal Nursing* 33(5): 554–60.

Kennedy HP (2000) A model of exemplary midwifery practice: results of a Delphi study. *Journal of Midwifery and Women's Health* 45(1): 4–19.

Kennedy HP (1995) The essence of nurse-midwifery care. The woman's story. *Journal of Nurse Midwifery* 40(5): 410–7.

Kirkham M (2000) Stories and childbirth. In Kirkham MJ, Perkins ER (eds) *Reflections on Midwifery*, Chapter 9. London, Bailliére Tindall, 183–204.

Kitzinger S (2005) Home birth: a social process, not a medical crisis. *The Practising Midwife* 8(4): 26–9.

Kosfeld M, Heinrichs M, Zak PJ, Fischbacher U, Fehr E (2005) Oxytocin increases trust in humans. *Nature*, 435: 673–6.

Leap N (2000) The less we do, the more we give. In Kirkham M (ed). *The Midwife–Mother Relationship*, Chapter 1. New York, Palgrave, 1–17.

Leap N, Hunter B (1993) *The Midwife's Tale: An Oral History from Handywoman to Professional Midwife*. Gateshead, Scarlet Press.

Lehrman EJ (1988) *A theoretical framework for nurse-midwifery practice*. Unpublished Doctoral Dissertation, University of Arizona.

Leonard VW (1994) A Heideggerian phenomenological perspective of the concept of person. *Interpretive Phenomenology. Embodiment, Caring, and Ethics in Health and Illness*. Thousand Oaks, Sage, 43–63.

Lennon J, McCartney P (1964) A hard day's night. Song and lyrics on album, *Let It Be*. London, Apple Records.

Lennon J, McCartney P (1970) The long and winding road. Song and lyrics on album. *Let it Be*. London, Apple Records.

Mackinnon K, McIntyre M, Quance M (2005) The meaning of the nurse's presence during childbirth. *Journal of Obstetric, Gynecologic, and Neonatal Nursing* 34: 28–36.

Malone R (2003) Distal nursing. *Social Science and Medicine* 56(11): 2317–26.

Odent M (1984) *What Birth Can and Should Be*. London, Souvenir Press.

RCM (2007) *Web Page on Careers: Midwifery as a Career: Your Opportunity to Make a Contribution to the Health of Mothers and Babies*. Royal College of Midwives. http://www.rcm.org.uk/career/pages/introduction.php?id=3. (Retrieved 5/12/07).

Reddy H, Burton R (1972) *I am Woman*. Los Angles, Capitol Records.

Sandelowski M (2002) Visible humans, vanishing bodies, and virtual nursing: complications of life, presence, place, and identity. *Advances in Nursing Science* 24(3): 58–70.

Shannon M, King TL, Kennedy HP (2007) Allostasis: a theoretical framework for understanding and evaluating perinatal health outcomes. *Journal of Obstetrical, Gynecologic, and Neonatal Nursing*. 36(2): 125–34.

Simkin P (1999) Just another day in a woman's life? Women's long term perceptions of their first birth experience. Part 1. *Birth* 18: 203–10.

Tavernier SS (2006) An evidence-based conceptual analysis pf presence. *Holistic Nursing Practice* 20(3): 152–6.

Taylor SE, Klein LC, Lewis BP, Gruenewald TL, Guring RA, Updegraff JA (2002) Behavioural responses to stress in females: tend and befriend, not fight and flight. *Psychology Review* 109(4): 745–50; discussion 751–3.

Uvnas-Moberg K (2003) *The Oxytocin Factor: Tapping the Hormone of Calm, Love and Healing*. Cambridge, Da Capo Press.

Chapter 8
Skills for Working
with (the Woman in) Pain

Rosemary Mander

Introduction

Few people would argue with the observation that for most women the
experience of healthy, physiological labour involves a certain degree of
pain. It might even be that, for some, the pain of labour is its defining
characteristic. Attitudes to that pain, though, appear to be evolving,
or may even be undergoing a revolution. This relates to the attitude
with which many women and many midwives are familiar. This is
a reference to the medical view of pain, which is determined by the
assumption that pain is invariably caused by disease or trauma.

> Pain is an unpleasant sensory and emotional experience associated
> with actual or potential tissue damage or described in terms of such
> damage.
>
> (IASP 1979)

Hence, this view is associated with the widespread assumption that
pain, including labour pain, is pathological and carries with it the imperative for intervention to treat it. Such assumptions are only affirmed by
the associated stereotypically masculine, medical and confrontational
analogies of fighting and battle. They seem to seek to persuade that
pain needs to be defeated, by whatever means are available. Hence,
the library catalogues titles such as *Defeating pain*, *The challenge of pain*,
The conquest of pain and *Victory over pain* (Robinson 1946; Fairley 1978;
Wall & Jones 1991; Melzack 1996).

Such warlike images are becoming less and less appropriate as
midwives and childbearing women come to realise that labour and
labour pain are not the one-dimensional, mechanistic processes which
we may have been led to believe. This realisation is not new but may

be a revelation to some in the health field. The library catalogues' hostile images reflect but one of the many meanings of pain. Some would argue, though, that pain, by its very nature, serves to obliterate meaning (Mander 2000). In spite of this, it is likely that the meaning of labour pain, like other aspects of childbearing, is unique to the woman experiencing it. I would suggest that it is the midwife's responsibility to come to understand and help the woman to recognise that meaning and to make good use of it.

For the midwife, as well as facilitating understanding, the experience of being with a woman in labour brings a number of other challenges (Vague 2004). These relate to both the midwife's professional competencies, as well as her human and womanly attributes. Occasionally, though, the midwife may inadvertently find herself reacting in a way which may not be helpful to the woman. An example would be the professional carer who demands of a woman with a failed epidural:

> Why are you making all this fuss? I had four without an epidural and I never made all this noise.
>
> (Mander 2004a, p. 68)

Such reactions may result from the woman's behaviour or, particularly, the words or sounds which the woman articulates or vocalises (Woollett *et al.* 1983). In order for the midwife to be able to rid herself of any of these spontaneous and unwanted responses, a different way of interpreting labour pain has been identified. This reinterpretation provides the basis of the skills which are essential to being able to work with the woman who is experiencing pain in labour.

This chapter begins with a consideration of how views about pain have developed to lead to the models which may now be becoming more appropriate to midwifery care. Leading on from these developments, it reviews some of the aspects which have been suggested as potential benefits of the experience of labour pain. The next part of this chapter is a consideration of who is likely to use these models of understanding pain and how they may be put into effect in the form of support in labour. Leading on from the crucial role of support, the chapter concludes with contemplation of a range of other skills which may help the woman and the midwife to work together with the pain of labour.

Models of pain

Because as human beings we are meant to be logical, we seek explanations for the world about and within us. These explanations are invariably derived from our current state of knowledge. Thus, the understanding of a phenomenon as universal as pain has already passed through a number of interpretations, and may still continue to move through yet more.

In prehistoric times magical influences were held to be responsible for painful experiences; faith in these influences was gradually superseded by trust in or fear of deities (Main & Spanswick 2001). In a similar way, these authors maintain that some cultures have attributed pain to the absence of balance, or to the frustration of desires. As knowledge increased, the ancient Greeks came to recognise the role of the brain, but the relative inputs of the senses and the heart were less clear. Galen, in ancient Rome, realised that nerve fibres were differentiated, but not what the different nerves did. Right through to the Middle Ages, the role of the spinal cord and nerve fibres in the sensation of pain was a subject for conjecture.

Cartesian theory in the 17th century argued that there was a division between the physical body, which experiences pain, and the rational soul, which was thought to control all functions. Thus, Descartes regarded the nerves as simply mechanical in their transmission of sensations, such as pain. The Cartesian legacy of the specificity theory of pain regarded specific nerves as transmitting impulses to the brain from receptors in the skin. This legacy was eventually dispelled by the gate control theory (Melzack & Wall 1965), which proposes that pain is psychophysiological in origin. Since its introduction, the gate control theory has been developed, and still remains largely accepted today. Thus, the understanding of general bodily pain has changed markedly over time.

In Judaeo-Christian societies, labour pain was traditionally regarded as 'God-given'. For this reason, the application of pain theory to childbearing did not present a problem, as no remedies could be contemplated. This situation began to change in the 19th century when James Young Simpson challenged the church's traditional teaching of the 'curse of Eve'. His objection led to a reinterpretation of biblical passages, and the use of ether, and later chloroform, in labour was permitted (Mander 1998a). With these changes, the pain of labour has become an uneasy bed-fellow with pathological, surgical and other traumatic forms of pain.

This way of viewing labour pain as just another 'dis-ease' provoked a backlash and paved the way for the introduction of 'natural childbirth' (Dick-Read 1933), psychoprophylaxis (Lamaze 1956) and psychosexual approaches to pain control (Kitzinger 1989b). The latter approaches were used to develop 'endorphin theory' by Odent. He argued that endogenous opioids, familiar to extreme sportspeople, serve to facilitate the woman's coping, as well as progress in labour (Robertson 1994). Whether the techniques derived from these models of pain have any more research-based authority than the influences held in awe by our prehistoric ancestors is not certain (Yildirim & Sahin 2004).

A major criticism of most models is their tendency to simplify the experience of pain, to the point where the model ceases to be relevant to the woman in labour. Mechanistic interpretations of labour and the accompanying pain have prevailed since science was first applied by William Smellie (1697–1763) to this most unscientific of human activities (Mander 2004b). The models' one-dimensional approaches fail to take account of processes as unimaginably complex as childbearing and the pain with which it is associated.

It was against this background of questionable science that a refreshingly different model of pain, drawing on midwifery expertise, was introduced. This model developed from an, albeit small, qualitative study involving a wide-ranging literature review and interviews with midwives experienced in attending births at home (Leap 1996). On the basis of this research, Leap proposed the existence of two paradigms which differ fundamentally from previous models. The two approaches which Leap described were entitled 'pain relief' and 'working with pain' (Leap 1997, 1998, 2000a; Leap & Anderson 2004).

While Leap makes every effort not to equate 'pain relief' with the medical model, her efforts are less than entirely convincing. 'Pain relief' involves the well-meant offering to the woman a menu of pain control methods early on; possibly during childbirth education or else at the beginning of labour. Although certainly not intended to do so, this menu persuades the woman that she will inevitably need this panoply of techniques and medications (Evans 2006). Thus, a self-fulfilling prophecy begins to manifest itself. One of the factors which is possibly causatively associated with the 'pain relief' model is a staff culture of difficulty in coping with a woman who is in pain and who is clearly articulating that pain:

> Some midwives give pethidine because they don't like the fuss and noise and the agitation and the fact that the woman won't settle down. I think that sometimes the midwife isn't coping with the pain either. They think that the woman isn't and actually they're not.
>
> (Leap 1996, p. 48)

This difficulty in coping is aggravated by a generally low tolerance for noise in labour areas. The result may be the midwife being reprimanded by her colleagues for any noise emanating from the room in which she is attending a woman.

Thus, the 'menu of pain relief' originates as well-meant, to the point of being humanitarian. This menu, though, insidiously carries subliminal messages. This well-meant approach metamorphoses to become increasingly directive, to the extent that pressure may be applied to the woman in labour to accept a hi-tech form of pain control. Such pressure may be applied by staff that, the woman had assumed, were sympathetic to her goals and ideals. In this way, the woman becomes doubly vulnerable to any pressure being applied, having been let down by those she assumed would support her.

In Leap's (1996) research, the midwives distinguished the 'pain relief' model from the paradigm which she entitled 'working with pain' (1996, p. 50). This concept emerged from the midwives' recognition that a certain degree of pain is a fundamental aspect of healthy labour. Recognising this reality meant that the midwives were able to accept that the woman's pain, and her expression of it, was not pathological and did not automatically require the midwives to either remedy it or remove it. The midwives were keen to differentiate the 'normal' pain of physiological labour, from what they regarded as the 'abnormal' pain of a labour which was becoming complicated leading to a deterioration in the woman's physical condition. There was no doubt in the midwives' minds that the recommendation of effective pain control medication was essential when attending such a complicated labour.

Fundamental to the 'working with pain' paradigm were the midwives' philosophical positions. Their philosophy was founded on their confidence in the ability of the woman and the woman's body to give birth spontaneously and physiologically. The midwives deplored the cultural phenomena which serve to diminish the woman's confidence in her body, her self and her close companions. The midwives perceived their crucial role as to create, to enhance or to re-establish that confidence:

> If you can build up confidence in women that they can definitely get on and do this, then I think they will.
>
> > (Leap 1996, p. 65)

Unsurprisingly, Leap's work on pain has made a major contribution to the midwifery campaign in the United Kingdom to regain or maintain the 'normality' of childbirth (Downe 2008).

Pain as transformatory

Childbirth may be regarded as one of the major transitions of a woman's life. This is when she moves from being relatively footloose and independent to taking on the awe-inspiring responsibility of nurturing a new human being. In other words, she becomes a mother. The extent to which western society currently understands the import of this transition is less than clear. Anthropologists, though, have long recognised the significance of birth as transitional in some cultures (van Gennep 1960).

The rituals surrounding these transitions have become the familiar 'rites of passage'. They manifest themselves at the critical, usually challenging, occasions in a person's life. These transitions, such as death or bereavement, committing to a partner, reaching maturity and giving birth carry a range of meanings, which need to be recognised by all who are close by.

The associated ritual varies between cultures, but will usually comprise three main phases (Helman 2007, p. 230). In the context of birth, the first is the separation or seclusion of the childbearing woman, which in western society tends to happen with the onset of labour and the woman's journey to hospital. Second is the transitional, liminal or marginal period, during which the woman is without status, having given up her previous independent role, but not yet assumed her new maternal role. This period is often regarded as a dangerous time, to both the woman and those around her. Traditionally, this danger has been attributed to the polluting effects of blood being shed. The liminal period frequently involves pain being inflicted and/or experienced. The third and final phase is the reincorporation of the woman back into society in her newly elevated social status, which is a cause for celebration. At this time the woman is likely to be specially privileged, respected or permitted to be excused from certain social obligations.

Rites of passage are often associated with some form of stress, which may need to be reduced; the anxieties of nearing adulthood are examples. Thus, rituals help individuals to cope with what would otherwise be challenging life transitions. This is clearly apparent following a death and may also apply when a life-partner is chosen. The stress of childbirth and new parenthood provides a further example.

As well as stress, personal growth may feature. This is obvious in maturation rituals associated with puberty. Growth may also be seen to apply in a person who is bereaved and who may change as a result.

It may be useful to consider the extent to which such personal growth occurs in the context of childbirth. This form of growth becomes apparent in the writing of Leap and Anderson (2008). The woman's experience of the pain of childbirth may be regarded as fundamental to such growth. It is through this experience of dealing with labour pain that the woman is able to become aware of the extent of her own ability to cope with an experience which many find challenging. Through her experience of labour, the woman is convinced that she is a fully mature person who, knowing that she can work though the pain of birth, is likely to be able to summon up sufficient resources to mother this new human being to whom she has given birth.

Thus, in this way, the woman's ability to 'work with the pain' of labour bestows on her a greater sense of maturity or achievement. She will be able to draw on this increased self-esteem when motherhood presents her with challenges. This is because her aspirations may have increased and she may be more confident in her relationships and her self-image. For these reasons, her ability to deal with labour pain may correctly be regarded as life-changing or transformatory.

If the pain of labour is able to have such life-changing effects, which serve to enhance the woman's self regard, what may threaten or jeopardise her ability to work with that pain? A variety of interventions may have the effect of interfering with the woman's personal growth through childbirth. These interventions, though, tend to relate to the undermining of the woman's confidence in her own ability. An example would be the effects of the 'menu of pain relief' which may be presented to the woman during pregnancy or at the beginning of labour. Another example would be the woman who has been persuaded of her inability to withstand the pain of labour and the need for the early setting up of an epidural. This woman might have been so persuaded that she does not even allow herself the opportunity to find out how she would cope with the pain of labour. Thus, it might be said that the anaesthetising of her labour would reduce the impact of her achievement and the associated opportunity for transformation (D. Walsh 2007, Personal communication).

Support at the birth

As is discussed below, the environment in which the woman gives birth is increasingly being recognised as crucial to her satisfaction with her experience of birth. The word 'environment', though, may be interpreted artificially and narrowly to include just the room, clinical area or building in which she labours. Here, the meaning of environment is broadened to encompass, as well, the other people and their behaviour towards the woman in labour. These people would be likely to include her partner and possibly family members as well as one or more of a range of professionals.

I would suggest that the most significant behaviour or activity of all of these people is their ability to offer effective support to the woman. That said, what is meant by support should be considered, because it is a phenomenon which brings different meanings to the same person at different times, and certainly different meanings to different people. The main types of support are far from discrete entities; but they include, first, emotional support, which shows concern, along with some degree of intimacy. Second, and more practical, is instrumental support which essentially lightens the load of difficulty with which the woman must contend; this may include a wide range of interventions intended to provide greater comfort. Third is informational support, which allows the woman to work out where she is in relation to her own goals and aspirations. The final aspect of support, enhancing self-esteem, plainly links the other three (Mander 2001).

The undoubted benefits of providing support to the woman in labour have been clearly demonstrated by a series of 14 randomised controlled trials (RCTs) (Hodnett 2001). Although the RCT may be regarded as a rather 'hard-edged' research approach for a subject as human as support in labour, it carries certain advantages. For example, it may serve to persuade those who might otherwise be resistant to new ideas, such as budget-holders. In the RCTs, the support was provided by women who were either experienced mothers or had been trained for a support role; that training, however, was often minimal and tended not to include midwives, because they rarely practised in the research settings. The focus was on the benefits of continuous support, although the extent of that continuity was often left undefined, as was the precise nature of the support itself. The RCTs have quite consistently shown a range of benefits, such as a reduction in both the length of labour and the use of pharmacological methods of pain control. Other interventions, such as birth assisted with instruments and Caesarean, were also less likely.

The environments in which the RCTs were undertaken varied little in how conducive they were to a satisfying birth experience, being largely sited in developing countries or those with highly medicalised systems of care in labour. For example, generally the settings provided barely adequate staffing and the woman was rarely permitted to bring her own companion, so she invariably laboured alone. It may be argued that, under such dire regimes, *any* intervention could only improve matters. Hence the benefits in more congenial settings would be proportionately greater.

This argument has been used to advance the development of the doula industry (Stockton 2003). The doula is a person whose sole focus is the support of one woman in labour, a role which contrasts markedly with the multiplicity of obligations of the typical midwife employed in the UK National Health Service. Perhaps for this reason, the support provided by the midwife has attracted less interest than that provided by the doula. For similar reasons, support of the midwife is also being recognised as deserving attention (Kirkham 1999).

Despite the pressure on the male partner to attend the birth, relatively little is known about his experience (Dellmann 2004). It is widely recognised that the labouring woman appreciates his presence (Somers-Smith 1999), but whether he is an effective source of support is less certain. The reason for this uncertainty is due to his anxiety, first, about his partner's well-being, second, about his inability to provide the depth of emotional support expected of him and, third, about his own limitations becoming apparent (Vehvilainen-Julkunen & Liukkonen 1998; Hallgren *et al.* 1999). It may be argued that as long as the father is able to conceal his profound anxiety from his partner, the fact that the anxieties exist is irrelevant. However, this argument clearly helps no one.

An alternative solution which is more realistic has been suggested by Anderson (1996). She proposes that the woman should be encouraged to select an appropriately experienced birth companion whose anxiety levels would be lower and unlikely to affect the childbearing woman. Experienced sisters and perhaps mothers would possibly make suitable companions, as shown by Madi and her colleagues (1999) working in Botswana.

Skills and other aspects of working with pain in labour

Learning any form of midwifery skill is far from straightforward. Because women and their experiences of childbearing are unique, a form of care which is effective for one woman may be little more than irritating to another. Further, the intimate nature of midwifery care means that the presence of a learner or observer, who constitutes a third party, may alter the crucial interpersonal dynamics which facilitate effective midwifery care. The avoidance of such an unintended intervention may be another of the advantages of the woman choosing to give birth at home (Vague 2004, p. 26). The intimacy of care, additionally, usually means that there is not another person present to witness the high-quality care offered by a particular midwife. This unobserved and unrecorded aspect of the midwife's practice is eloquently summarised by Seibold *et al.* (1999) and her colleagues:

> the literature is relatively silent on how the majority of midwives actually practice.
>
> (1999, p. 22)

In order to overcome this challenge, Vague (2004) suggests that midwives should share the stories of their practice with their colleagues (2004).

Before considering in detail what assists working with the woman in pain, it is necessary to mention two closely linked phenomena which may or may not be helpful. The first is the management of time, the midwife's re-interpretation of which emerged as a major theme in the study by Vague (2004). In this research, the midwives used a range of strategies to make the duration of labour, and hence the pain, more manageable for the woman. These include the 'one-contraction-at-a-time' strategy, which involves the limitation of the horizon by breaking time into more manageable 'bite-sized' chunks (2004, p. 24).

This creative 'working with time' (Vague 2004, p. 24) contrasts markedly with one of the traditional complaints of the woman giving birth in hospital. This is that the environment, and hence her experience, is dominated by the clock. This tyrannical dominance is both exemplified and compounded by the current ubiquitous subservience to the partograph.

The people

The fundamentally important relationship between the midwife and the labouring woman is widely recognised. The development of this relationship over the weeks and months of pregnancy is much sought after. Yet all too often, the organisation of the maternity services means that this is an elusive ideal. The term 'partnership' has been used to emphasise the equality of the woman–midwife relationship (Pairman 2000). The benefits of the partnership manifest themselves very clearly when the woman is approaching the actual birth. Seibold *et al.* (1999) and her colleagues recount how the woman may panic, requiring the midwife to assume a 'head-coach' (1999, p. 25) role based on her established knowledge of the woman's aspirations. This dynamic role resonates with 'external control', by which the woman confidently relinquishes her own control to the trusted midwife (Green & Baston 2003). These authors have shown this role to be highly valued.

It may be that an even deeper level of sharing is required to achieve a truly satisfying birth experience. This depth takes the form of a shared understanding of the meaning of the woman's pain. Thus, a congruence of interpretation of that meaning facilitates appropriate care and the woman's long-term satisfaction (Vague 2004, p. 26).

The fundamentally deep relationship between the woman and the midwife may emerge in another, possibly more familiar, form. This is when the midwife uses her gut feeling to offer care which verges on the intuitive by behaving in a candidly motherly way. Anderson (2000) summarises this form of care as 'a firm-handed mother figure who has to be obeyed' (2000, p. 100).

Probably in the same way as the childbearing woman behaves differently in differing circumstances, Walsh (2006) recounts this motherly or 'matrescent' care in somewhat different terms (2006, p. 82). For Walsh (2006), this motherly role of the midwife is more 'protective, nurturing' (2006, p. 103), offering calm reassuring security, like a warm embrace.

Yet another view of the relationship between the woman and the midwife is to be found in the ideas of Cronk (2000, 2005). She argues that one effect of the advent of the UK National Health Service was to break the direct contractual relationship between the woman and her midwife. This, Cronk maintains, has severed the connection between the midwife and the one who was formerly her employer and has, effectively, demoted or disempowered the childbearing woman. Cronk suggests that if women are to assume the responsibility which becoming a mother inevitably brings with it, the midwife should regard herself as offering a service, that is, by taking on the role of a servant.

As mentioned above, although the presence of the woman's partner at the birth is widely regarded as relatively routine, his input has yet to be evaluated to demonstrate who benefits (Mander 2004b).

The place

The woman's relationships constitute one crucial aspect of her birthing environment. It is necessary to consider other aspects of that environment because the link between the experience of labour pain and place of birth is too strong to be ignored. On the one hand, there is the confidence-busting effect of the traditional labour ward, where the woman's choices are at best 'considerably limited' (Seibold *et al.* 1999). On the other hand, women planning to give birth at home have been found to use the least invasive approaches to cope with their pain and, of these women, a large proportion use no external intervention or agent (Jowitt 2000). This finding may be associated with the woman's reduced perception of pain if she gives birth at home (Morse & Park 1988). While these Canadian authors' authoritative study found that women giving birth at home anticipated less pain, Kitzinger (1989a) concludes that the woman's control is the key. This link between place of birth and pain medication is further endorsed by a more recent quantitative study involving 10 695 women of whom 5971 planned a home birth (Chamberlain *et al.* 1997). According to the authors, the women who gave birth at home were more likely not to use any method of pain control (18.8%), compared with those who planned to give birth in hospital (8.6%).

The practices

The repertoire of interventions on which the midwife is able to draw to help the woman in pain is probably infinite. Banks (2000) summarises the possibilities as ranging from 'Do Nothing' to the extremely interventive 'Break and Enter' (2000, p. 136). The midwifery practices are more usually divided into the non-pharmacological and the pharmacological. Because of their interest to medical practitioners, the pharmacological methods are well known in terms of both their benefits and their potential for harm (Mander 1998b).

Of the non-pharmacological approaches to labour pain, many require the input of a specialist practitioner at some stage, if only to teach the woman how to apply the technique for herself. Such methods include hypnotherapy, guided imagery, biofeedback, acupressure and acupuncture. Of course, this specialist practitioner and teacher may also be the woman's midwife. The research into the effectiveness of the non-pharmacological approaches has tended to focus on those methods which require specialist techniques or equipment, such as transcutaneous electrical nerve stimulation (TENS), acupuncture and intradermal injections of sterile water. The evidence base for the non-pharmacological approaches, though, still remains relatively weak (Smith *et al.* 2006).

In spite of this generally scant research evidence base, the midwife would be justified in discussing with the woman the least invasive and lowest-tech approach to helping her cope with labour pain. In their book on facilitating progress in labour, Simkin and Ancheta (2000) discuss and illustrate a wealth of minimally invasive interventions. The woman's relaxation, posture, position and ambulation may be adjusted in order to facilitate progress in labour and also to assist her in coping with pain. 'Slow dancing' (2000, p. 157) is an example of a technique which provides the woman with both emotional and physical support, while providing an element of relaxation and distraction through the music. Simkin and O'Hara (2002) suggest that such relatively simple interventions are effective in increasing comfort while enhancing progress.

Marginally more complex approaches to assisting the woman to cope with her pain include heating or cooling agents and water (in a birthing pool or shower), which may be combined. Hydrotherapy in the form of baths rather than showers has been shown to be effective later in labour and safe if the water is not hotter than body temperature (Simkin & O'Hara 2002).

The problem of back pain brings its own unique challenges and may be remedied by some of the techniques mentioned already. Of particular value, though, is the use of massage or counter-pressure, more often known as *back-rubbing* (Simkin & Ancheta 2000).

The essential role of support as a midwifery skill which has been shown to be an effective approach to pain has been discussed already (please see 'Support at the birth', above).

Being with

The midwife's fundamental and unique role of being 'with woman' may have been publicised to the point of becoming a cliché. In the context of the woman's pain, though, this crucial aspect of midwifery practice is being recognised as increasingly significant. In nursing, the synonym 'presence' has attracted more attention, and over a longer period. It has been described in terms of mutuality, reciprocity, availability and spontaneity (Paterson & Zderad 1976). This midwifery concept verges on the *Gestalt*, that is, the whole being greater than the sum of the parts, in the form of:

> The less we do, the more we give.
>
> (Leap 2000b, p. 1)

Thus, the emphasis on 'being' emerges loud and clear, contradicting any 'doing' through interventive, task-oriented or meddlesome practices. On the contrary, links have been shown between presence and stillness and the need to be able to judge if and when activity is permissible (Lundgren 2004). This research indicated that in midwifery, 'being with' requires not only physical, but also emotional, physiological, spiritual and psychological presence (2004, p. 371).

Although such practice is widely endorsed, Haraldsdottir's (2007) research indicates that matters are less straightforward (2007). In a nursing setting, she found that the reality of 'being with' is far more difficult to achieve than is generally recognised. This difficulty deserves more attention. It does, however, indicate that 'doing' is often far more comfortable for the practitioner than 'simply' being present. It may be that the midwife's comfort or otherwise with such 'masterly inactivity' may be perceived by the woman. In such a situation the potential for the midwife's presence to become an intervention turns into a reality. Thus, 'being with' may assume the possibility of influencing the course of labour, either positively or negatively.

Conclusion

This chapter is an attempt to show the relevance of working with the woman in pain to maintaining labour as a healthy, physiological experience. This principle has been shown to operate at theoretical, clinical and interpersonal levels. Of fundamental importance to working with the woman in pain is the maintenance, establishment or re-establishment of confidence. The confidence which is needed applies to the woman's and the midwife's confidence in themselves, as well as in each other. It has been suggested that the experience of working with pain may be transformatory for the woman. I venture to suggest that this transformation may also apply to the midwife. Such a transformation would increase the midwife's confidence in both her own clinical skills and the woman's ability to give birth healthily and spontaneously.

References

Anderson T (1996) Support in labour. *Modern Midwife* 6(1): 7–11.

Anderson T (2000) Feeling safe enough to let go: the relationship between the woman and her midwife during the second stage of labour. In Kirkham M (ed) *The Midwife–Mother Relationship* Chapter 5 London, Macmillan, 92.

Banks M (2000) *Home Birth Bound Mending the Broken Weave*. Hamilton, Birthspirit.

Chamberlain G, Wraight A, Crowley P (1997) *Home Births: The Report of the 1994 Confidential Enquiry by the National Birthday Trust Fund*. Carnforth, Parthenon.

Cronk M (2000) The midwife: a professional servant? In Kirkham M (ed) *The Midwife–Mother Relationship*. London, Macmillan.

Cronk M (2005) Guest editorial. Midwives: professional servants? *RCM Midwives* 8(6): 240.

Dellmann T (2004) "The best moment of my life": a literature review of fathers' experience of childbirth. *Australian Midwifery* 17(3): 20–6.

Dick-Read G (1933) *Natural Childbirth*. London, W Heinemann.

Downe S (2008) *Normal Childbirth: Evidence and Debate*. Edinburgh, Churchill Livingstone.

Evans M (2006) The 'pain relief talk': is it informing, frightening or empowering – time to re-evaluate the focus. *MIDIRS Midwifery Digest* 16(2): 265–8.

Fairley P (1978) *The Conquest of Pain*. London, Joseph.

van Gennep A (1960) In Vizedom MB, Caffee GL (eds) *The Rites of Passage Trans.* London, Routledge & Kegan Paul.

Green JM, Baston HA (2003) Feeling in control during labor: concepts, correlates, and consequences. *Birth* 30(4): 235–47.

Hallgren A, Kihlgren M, Forslin L, Norberg A (1999) Swedish fathers' involvement in and experiences of childbirth preparation and childbirth. *Midwifery* 15(1): 6–15.

Haraldsdottir E (2007) *The constraints of the ordinary: 'Being with' patients in a hospice in Scotland*. Unpublished PhD Thesis, University of Edinburgh.

Helman C (2007) *Culture, Health and Illness*, 5th edition. London, Hodder-Arnold.

Hodnett E (2001) Caregiver support for women during childbirth. *The Cochrane Library*, Issue 1. Oxford, Update Software.

IASP (1979) Pain terms: a list with definitions and notes on usage. *Pain* 6: 249–52.

Jowitt M (2000) Association of radical midwives pain in labour – is it insufferable? *Midwifery Matters* Summer (85): 10–11.

Kirkham M (1999) The culture of midwifery in the National Health Service in England. *Journal of Advanced Nursing* 30(3): 732–9.

Kitzinger S (1989a) *Giving Birth*. London, Farrar, Straus & Giroux.

Kitzinger S (1989b) Perceptions of pain in home and hospital births. In Van Hall EV, Everaerd W (eds) *The Free Woman: Women's Health in the 1990s*. Carnforth, Parthenon, 90–100.

Lamaze F (1956) *Painless Childbirth: Psychoprophylactic Method*. Chicago, Regnery.

Leap N (1996) *A midwifery perspective on pain in labour*. Unpublished MSc Dissertation, South Bank University, London.

Leap N (1997) Birthwrite. Being with women in pain – do midwives need to rethink their role? *British Journal of Midwifery* 5(5): 263.

Leap N (1998) A fresh approach to pain in labour. *New Zealand College of Midwives Journal* 19: 17–8.

Leap N (2000a) Pain in labour: towards a midwifery perspective. *MIDIRS Midwifery Digest* 10(1): 49–53.

Leap N (2000b) The less we do, the more we give. In Kirkham M (ed) *The Midwife–Mother Relationship*, Chapter 1. London, Macmillan, 1.

Leap N, Anderson T (2004) The role of pain in normal birth and the empowerment of women. In Downe S (ed) *Normal Childbirth: Evidence and Debate*, Chapter 2. Edinburgh, Churchill Livingstone, 25.

Leap N, Anderson P (2008) The role of pain in normal birth and the empowerment of women. In Downe S (ed) *Normal Childbirth: Evidence and Debate*. London, Churchill Livingstone.

Lundgren I (2004) Releasing and relieving encounters: experiences of pregnancy and childbirth. *Scandinavian Journal of Caring Sciences* 18(4): 368–75.

Madi BC, Sandall J, Bennett R, Macleod C (1999) Effects of female relative support in labor: a randomized controlled trial. *Birth* 26(1): 4–10.

Main CJ, Spanswick CC (2001) Models of pain. In Strong J, Unruh A, Wright A, Baxter GD (eds) *Pain: A Textbook for Therapists*, Chapter 1. Edinburgh, Churchill Livingstone.

Mander R (1998a) A reappraisal of Simpson's introduction of chloroform. *Midwifery* 14(3): 181–90.

Mander R (1998b) *Pain in Childbearing and its Control*. Oxford, Blackwell Scientific.

Mander R (2000) The meanings of labour pain or the layers of an onion? A woman oriented view. *Journal of Reproductive and Infant Psychology* 18(2): 133–42.

Mander R (2001) *Supportive Care and Midwifery*. Oxford, Blackwell Science.

Mander R (2004a) Failure to deliver – ethical issues relating to epidural analgesia in uncomplicated labour. In Frith L, Draper H (eds) *Ethics and Midwifery: Issues in Contemporary Practice*, 2nd edition. Edinburgh, Books for Midwives.

Mander R (2004b) *Men and Maternity*. London, Routledge.

Melzack R (1996) *The Challenge of Pain*, 2nd edition. London, Penguin.

Melzack R, Wall PD (1965) Pain mechanisms: a new theory. *Science* 150: 971–9.

Morse JM, Park C (1988) Home birth and hospital deliveries: a comparison of the perceived painfulness of parturition. *Research in Nursing Health* 11(3): 175–81.

Pairman S (2000) Woman-centred midwifery: partnerships or professional friendships?. In Kirkham M (ed) *The Midwife–Mother Relationship*, Chapter 10. London, Macmillan, 207–26.

Paterson JG, Zderad LT (1976) *Humanistic Nursing*. New York, John Wiley.

Robertson A (1994) *Empowering Women: Teaching Active Birth in the '90s Camperdown*. Australia, ACE Graphics.

Robinson V (1946) *Victory Over Pain: A History of Anesthesia*. New York, Schuman.

Seibold C, Miller M, Hall J (1999) Midwives and women in partnership: the ideal and the real. *Australian Journal of Advanced Nursing* 17(2): 21–7.

Simkin P, Ancheta R (2000) *The Labor Progress Handbook*. Oxford, Blackwell Science.

Simkin P, O'Hara M (2002) Nonpharmacologic relief of pain during labor: systematic reviews of five methods. *American Journal of Obstetrics and Gynecology* 186(5): S131–59.

Smith CA, Collins CT, Cyna AM, Crowther CA (2006) Complementary and alternative therapies for pain management in labour. *Cochrane Database of Systematic Reviews* (4), Art. No: CD003521. DOI: 10.1002/14651858. CD003521.pub2.

Somers-Smith MJ (1999) A place for the partner? Expectations and experiences of support during childbirth. *Midwifery* 15(2): 101–8.

Stockton A (2003) Doulas – the future guardians of normal birth? *MIDIRS Midwifery Digest* 13(3): 347–50.

Vague S (2004) Midwives' experiences of working with women in labour: interpreting the meaning of pain. *New Zealand College of Midwives Journal* 31: 22–6.

Vehvilainen-Julkunen K, Liukkonen A (1998) Fathers' experiences of childbirth. *Midwifery* 14(1): 10–7.

Wall PD, Jones M (1991) *Defeating Pain: The War Against a Silent Epidemic.* New York, Plenum.

Walsh D (2006) 'Nesting' and 'Matrescence': distinctive features of a free-standing birth centre. *Midwifery* 22(3): 228–39.

Woollett A, Lyon L, White D (1983) The reactions of East London women to medical interventions in childbirth. *Journal of Reproductive and Infant Psychology* 1: 37–46.

Yildirim G, Sahin NH (2004) The effect of breathing and skin stimulation techniques on labour pain perception of Turkish women. *Pain Research and Management* 9(4): 181–2.

Chapter 9
Complementary Therapies in Labour: A Woman-Centred Approach

Denise Tiran

Introduction

Women increasingly use complementary therapies as a means of retaining control over their childbearing experiences and as additional choices for managing antenatal symptoms and intrapartum comfort and progress. This has led many midwives to incorporate different strategies from various therapies into their practice. However, 'complementary medicine' is not *a single* entity; there are over 300 different therapies or aspects of therapies, with at least 20 commonly used in the United Kingdom. Many are nationally regulated with an ever-growing body of research evidence whilst many more remain unregulated, with superficially trained practitioners. Generally, it appears that midwives choose to use one or two related therapies, most commonly massage–aromatherapy–reflexology or, less frequently, acupuncture–acupressure–shiatsu as an overall adjunct to conventional maternity care, whilst a few use hypnotherapy or herbal, homeopathic or Bach flower remedies.

However, a *woman-centred* perspective on intrapartum care may require a 'fusion' approach, in which several therapies are used either in isolation or in combination, ensuring that the mother's needs are met to ease pain, anxiety and fear, to facilitate progress, to prevent or manage complications, or for any other indications. Midwives can learn to apply a selected range of complementary strategies and to advise on natural remedies to aid the mother's well-being and progress in labour, in accordance with professional regulations and responsibilities. Alternatively, a woman may have been receiving antenatal therapy from an independent practitioner whom she wishes to accompany her in labour. Additionally, the increase in the number of doulas supporting women may mean that mothers receive non-conventional care whilst in labour, with or without the knowledge of the midwife who, of course, retains legal responsibility for her care.

Key evidence

Although the evidence base of complementary medicine is still emerging, it is easy for sceptics to dismiss it as poorly researched. There is a growing body of research on many commonly used therapies, but maternity professionals need to know where to find it, since the conventional medical, midwifery and nursing research databases do not include many complementary medicine studies. The majority of these have been conducted only in the last decade and are not always published in mainstream journals. Unfortunately, the National Institute for Health and Clinical Excellence (NICE) in its guideline on routine care of the healthy pregnant woman (National Collaborating Centre for Women's and Children's Health 2003) suggested that there is 'insufficient evidence of either safety or efficacy' of complementary therapies during pregnancy and advocated actively discouraging women from using them. The more recent guideline on care of women in normal labour similarly fails to acknowledge complementary medicine as sufficiently well researched to merit its use in intrapartum care (NICE 2006, 2007), simply because most studies fail to meet the methodological 'gold standard' of being randomised controlled trials (RCTs). However, this is unhelpful and potentially liable to drive women to use natural remedies clandestinely, a fact which may endanger the health of both mother and fetus (Tiran 2005).

Although there are some RCTs in complementary medicine research, it may be necessary for midwives to relate generic findings to labour physiology. An example of this would be applying the results of studies on healthy volunteers in which massage is found to reduce blood pressure (Olney 2005; Cambron *et al.* 2006) to the physio-pathological factors, which affect intrapartum blood pressure, such as epidural anaesthesia. Where RCTs have not been undertaken, there may be other types of large-scale empirical studies, which contribute to a deeper understanding of the mechanisms of action, efficacy and safety of different complementary therapies. However, it is vital to balance the studies, which appear to offer positive results with those in which a positive clinical hypothesis is not proven. Furthermore, midwives should not take at face value those studies demonstrating efficacy without considering safety. An example of this in pregnancy is the common practice of midwives to advise women with nausea and vomiting to take ginger, without appreciating the potential dangers of inappropriate administration (Tiran & Budd 2005). Ginger can exacerbate symptoms and trigger new problems such as heartburn in some women. More significantly, ginger has anticoagulant effects if taken in doses of more than 1 g per day, or for longer than 3 weeks continuously. Women with clotting disorders, or on medication with similar effects, including warfarin, aspirin and non-steroidal anti-inflammatories should not take ginger at all (Shalansky *et al.* 2007).

Helping mothers to cope with contractions

Midwives have traditionally used touch to ease pain in labour. In recent years, some have formally incorporated *massage* and *aromatherapy* into antenatal and intrapartum care (Tiran 2003a; Mousley 2005). Several investigations into touch therapies have demonstrated positive effects on pain, anxiety and reducing stress hormones, all of which rebalance homeostasis sufficiently to facilitate adequate oxytocin release. A pilot study by McNabb *et al.* (2006) explored the impact of late pregnancy massage, breathing and relaxation techniques, on pain perception in labour. This study found that, although cortisol levels were similar to those recorded in other studies in which no massage was used, Visual Analogue Scale (VAS) pain scores at 90 minutes post-delivery were significantly lower than scores recorded in other studies at 2 days post-partum; a larger scale trial is planned to attempt to confirm these findings (Kimber 2007, Personal communication). Similarly, numerous studies at the Miami Touch Research Institute suggest that antenatal massage decreases intrapartum cortisol and norepinephrine levels and increases serotonin and dopamine, resulting in fewer intrapartum and neonatal complications (Field *et al.* 1999, 2004, 2005). In another UK study, (McNeill *et al.* 2006), reflexology was offered to women from 36 weeks' gestation and demonstrated a reduced use of Entonox™ in labour, although there was no significant difference in duration of pregnancy or labour between groups, and there were more forceps deliveries in the reflexology group than in the control group. Unfortunately, this study lacked rigour, as some assumptions were made regarding the effects of antenatal reflexology on labour. In particular, there was no real consistency in the number of treatments, some women having as few as a single reflexology session prior to labour onset. Other studies have demonstrated reduced pain-relief requirements and increased normal delivery outcomes following intrapartum reflexology (Feder *et al.* 1993; Motha & McGrath 1993). Anecdotal experience and communication with many midwives, suggests that touch – massage, aromatherapy and reflexology – is increasingly being used to good effect, improving maternal satisfaction and progress and reducing the need for pharmacological or surgical intervention (see Case Study 9.1).

Case Study 9.1

Student midwives from a UK university were fortunate enough to participate in an exchange programme, in which they went to work in a hospital in Lille, France, whilst some of the French students came to Britain. Two of the UK students were working with a French midwife caring for a mother in established labour. Over the next few hours she became increasingly distressed, to the point where contractions were slowing; intramuscular analgesia had been administered but appeared ineffective. Vaginal examination showed that cervical dilatation was 8 cm and the fetal head was 1 cm below the ischial spines. The mother was thrashing around and was unable to listen to advice about positioning, nor was she able to make any objective decisions about pain relief. The French midwife seemed unsure of how to manage the situation and was considering requesting medical intervention to expedite delivery. The students had attended some workshops on complementary therapies (with this author) and asked the midwife and the mother if they could try a simple technique, using a reflexology relaxation point on the hands. They each took hold of one of the mother's hands and gently massaged the relevant point on her palms, for about 5 minutes. Gradually the mother calmed down. Following this, contractions accelerated again and the mother reached the second stage unaided by medical intervention, proceeding to a normal delivery of a beautiful baby boy.

One of the largest clinical aromatherapy studies was conducted in the delivery suite of the John Radcliffe Hospital in Oxford, UK (Burns *et al.* 2000) although it was not an RCT and was therefore omitted from the NICE guidelines on intrapartum care (NICE 2006, 2007). In this 9-year study, a self-selected group of over 8000 women received aromatherapy in first-stage labour, for relief of pain and discomfort, anxiety, nausea and for general relaxation. A statistically significant reduction in the use of opioid analgesics and oxytocic augmentation was demonstrated with less than 1% of maternal side effects and no adverse fetal–neonatal reactions. Maternal satisfaction scores were high and, interestingly, midwifery recruitment and retention were later found, incidentally, to be better than before the trial started. Although the authors admit to some methodological inadequacies, a more recent Italian RCT compared 251 labouring women who received midwife-administered aromatherapy with 262 women who received standard midwifery care (Burns *et al.* 2007). There was no significant difference between the two groups in terms of duration of labour, requirements for augmentation or the incidence of spontaneous or operative delivery, but there were more neonatal intensive-care admissions in the control group. It was postulated by the study team that this may have been due to perceived maternal pain levels remaining higher than in the trial group, despite the use of opiate analgesia and epidural anaesthesia. This study was, however, valuable in that it demonstrated that RCTs can be used to investigate the use of intrapartum aromatherapy, and provided useful guidance for future studies.

In an attempt to determine the physiological reasons behind the apparent success of aromatherapy in labour, Hur *et al.*'s (2005) Taiwanese RCT investigated the use of essential oils on responses to labour stress and anxiety, and to stress in the early post-partum period in 24 primiparae at term who were compared to 24 control subjects. Stress hormone levels were found to be significantly lower in the trial group, although there was no reported difference in the women's own perceptions of their stress status. Other studies have also demonstrated significant pain relief and reduction in stress hormone levels in labouring mothers receiving massage, with or without essential oils (Chang *et al.* 2002, 2006; Yildirim & Sahin 2004). Lis-Balchin's (1999) research on rats investigated the possible dangers of essential oils and postulated that, as tea tree oil may cause smooth muscle relaxation, it should be avoided in labour. Whilst it is not possible to apply the findings from animal studies directly to humans, these studies do provide the rudiments of a developing body of knowledge which should not be ignored. Similarly, although there has been one small study undertaken on the potential use of ginger essential oil to accelerate labour (Calvert 2005) it must be emphasised that this would not be a universally acceptable oil, since ginger, in Chinese medicine terms, is a 'hot' remedy and not therefore suited to women who are already too '*yang*' or 'hot' during labour; inappropriate use of this or other herbal remedies or essential oils could be both counterproductive to the progress of labour and potentially harmful to mother and fetus (Langmead & Rampton 2001; Kuczkowski 2006). This latter study highlights the problems of combining therapies which work on different philosophies, without comprehensive understanding of the possible interactions between them.

Hypnotherapy is currently enjoying a contemporary popularity as a means of coping with labour pain, partly due to the active marketing by some commercial organisations, which have designed specific programmes for pregnancy preparation and intrapartum use. Hypnotherapy has been used to beneficial effects to reduce fear, anxiety and pain in women at term (Mehl-Madrona 2004; Cyna *et al.* 2006; VandeVusse *et al.* 2007) as well as in those undergoing first trimester abortion for fetal abnormality (Marc *et al.* 2007). Hypnosis may also prevent the onset of cervical dilatation in women threatening preterm labour (Brown & Hammond 2007).

Many RCTs have investigated the value of acupuncture–acupressure on pain relief in labour, with the secondary outcome measures being onset and duration of the first stage. Hantoushzadeh *et al.* (2007) found a positive correlation between acupoint stimulation and all three outcome measures, whereas, although Chung *et al.* (2003) demonstrated positive effects of acupuncture on pain perception, no significant effects on the onset or duration of labour were observed. It is interesting to note that Hantoushzadeh's team compared true acupuncture with minimal (sham or false) acupuncture, whilst other studies compared acupuncture with no treatment. The practice of using sham acupuncture points is thought to reduce the placebo effect, for which complementary therapy studies are so often dismissed. Ramnerö *et al.*'s (2002) Swedish study showed a generalised reduction in opioid use, while Nesheim *et al.*'s (2003) randomised, controlled, non-blinded study specifically demonstrated a decreased use of meperidine. Intrapartum electro-acupuncture has also been found to have an analgesic and relaxation effect (Qu & Zhou 2007). It may also be possible to use transcutaneous electrical nerve stimulation (TENS) for analgesia on specific acupuncture points more commonly used to facilitate uterine action (Chao *et al.* 2007).

Facilitating uterine action

Several studies have shown promising results for using acupuncture and/or acupressure for induction and acceleration of contractions, which may offer alternative options for women requiring medical or surgical augmentation of labour. Commonly, the acupoints used to stimulate myometrial action include Spleen 6 (Sp6), a point on the inner aspect of the leg, just above the ankle bone, Large Intestine 4 (LI4) in the webbing between thumb and forefinger, and Gall Bladder 21 (GB21) on the dorsal aspect of the shoulders, immediately below the trapezius muscle. Stimulation is usually by needling (acupuncture) or thumb pressure (acupressure–shiatsu); occasionally, electro-acupuncture (TENS) is applied at the relevant points. Ingram *et al.* (2005) designed a collaborative pilot audit in which 66 women at 40-weeks' gestation who received shiatsu stimulation to the Sp6, LI4 and GB21 acupoints were found to be more likely to commence labour spontaneously and to achieve a normal birth than those in a control group who did not. This is an interesting study in that it was undertaken with UK midwives trained in shiatsu, and highlights the ease with which this treatment could be incorporated into midwifery practice, thus possibly reducing the need for, and clinical and psychosocial problems associated with, medical induction for post-dates pregnancies.

Gaudernack *et al.*'s (2006) acupuncture study allocated 100 women with spontaneous membrane rupture at term to receive Sp6 stimulation or to act as a control. In the study group, there was a significantly shorter duration of labour than in control subjects and less need for oxytocic acceleration; in those who did require pharmacological augmentation, the duration of the latent phase was significantly shorter than in similar women in the control group. Acupuncture stimulation applied to the Sp6 and LI4 points on alternate days commencing from the due date also appears to facilitate cervical ripening and reduce the interval between the expected date of delivery and the onset of spontaneous labour (Rabl *et al.* 2001). Similarly, Harper *et al.*'s (2006) RCT using LI4, Sp6 and other acupoints in 56 primigravidae at term showed shorter first-stage labours and less incidence of Caesarean section in the acupuncture group than the control, although the findings did not reach statistical significance. Replicated studies by Lee *et al.* (2004) and Chang *et al.* (2004) reached similar conclusions, with shorter first stages, fewer Caesareans and greater pain relief following Sp6 acupressure than in controls.

Several herbal remedies are traditionally thought to aid progress in labour, but these are not without considerable risk in untrained hands. Midwives should be extremely cautious about advising women on herbal remedies unless their information is reliable, accurate, comprehensive and evidence-based (Tiran 2003b; Marcus & Snodgrass 2005). Many herbal medicines are contraindicated during pregnancy as they may potentially cause fetal malformations, whilst both ante- and intrapartum use may interfere with normal physiology or cause interactions with prescribed drugs (Vaes & Chyka 2000; Ang-Lee *et al.* 2001; Scott & Elmer 2002). Raspberry leaf tea is perhaps the most well-known pregnancy remedy, thought to tone the myometrium, facilitate cervical ripening and uterine contractions and, indirectly, to reduce pain. However, evidence from RCTs in Australia is rather inconclusive (Parsons *et al.* 1999; Simpson *et al.* 2001), whilst Rojas-Vera *et al.*'s (2002) study on guinea pigs suggests the effects are dose-related; researchers generally agree that further studies are needed. It is of increasing concern that midwives frequently support women's *routine* use of raspberry leaf without checking first whether they have any contraindications, such as a previous Caesarean section, precipitate or preterm labour, or medical or obstetric complications or advising women to reduce the dose in the event of excessive Braxton Hicks contractions.

Another herbal remedy of dubious safety is *Blue cohosh* (*Caulophyllum thalictroides*), which is thought to increase uterine efficiency in labour. However, certain constituents appear to be vasoconstrictive and cardiotoxic (Irikura & Kennelly 1999), and fetal hypoxia, neonatal myocardial infarction and congestive cardiac failure have been reported (Jones & Lawson 1998; Gunn & Wright 1996). The use of blue cohosh by UK medical herbalists has now been discontinued (McIntyre 2001), yet it continues to be used by American nurse-midwives (McFarlin *et al.* 1999; Refuerzo *et al.* 2005) and remains accessible to UK women via the Internet. Even black cohosh (*Cimicifuga racemosa*) should be used with caution in pregnant and childbearing women, since it has known uterine-stimulating and labour-inducing properties (Dugoua *et al.* 2006).

These issues do not generally apply to homeopathic remedies, which bear the same Latin name as the herbal remedies (i.e. *caulophyllum* or *cimicifuga*). Whilst herbal medicine acts pharmacologically, homeopathy is thought to be a form of energy medicine and the remedies do not act chemically. Homeopathic remedies are prepared by diluting the relevant substance in water and vigorously shaking it (called *succussing*); it is believed that the shaking releases the active ingredient into the water, which is then further diluted and succussed many times. The more dilute a remedy, the further from the original substance it becomes chemically, which is important given that some substances are potentially toxic in their original format, e.g. arsenic.

However, correct prescription of homeopathic remedies is essential to avoid a *reverse proving* in which prolonged incorrect use can begin to trigger the symptoms which the wrongly used remedy is designed to treat, without resolving the presenting symptoms. It is inappropriate for midwives to advocate remedies such as caulophyllum for women who are post-dates, unless they have a comprehensive understanding of homeopathic theory. Furthermore, Cuesta Laso and Alfonso Galán's (2007) review questioned the ethics of remedies labelled as 'homeopathic' which are not sufficiently highly diluted nor vigorously *succussed*, increasing the risk of pharmacological interaction with prescribed medications. Ernst (2005) agrees that this modality is not without risk and suggests that, with the paucity of research, the hazards outweigh the benefits of homeopathic remedies. Even trials of the ubiquitous arnica, a homeopathic remedy often used to combat bruising, trauma and stress following delivery, have produced inconclusive results (Vickers *et al.* 1998; Stevinson *et al.* 2003; Brinkhaus *et al.* 2006). Conversely, homeopathy is a gentle form of medicine, which appears to have positive benefits for some women, although whether this is a placebo effect has not yet been clarified.

Implications for midwifery practice

Women frequently use complementary therapies prior to and during pregnancy, although many refrain from informing their midwives, which may increase the risks of interactions with drugs or exacerbation of complications, particularly during labour. Midwives should ask all women at booking and again, towards term, about their actual or intended use of complementary therapies, since inappropriate use may be detrimental to mother and/or baby. Whilst complementary therapies can be extremely beneficial in labour, helping the mother to cope with contractions and offering alternatives for acceleration of labour, natural remedies and complementary techniques may constitute as much of an intervention as pharmacological substances and surgical procedures, with similar risks and dangers. For example, the concomitant use of hypotensive aromatherapy oils such as lavender with epidural anaesthesia would be inappropriate unless the midwife was aware of the possible effect on the blood pressure. Similarly, the anti-coagulant risks of many herbal medicines preclude their use prior to or during surgery; any mother due to have an elective Caesarean section should discontinue all herbal remedies for at least 2 weeks prior to the date of surgery (Vaes & Chyka 2000). It is also unacceptable for midwives to condone the contemporary trend for mothers to ask their independent practitioner (most commonly, reflexologists or acupuncturists), to 'start labour off' *before* term, in the mistaken belief that this is preferable to medical induction for post-dates pregnancies. Inadvertent overstimulation of the uterus can occur when enthusiastic therapists attempt to induce labour, without a full understanding of pregnancy and labour physiology, in general, and of the individual mother's circumstances, in particular.

Mothers who choose to self-administer natural remedies in labour are at liberty to do so, but the midwife should document this and if in doubt about the safety of a particular substance, should counsel the mother accordingly and seek advice from a suitably qualified therapist (NMC 2004), preferably one who is experienced in caring for pregnant and labouring mothers. Women may have consulted an independent therapist antenatally about remedies such as aromatherapy essential oils, herbal, homeopathic or Bach flower remedies, but may need help to select appropriate remedies during the dynamic events of labour. The midwife remains accountable for the mother's care and should document any discussions she or he may have about these remedies, stressing to the parents that they are not without risks if used inappropriately.

Some mothers wish to be accompanied in labour by a complementary therapist, doula or other birth supporter who uses natural remedies or complementary techniques. The independent practitioner should acknowledge the midwife's legal responsibility for the mother's care, preferably in writing. In some trusts, the therapist may be asked to produce documentary evidence of appropriate personal indemnity insurance cover. Whilst the midwife cannot be held responsible for the actions of another, she or he should, where possible, record in the mother's notes, and on the cardiotocograph printout, the timing of natural substances administered by the accompanying practitioner.

A unit policy, specifying the expected lines of communication between midwife, therapist and obstetrician, should be developed to outline midwifery responsibilities if women are accompanied in labour by an independent therapist.

Midwives may use complementary therapies in their own practice and are permitted to do so if it is in the best interests of the woman and with her fully informed consent (NMC 2004). The midwife must be trained to use complementary therapies, although it is not essential to be a formally qualified practitioner – elements of therapies, for example specific techniques to accelerate labour, can be learned and applied to midwifery practice. Conversely, midwives who are qualified in a particular therapy should not assume that they are appropriately prepared to use it within midwifery practice without further education to enable them to apply principles to practice, and must have the permission of their employing authority to use complementary therapies within their midwifery practice. They must be able to justify their actions in the same way as any other element of midwifery care, and should not continue to use a therapy when medical management is more appropriate.

Case Study 9.2

A multiparous mother at 41 + 5 gestation had brought with her into the delivery suite a selection of homeopathic remedies, with written instructions, from a homeopath, for use in labour. She was using caulophyllum, a remedy often used to accelerate labour, especially after the estimated date of delivery (Tiran 2008). She was being cared for by a midwife with no complementary therapy training, but who assumed that the instructions given to the mother were accurate. The midwife documented the mother's self-administration of tablets, in the notes. After 2 hours, labour was established and the mother was progressing well and coping with the contractions. She continued to self-administer the caulophyllum, but after another 3 hours had passed, the contractions began to slow down, although there was no apparent physiological reason. The midwife asked the mother about her continued use of the caulophyllum and read the instructions that caulophyllum may not be appropriate once labour was established. The midwife therefore decided to consult a colleague who was experienced in complementary therapies, who suggested that the mother should now discontinue the homeopathic remedy to avoid a 'reverse proving'. The midwife documented this recommendation and her discussion with the mother, who agreed to stop taking the tablets. After this, contractions recovered and the mother progressed to full cervical dilatation about 3 hours later.

Case Study 9.3

A mother had a prolonged third stage of labour but, despite administration of oxytocic drugs, the uterus remained poorly contracted. The midwife, a qualified therapist, decided to try reflexology although she did not have permission to use reflexology in her midwifery practice. She stimulated the foot zone corresponding to the pituitary gland, in an attempt to stimulate oxytocin production to facilitate placental separation and the third stage was completed spontaneously. When another mother had a prolonged third stage the midwife used the same reflexology technique but there was no progress. She had failed to realise that, in this case, as placental separation had already occurred and the uterus was well contracted, reflexology to the zone for the pituitary gland (to trigger oxytocin release) was not required and had, in fact, compounded the problem, causing the cervix to constrict around the placenta. (This situation actually required her to use a technique to sedate the foot zone for the cervix to relax and dilate it so that the placenta could be expelled).

Implications for midwifery education

All midwives should have a basic appreciation of complementary therapies for use in labour, particularly as this is a time when the mother may wish to use her own remedies for pain relief. Student midwives should receive an introduction to the subject, with further education available after qualifying, should they so desire. Where possible, this subject matter should be cross-related to standard subjects within the curriculum. For example, whilst a session on 'complementary therapies in midwifery' is useful, some examples should be incorporated into each of the sessions on subjects like 'helping the mother to cope with contractions in labour' or 'management of retained placenta'. Practising midwives who wish to incorporate complementary therapies into their practice and who may choose to qualify in a particular therapy must be able to apply generic principles to midwifery but may need help to do this. Post-qualifying courses should be available specifically for midwives, perhaps as modules within further education programmes.

Additionally, at least one midwifery lecturer in each educational establishment should possess a rudimentary knowledge of a range of complementary strategies that may be useful – or indeed possibly harmful – in pregnancy and labour. The lecturer should be able to apply principles to practice, encompassing the risks and benefits of complementary therapies in childbirth and relating them to the professional accountability of midwives. It may be interesting to invite visiting lecturers who are qualified in one or more therapies to speak to students, followed by seminar work or guided discussion by midwives to facilitate students to appreciate the boundaries within which they are permitted to work.

Managers and supervisors should be aware of the actions of their midwifery staff–supervisees in relation to complementary therapies; indeed, it may be necessary for supervisors to have some knowledge of complementary therapies in order to supervise midwives appropriately.

Implications for strategic policy

Where maternity units are considering implementing complementary therapies, for example to normalise birth, reduce intervention rates and improve maternal and staff satisfaction, it is essential to investigate the calibre of courses offered to ensure that they are relevant to the practice of midwives within a National Health Service (NHS) trust. Whilst a degree of cascade training is acceptable, it must be acknowledged that this will, of necessity, dilute the content so that those to whom the information is being imparted may be less well prepared to use complementary therapies than those who have undertaken complete maternity-related therapy courses. Conversely, in order to focus on the woman-centred approach, it may be preferable to incorporate complementary techniques as additional options for dealing with situations faced by mothers and midwives, for instance including the use of moxibustion on a day devoted to breech presentation, or acupressure techniques when debating induction and acceleration.

The Nursing and Midwifery Council (NMC) supports the use of complementary therapies by midwives, subject to adherence to Council regulations on practice, as detailed above. The NMC can only regulate the practice of complementary therapies when they are used in conjunction with an individual's NMC registration, either in employment or independently, and midwives should make themselves aware of the relevant guidelines and directives, which inform practice. However, the increasing use of complementary therapies, both by consumers and NMC-registered practitioners, suggests that further monitoring and guidance by the NMC may be required to ensure fitness to practice (Tiran 2007).

Unfortunately, strategic organisations concerned with conventional health care, frequently include erroneous statements in their literature and on their websites, usually due to lack of understanding of this specialist field. The NMC's website, in its advice sheets for registrants, contains one on 'Complementary alternative therapies and homeopathy'. The content indicates that the author(s) have no understanding of the mechanism of action of homeopathy, nor any appreciation of the diverse nature of 'complementary medicine' in which individual therapies cannot easily be singled out within a general advice sheet (NMC 2008). Furthermore, the working parties, which devised the NICE guidelines on pregnancy and childbirth (National Collaborating Centre for Women's and Children's Health 2003), omitted many studies on pregnancy and labour complementary therapies, either because they were not RCTs, or because the working party had not searched the relevant complementary medicine databases.

Conclusion

The use of complementary therapies should be perceived as a specialist area of midwifery practice, in the same way as some midwives choose to specialise in care of women with high-risk pregnancies, or specific client groups such as those suffering domestic violence. Whilst all midwives should have a basic understanding of the possible uses of complementary therapies in pregnancy, it is not professionally acceptable for individuals to offer advice or provide treatment unless it is based on a comprehensive knowledge and understanding of the relevant complementary discipline.

Although the status of complementary medicine in general has improved, there is still a way to go before it is accepted by orthodox medicine as an equal component of health care. However, when major strategic organisations choose to discuss the use of complementary therapies in relation to specific client groups or clinical specialities, it is of concern that they should offer incomplete and erroneous information. Contemporary evidence-based medicine, which is largely based on risk management strategies, suggests that it is now timely to consider the appointment of specialist advisors in complementary medicine to ensure that regulatory, professional and health advisory organisations are able to comment authoritatively on an increasingly academic area of health care.

Complementary therapies offer an invaluable aid to returning to normal birth and being 'with woman' and can improve satisfaction for both mothers and midwives. They provide additional choices and tools for aiding relaxation, easing anxiety, reducing stress and pain and facilitating progress. Used correctly, they are usually at least as effective and often much safer than conventional medical interventions and deserve to be further incorporated into normal maternity care options. As a profession, midwives should embrace complementary therapies as a realistic and pleasant range of strategies for enhancing care in labour.

Glossary

Acupuncture/acupressure: An aspect of Chinese medicine based on energy lines (meridians) which link different parts of the body to each other. Ill health or physical, emotional or spiritual stress may cause blockages or excesses of energy at certain points – specific points along the meridians are either stimulated or sedated with needles (acupuncture) or thumb pressure (acupressure) to rebalance energy flow and assist in a return to full health.

Aromatherapy: Uses concentrated plant essential oils for their therapeutic properties, obtained from various chemical constituents, administered in massage, in the bath, by inhalation, in creams, compresses or occasionally heat on skin.

Hypnotherapy hypnosis: Induction of deep relaxation or trance-like state to cause changes in behaviour.

Massage: Systematic stroking or kneading of the body to aid relaxation, stimulate circulation and excretion and lower blood pressure.

Reflexology, reflex zone therapy: Manual therapy in which the feet (or hands) represent a map of the whole body so that conditions in areas distal to the feet can be treated.

Shiatsu: Modern-day Japanese manual therapy, similar to acupressure, involving thumb and finger pressure applied to specific points to re-balance the internal energies and aid return to optimum health.

References

Ang-Lee MK, Moss J, Yuan CS (2001) Herbal medicines and perioperative care. *Journal of the American Medical Association* 286(2): 208–16.

Brinkhaus B, Wilkens JM, Lüdtke R, Hunger J, Witt CM, Willich SN (2006) Homeopathic arnica therapy in patients receiving knee surgery: results of three randomised double-blind trials. *Complementary Therapies in Medicine* 14(4): 237–46.

Brown DC, Hammond DC (2007) Evidence-based clinical hypnosis for obstetrics, labor and delivery, and preterm labor. *The International Journal of Clinical and Experimental Hypnosis* 55(3): 355–71.

Burns EE, Blamey C, Ersser SJ, Barnetson L, Lloyd AJ (2000) An investigation into the use of aromatherapy in intrapartum midwifery practice. *The Journal of Alternative and Complementary Medicine* 6(2): 141–7.

Burns E, Zobbi V, Panzeri D, Oskrochi R, Regalia A (2007) Aromatherapy in childbirth: a pilot randomised controlled trial. *British International Journal of Obstetrics and Gynaecology* 114(7): 838–44.

Calvert I (2005) Ginger: an essential oil for shortening labour? *The Practising Midwife* 8(1): 30–4.

Cambron JA, Dexheimer J, Coe P (2006) Changes in blood pressure after various forms of therapeutic massage: a preliminary study. *The Journal of Alternative and Complementary Medicine* 12(1): 65–70.

Chang MY, Chen CH, Huang KF (2006) A comparison of massage effects on labor pain using the McGill Pain Questionnaire. *The Journal of Nursing Research* 14(3): 190–7.

Chang MY, Wang SY, Chen CH (2002) Effects of massage on pain and anxiety during labour: a randomized controlled trial in Taiwan. *Journal of Advanced Nursing* 38(1): 68–73.

Chang SB, Park YW, Cho JS, Lee MK, Lee BC, Lee SJ (2004) Differences of cesarean section rates according to San-Yin-Jiao(SP6) acupressure for women in labor. *Taehan Kanho Hakhoe Chi* 34(2): 324–32.

Chao AS, Chao A, Wang TH *et al.* (2007) Pain relief by applying transcutaneous electrical nerve stimulation (TENS) on acupuncture points during the first stage of labor: a randomized double-blind placebo-controlled trial. *Pain* 127(3): 214–20.

Chung UL, Hung LC, Kuo SC, Huang CL (2003) Effects of LI4 and BL 67 acupressure on labor pain and uterine contractions in the first stage of labor. *The Journal of Nursing Research* 11(4): 251–60.

Cyna AM, Andrew MI, McAuliffe GL (2006) Antenatal self-hypnosis for labour and childbirth: a pilot study. *Anaesthesia and Intensive Care* 34(4): 464–9.

Dugoua JJ, Seely D, Perri D, Koren G, Mills E (2006) Safety and efficacy of black cohosh (Cimicifuga racemosa) during pregnancy and lactation. *The Canadian Journal of Clinical Pharmacology* 13(3): e257–61.

Ernst E (2005) Is homeopathy a clinically valuable approach? *Trends in Pharmacological Science* 26(11): 547–8.

Feder E, Liisberg GB, Lenstrup C *et al.* (1993) Zone therapy in relation to birth. *Proceedings of the International Confederation of Midwives 23rd International Congress* 2: 651–6.

Field T, Diego MA, Hernandez-Reif M, Schanberg S, Kuhn C (2004) Massage therapy effects on depressed pregnant women. *Journal of Psychosomatic Obstetrics and Gynaecology* 25(2): 115–22.

Field T, Hernandez-Reif M, Diego M, Schanberg S, Kuhn C (2005) Cortisol decreases and serotonin and dopamine increase following massage therapy. *International Journal of Neuroscience* 115(10): 1397–413.

Field T, Hernandez-Reif M, Hart S, Theakston H, Schanberg S, Kuhn C (1999) Pregnant women benefit from massage therapy. *Journal of Psychosomatic Obstetrics and Gynaecology* 20(1): 31–8.

Laso C, Galan A (2007) Possible danger for patients using homeopathy: may a homeopathic medicinal product contain active substances that are not homeopathic dilutions? *Medical Law* 26(2): 375–86.

Gaudernack LC, Forbord S, Hole E (2006) Acupuncture administered after spontaneous rupture of membranes at term significantly reduces the length of birth and use of oxytocin: a randomized controlled trial. *Acta Obstetrica Gynecology Scandinavia* 85(11): 1348–53.

Gunn TR, Wright IM (1996) The use of black and blue cohosh in labour. *The New Zealand Medical Journal* 109: 410–41.

Hantoushzadeh S, Alhusseini N, Lebaschi AH *et al.* (2007) The effects of acupuncture during labour on nulliparous women: a randomised controlled trial . *Australian and New Zealand Journal of Obstetrics and Gynaecology* 47(1): 26–30.

Harper TC, Coeytaux RR, Chen W *et al.* (2006) A randomized controlled trial of acupuncture for initiation of labor in nulliparous women. *The Journal of Maternal-Fetal and Neonatal Medicine* 19(8): 465–70.

Hur MH, Cheong N, Yun H, Lee M, Song Y (2005) Effects of delivery nursing care using essential oils on delivery stress response, anxiety during labor, and postpartum status anxiety. *Taehan Kanho Hakhoe Chi* 35(7): 1277–84.

Ingram J, Domagala C, Yates S (2005) The effects of shiatsu on post-term pregnancy. *Complementary Therapies in Medicine* 13(1): 11–5.

Irikura B, Kennelly EJ (1999) Blue cohosh: a word of caution. *Alternative Therapies in Womens Health* 1: 81–3.

Jones TK Lawson BM (1998) Profound neonatal congestive heart failure caused by maternal consumption of blue cohosh herbal medication. *Journal of Pediatrics* 132: 550–2.

Kuczkowski KM (2006) Labor analgesia for the parturient with herbal medicines use: what does an obstetrician need to know? *Archives of Gynaecology and Obstetrics* 274(4): 233–9.

Langmead L, Rampton DS (2001) Review article: herbal treatment in gastrointestinal and liver disease – benefits and dangers. *Alimentary Pharmacology* 15(9): 1239–52.

Lee MK, Chang SB, Kang DH (2004) Effects of SP6 acupressure on labor pain and length of delivery time in women during labor. *Journal of Alternative and Complementary Medicine* 10(6): 959–65.

Lis-Balchin M (1999) Possible health and safety problems in the use of novel plant essential oils and extracts in aromatherapy. *Journal of the Royal Society of Health* 119(4): 240–3.

Marc I, Rainville P, Verreault R, Vaillancourt L, Masse B, Dodin S (2007) The use of hypnosis to improve pain management during voluntary interruption of pregnancy: an open randomized preliminary study. *Contraception* 75(1): 52–8.

Marcus DM, Snodgrass WR (2005) Do no harm: avoidance of herbal medicines during pregnancy. *Obstetrics and Gynaecology* 105(5 Pt 1): 1119–22.

McFarlin BL, Gibson MH, O'Rear J, Harman P (1999) A national survey of herbal preparation use by nurse-midwives for labor stimulation. Review of the literature and recommendations for practice. *Journal of Nurse-Midwifery* 44: 205–16.

McIntyre M (2001) Traditional medicine and childbirth. Paper presented at Forum on Maternity and the Newborn Conference on Complementary Therapies for Mothers and Babies Royal Society of Medicine, London, 8th November 2001.

McNabb MT, Kimber L, Haines A, McCourt C (2006) Does regular massage from late pregnancy to birth decrease maternal pain perception during labour and birth? A feasibility study to investigate a programme of massage, controlled breathing and visualization, from 36 weeks of pregnancy until birth. *Complementary Therapies in Clinical Practice* 12(3): 222–31.

McNeill JA, Alderdice FA, McMurray F (2006) A retrospective cohort study exploring the relationship between antenatal reflexology and intranatal outcomes. *Complementary Therapies in Clinical Practice* 12(2): 119–25.

Mehl-Madrona LE (2004) Hypnosis to facilitate uncomplicated birth. *The American Journal of Clinical Hypnosis* 46(4): 299–312.

Motha G, McGrath J (1993) The effects of reflexology on labour outcomes. *Journal of the Association of Reflexologists*: 2–4.

Mousley S (2005) Audit of an aromatherapy service in a maternity unit. *Complementary Therapies in Clinical Practice* 11(3): 205–10.

National Collaborating Centre for Women's and Children's Health (2003) *Antenatal Care: Routine Care for the Healthy Pregnant Woman*. London, RCOG Press.

National Institute for Health and Clinical Excellence (2006) *Final Draft Guidelines for Consultation: Intrapartum Care: Care of Healthy Women and their Babies during Childbirth*, available from: http://www.nice.org.uk/page.aspx?o=334322 (accessed 14/08/09).

Nesheim BI, Kinge R, Berg B *et al.* (2003) Acupuncture during labor can reduce the use of meperidine: a controlled clinical study. *The Clinical Journal of Pain* 19(3): 187–91.

NMC (2004) *Midwives' Rules and Standards 05-04*. London, NMC.

NMC (2008) *Advice Sheet: Complementary Alternative Therapies and Homeopathy*, available from: http://www.nmc-uk.org/aFrameDisplay.aspx?DocumentID =4023 (accessed 15/07/08).

Olney CM (2005) The effect of therapeutic back massage in hypertensive persons: a preliminary study. *Biological Research for Nursing* 7(2): 98–105.

Parsons M, Simpson M, Ponton T (1999) Raspberry leaf and its effect on labour: safety and efficacy. *Journal of the Australian College of Midwives* 12(3): 20–5.

Qu F, Zhou J (2007) Electro-acupuncture in relieving labor pain. *Evidence Based Complementary and Alternative Medicine* 4(1): 125–30.

Rabl M, Ahner R, Bitschnau M, Zeisler H, Husslein P (2001) Acupuncture for cervical ripening and induction of labor at term: a randomized controlled trial. *Wiener Klinische Wochenschrift* 113(23-24): 942–6.

Ramnerö A, Hanson U, Kihlgren M (2002) Acupuncture treatment during labour: a randomised controlled trial. *British International Journal of Obstetrics and Gynaecology* 109(6): 637–44.

Refuerzo JS, Blackwell SC, Sokol RJ *et al.* (2005) Use of over-the-counter medications and herbal remedies in pregnancy. *American Journal of Perinatology* 22(6): 321–4.

Rojas-Vera J, Patel AV, Dacke CG (2002) Relaxant activity of raspberry (Rubus idaeus) leaf extract in guinea-pig ileum in vitro. *Phytotherapy Research* 16(7): 665–8.

Scott GN, Elmer GW (2002) Update on natural product-drug interactions. *American Journal of Health-System Pharmacy* 59(4): 339–47.

Shalansky S, Lynd L, Richardson K, Ingaszewski A, Kerr C (2007) Risk of warfarin-related bleeding events and supratherapeutic international normalized ratios associated with complementary and alternative medicine: a longitudinal analysis. *Pharmacotherapy* 27(9): 1237–47.

Simpson M, Parsons M, Greenwood J, Wade K (2001) Raspberry leaf in pregnancy: its safety and efficacy in labour. *Journal of Midwifery and Women's Health* 46(2): 51–9.

Stevinson C, Devaraj VS, Fountain-Barber A, Hawkins S, Ernst E (2003) Homeopathic arnica for prevention of pain and bruising: randomized placebo-controlled trial in hand surgery. *Journal of the Royal Society of Medicine* 96(2): 60–5.

Tiran D (2003a) Implementing complementary therapies into midwifery practice. *Complementary Therapies in Nursing and Midwifery* 9(1): 45–8.

Tiran D (2003b) The use of herbal remedies in pregnancy: a risk-benefit assessment. *Complementary Therapies in Nursing and Midwifery* 9(6): 176–81.

Tiran D (2005) Complementary therapies in maternity care: NICE guidelines do not promote clinical excellence. *Complementary Therapies in Clinical Practice* 11(2): 50–2.

Tiran D (2007) Complementary therapies: time to regulate? *The Practising Midwife* 10(3): 14–9.

Tiran D (2008) Homeopathy in pregnancy: issues for midwives. *The Practising Midwife* 11(5): 14–21.

Tiran D, Budd S (2005) Ginger is not a universal remedy for nausea and vomiting in pregnancy. *MIDIRS* 15(3): 335–9.

Vaes LP, Chyka PA (2000) Interactions of warfarin with garlic, ginger, ginkgo or ginseng: nature of the evidence. *Annals of Pharmacology* 34(12): 1478–82.

VandeVusse L, Irland J, Healthcare WF, Berner MA, Fuller S, Adams D (2007) Hypnosis for childbirth: a retrospective comparative analysis of outcomes in one obstetrician's practice. *The American Journal of Clinical Hypnosis* 50(2): 109–19.

Vickers AJ, Fisher P, Smith C, Wyllie SE, Rees R (1998) Homeopathic Arnica 30x is ineffective for muscle soreness after long-distance running: a randomized, double-blind, placebo-controlled trial. *The Clinical Journal of Pain* 14(3): 227–31.

Yildirim G, Sahin NH (2004) The effect of breathing and skin stimulation techniques on labour pain perception of Turkish women. *Pain Research and Management* 9(4): 183–7.

Further resources

www.expectancy.co.uk, Information, advice, consultancy and education on safe use of complementary therapies in pregnancy and childbirth.

www.nccam.nih.gov/camonpubmed, Joint UK/USA research initiative with a comprehensive database of research abstracts on complementary and alternative medicine.

Chapter 10
Midwifery Skills for Normalising Unusual Labours

Verena Schmid and Soo Downe

Introduction

From a 'normal science' perspective (Kuhn 1962), it might be assumed that definitions of normal childbirth are relatively invariant over time, given that physiological processes do not change rapidly across generations. However, beliefs about the nature of normality in childbirth have been subject to a multitude of definitions, interpretations and debates (Jordan 1993). In resource-rich countries, this debate has most recently been influenced by ideas of choice, control and consumerism (Zadoroznyj 2001), and by a society that is focused on risk identification and avoidance (Beck 1992). This tendency has repercussions for health-care system design and delivery (see Chapter 2). As one of us has commented previously, 'abnormality is increasingly defined as a deviation from the average, with the potential for pathology, rather than as a pathological entity in its own right' (Downe 2004a).

This issue at stake is whether normality thinking can be decoupled from what is seen as most common, or average. To do this, we need to move from seeing potential abnormality in all cases, and to move towards thinking 'are this woman and baby actually at imminent risk in this specific situation – or, although what is happening is unusual, could it be normal for them?' In an attempt to provide some tools to support this approach, this chapter addresses two issues. Firstly, we return to the fundamental nature of the physiology of labour and birth. Secondly, we summarise insights and techniques from the formal and the informal literatures, and from midwifery anecdotes, as a way of helping midwives and other labour carers to recognise when unusual labours and births are physiological (as opposed to pathological). Some of these experiences and accounts also provide possible techniques for ensuring mother and baby stay well, and for protecting them from unnecessary (and possibly harmful) just-in-case interventions in these circumstances of unusual physiological labour and birth.

Understanding labour physiology

This section is focused mainly on hormonal rather than mechanical aspects of labour physiology. The mechanical processes of labour are described in most midwifery and obstetric textbooks. However, the hormonal impact on labour progression is rarely discussed in detail in these texts. Indeed, the cyclical relationship between hormonal activity, emotion, bodily function and neuro-psycho-physiological response is a recently expanding field in all areas of health (Sternberg 2000). We begin an exploration of this field in this chapter. Sarah Buckley continues this process in Chapter 12.

The science of physiology describes how an individual works within the body, and in relationship with the environment. It takes a whole systems approach. The laws of physiology are the same in all women all over the world. They are ruled by the unconscious functions of the brain. Cultural, cognitive aspects interact with the physiologic aspects, changing them basically in two ways: they can change the direction of the physiologic systems towards a major contraction (shutting down physiological response) or a major expansion (increasing the capacity and potential of the physiological response).

The birth process can thus be defined as a process of dialogue and communication between physiological systems; between biology and consciousness; between the person and her environment; between the mother and baby; between the mother–baby dyad (or triad or more) and her birth companion(s) and attendants.

All the physiologic systems work in a rhythm of polarity. Normally the polarity is between expansion and contraction. The dynamic between these two poles creates a constant tension tending to homeostasis, but always ready to move in one or the other direction, answering to the stimuli arriving from the body and the environment. Sometimes systems become more contracted (as evidenced in the fight–flight reaction, in response to the stimulus of the sympathetic nervous system), and sometimes they are more expansive and relaxed (when the parasympathetic nervous system is dominant). Balance (health) is a dynamic, not a static condition. Labour requires an exquisite balance between the two systems.

Hormones

Hormones act to trigger transformations in the mother's and baby's body: in pregnancy, during birth, during breastfeeding. The main task for the carer is to create an environment in which hormones that support the labour process can flow freely and abundantly. Hormones work in dyads, with each pair generating opposing effects. When they are in balance, allostasis occurs (Bruce *et al.* 2003). They are the messengers in the body, and, with hormone receptors, they develop an intelligent language of the body. Hormones are triggered by, and trigger, emotional states, and transform them into physiological reactions (Young 2009). So, instead of concentrating on the effect of a specific hormone, it is important to be aware of the whole suite of active neurophysiological agents that orchestrate labour progress if they are allowed to work in harmony. The problem with synthetic hormones, such as artificial oxytocin, is that they play alone.

Labour hormones, such as endogenous oxytocin, endorphins and prolactin have an additional function in protecting the baby from danger and helping the fetal–neonatal adaptation process during and after birth (Carter *et al.* 1999; Soltis *et al.* 2005; Winberg 2005). The expression of prolactin, in particular, seems to vary by mode of birth for term infants (Heasman *et al.* 1997). These hormones are instrumental in that they prepare the process of bonding, love, happiness and well-being that form the ground on which the child can grow. Moreover, they activate a protecting behaviour in the parents towards the child, and damp down aggression. It has been demonstrated in rats that under the influence of high levels of endorphins and oxytocin, circuits of empathy and social capacities become activated in the maternal and neonatal brain (Pedersen & Boccia 2002). Recent research has identified new neurological entities, called 'mirror neurons' that seem to allow the reflection and development of socialising behaviour in children, and between adults (Rizzolatti & Sinigaglia 2007). The mirror-neuron system seems to develop fully over the first 12 months of a child's life. It is possible that, at the time when the awake and present mother meets her awake and present child for the first time, countless mirror neurons start to build up and work in the baby's brain. This may be part of the process that enables the child to feel empathy later in life, and in the development of social intelligence.

Prolactin reaches very high levels during labour and in the first period after birth. It helps to protect the baby's metabolism during birth, and it prepares the lungs for breathing (Scaglia *et al.* 1981; Tolino *et al.* 1983). Prolactin slows down aggressiveness towards others and activates defensive behaviours (such as those that might be used to defend the child) (Heasman *et al.* 1997; Soltis *et al.* 2005). It has been identified in men who attend birth (Fleming *et al.* 2002).

This overview indicates that the hormonal biology of labour and birth facilitates the complicated processes of change and adaptation, and, possibly, acts as a catalyst for social behaviours and effective relationships. For this reason, it is important to try to maximise the action of these hormones even where the labour of an individual woman is unusual. The emphasis should be on preserving physiological processes as much as possible. Where this is not possible, it is important to utilise techniques that maintain the woman's confidence and faith in her body, and that allow her to work as much as possible with the labour. These techniques include massage, counselling, changing position to maximise rotation, nutrition where possible, and crucially, maintaining confidence and belief in the woman among her caregivers. In general, continuity of supportive care in labour is shown to be beneficial, particularly if it is carried out by a non-professional woman (Hodnett *et al.* 2007). If this is not possible, either by the lay supporter or the clinical professional, because the caregiver is tired, hungry or demoralised, it is important for the individual to recognise this, and to hand over care to another attendant who is fresh and confident and able to support the woman effectively even if this is only until the primary caregiver is rested and recovered (Scott *et al.* 2006). Continuity of carer when the caregiver is tired and demoralised might be counterproductive. The woman will identify the emotional state of the caregiver, and this can trigger a mood change for her, with adverse hormonal and physiological consequences. The lift in mood that can be brought by a new attendant who is positive about the labour can be very noticeable.

The nervous system

There is communication between the neocortex and the cortex, and between the sympathetic and parasympathetic nerve systems. This link is specifically mediated by the limbic system. The limbic system includes centres such as the hypothalamus, amygdala and hippocampus that trigger emotional responses, sexual arousal, and unconscious memory. The high concentration of hormones released in labour is regulated by the hypothalamus, and this activates specific elements in the autonomic nerve system. During normal labour, under this hormonal control, the neocortex is depressed, and the parasympathetic nervous system is dominant. If she is left to work with her bodily responses, the woman tends to respond in an unconscious, emotional and instinctive manner. In these circumstances, birth is an unintentional, involuntary and uncontrollable process that cannot be predicted for an individual woman. It also carries the potential of unknown resources generated by the dominance of unconscious reflexes and responses. One of these resources is the response to labour pain. This is described in detail in Chapter 8.

An example of how this neurohormonal system works is given below.

Stimulus: This is generated from inside the body, such as by muscular activity, or from external environmental sources; during birth, this could be the pain of a contraction.

Neurohormonal response: The stimulus activates adrenocorticotrophic hormone, and the sympathetic nervous system. This then results in activation of the adrenal gland, and production of cortisone, and cate-cholamines including adrenaline. In female biology, after the first wave of adrenalin, there can be a wave of oxytocin and prolactin, especially if the stress stimulus concerns relationships and offspring (Taylor 2003). This is what happens in labour. Michel Odent calls *it* 'the paradoxical reflex of oxytocin in answer to a peak of adrenalin'.

Preparation to react: The whole body response to this hormonal stimulus is *arousal*, contraction of muscles (ready to fight or flee), mobilisation of energy sources, and a consequent rise in blood sugar.

Action: (Instinctive) movement takes place to enable the body to meet any threat, or to escape from it. In birth, the woman is stimulated to move, usually in a way that optimises the progress of the baby (see below for more discussion of this).

Release of tension: The heightened responses are active for as long as is necessary, and are often accompanied by vocal expression as well as movement.

Back to balance: In the final phase of the cycle, once the crisis is over, the stimulus is withdrawn, and the body pauses. If no further stimulus occurs, it enters a state of relaxation, governed by the parasympathetic nervous system.

During birth, this pattern repeats itself on a micro level during every contraction, and, on a macro level, across the whole labour. In order to be able to cope with the stresses of the 'fight' reaction and in order to let go and to open up to the coming of the baby, the woman needs to know and to be able to face the stimulus event (the process of birth), to be sure of having the right tools to face it (coping tools), and feel confident in the environment she is in, and in those she is trusting to help her through. If she lacks these tools, she can easily revert to a flight reaction, causing the sympathetic nervous system to close down her bodily reactions, slow down contractions as a consequence of exhaustion, and causing her to become fearful and passive. This reaction can lead to a feedback mechanism that produces high levels of cortisol to counter the up-regulation of adrenaline caused by the initial stimulus. Different modes of birth and/or lengths of labour are associated with variation in neonatal cortisol production (Taylor *et al.* 2000). Infants born after elective Caesarean section produce lower levels of salivary cortisol in response to stress (such as immunisation). Low levels of cortisol in adults who have been exposed to traumatic events have been associated with a higher tendency to experience post-traumatic stress disorder some time after the event (Pervanidou 2008). While it is not clear if these are cause or effect relationships, it does appear that excessive or minimal cortisol production in labour might not be optimal physiologically.

Mother–baby bond and the fetal–placental system

The fetal–placental system has two distinctive methods of functioning. One is autonomous. In this case, the baby is the main producer of hormones. These hormones work in a paracrine manner (from cell-to-cell) inside the uterus. The baby's placenta can carry out many of the functions of the adult body, and the baby is able to produce its own oxytocin and endorphins and, at the end of pregnancy and during birth, high levels of fetal adrenalin. At the same time, the fetal–placental system is enclosed in the mother's body, and works in symbiosis with it. The mother's biological systems reinforce those of the baby. Maternal oxytocin production appears to be protective for the fetal brain in labour, acting to temporarily block fetal neurotransmitters (Tyzio 2006).

Disruption to the maternal physiological processes of labour and birth (such as that secondary to epidural analgesia or Caesarean section) may impact on the optimum functioning of the fetal neurohormonal system, with unknown consequences. As noted above, we do know that different modes of birth and/or lengths of labour are associated with variation in the neonatal stress response. As the stress response is linked to the immune response (Soloman 1985), this may have consequences for infant well-being in the short- and longer term. There are important questions here that need to be answered in future research.

Physiological aspects of the baby

The baby is an important protagonist of labour. Specific motor patterns are developed during pregnancy that aid effective birth movements. The fetus can flex and deflex its spine, push with its feet, and rotate its head. It is possible that labour is also a learning process for the baby, as his body flexes and moves through the process of birth, and as his brain is primed with hormones that stimulate love and trust (oxytocin, endorphins and prolactin).

The baby, at the moment of birth and in the first months of life, carries out one of the most difficult adaptation processes of its whole life. For this reason, it is of vital importance that mother and baby are allowed to follow through their instinctive behaviours. Furthermore, a stress-free, close relationship between mother and baby in these early stages, under the influence of priming hormones like oxytocin and prolactin, creates responsive connectivity between mother and baby that is the basis for mutual responsiveness in the neonatal period and beyond (Carter *et al.* 1999; Pedersen & Boccia 2002).

The pillars of health

One-way of moving from a predominantly pathological focus on birth is to reframe the process in terms of salutogenic thinking (Antonovsky 1987; Downe & McCourt 2004; Schmid 2007). This concept is explored in more depth in Chapter 16. In summary, salutogenic thinking focuses on what makes things go well, as opposed to what makes them go wrong. In this model of care, practitioners search for signs of health, and of personal resources, rather than for signs of risk and pathology. This can be done by paying attention to the labouring woman on three levels: the physical expressions of her body; her behaviour and lifestyle; and in her emotional and psychosocial responses. These observations can be assessed against the following pillars of health:

- Dynamic communication between and effective activity of the autonomic nervous system
- Dynamic communication between and effective activity of the hormonal system
- Dynamic communication between and effective activity of the mother and the fetus (including the fetal–placental unit)
- Dynamic communication between the woman and her environment (human, social and material)

Signs of health will be evident if the rhythms in lifestyle and physical function of the woman alternate regularly between moments of crisis and activity and moments of well-being and rest. If the latter prevails at least a bit over the former, then the woman is likely to be in good health, and her resources are likely to be sufficient for a successful pregnancy and labour.

Caregivers can support this process by recognising the rhythmic nature of health, as modulated by the polarity in the autonomic nervous system, as opposed to expecting linear, regular, predictable development and responses through pregnancy and labour, and the post-natal period. There is some evidence that behavioural therapy can modulate the response of the autonomic nervous system in the case of pain (Andrasik & Rime 2007). Based on this emerging field of work, it is possible that the hormonal system can be stimulated or down-regulated through relaxation, visualisations, exchanging experiences, verbal expression, singing, shouting and structured breathing, all of which seem to make a difference to maternal behaviour and bodily responses in clinical practice. The fetal–maternal system can be optimised through active and holistic nutrition of the baby (and of the mother of course), both in terms of nutrition, in terms of positive thinking about labour and birth, and about the coming baby, and by way of sensory feedback to the baby, which stimulates brain development. The final pillar of health can be built via a good therapeutic relationship between the midwife and other caregivers and the woman, in an environment that offers space for self-expression, a sense of physical and emotional safety, choice and empowerment. This includes the creation of a space where positive, trusting communication can take place. Such communication creates a situation where the woman can be free from concern about external interference, and, as a consequence, allow her parasympathetic nervous system to activate oxytocin and endorphins and, therefore, an optimal development of pregnancy, and labour progress. In a feedback loop, this up-regulation of hormonal activity can reinforce trust in the caregivers (Zak *et al.* 2005). However, this may not be possible where the caregiver is feeling stressed and under scrutiny, or where they sense they might be judged unfavourably by their colleagues for supporting an unusual normal labour.

It has been noted that teams with greater cohesiveness have better outcomes (Grumbach & Bodenheimer 2004), and that effective team work is one of the characteristics of maternity care services with optimal rates of spontaneous birth, and Caesarean section (Ontario Womens Health Council 2001). Progress is clearly disrupted where the woman senses that the attending team does not trust each other, and there is even evidence that this might be associated with maternal morbidity and mortality (Health Care Commission 2006). In this circumstance, the woman has to switch back on her sympathetic nervous system in preparation to fight or run. This blocks the complementary activity of the parasympathetic system, shuts down the process of labour, and risks labour dystocia. It is for this reason that some assumptions about women may become a self-fulfilling prophecy. Caregivers should never assume that a labour will not progress unless there is evidence that this is the case. Politically, it is important that caregivers seek to build effective and authentically trusting relationships between each other to ensure that women have the best chance of labouring salutogenically.

The laws of physiology in labour

Pregnancy as preparation (foundation)

Pregnancy is the first aspect to take into consideration in labour physiology. During pregnancy the most important precursors of labour are prepared: the hormonal orchestra, the softening of the body's tissues and the pelvis, the receptors for oxytocin in the uterus, the receptors for endorphins, the health and reactivity of the baby, the mother's competency for active adaptation to the changes, the bonding process, the appearance of uterine contractions in the third trimester, the ripening of the baby's lungs and other physiological systems, and the developing biological symbiosis between mother and child. All of these processes will guide and protect the mother and baby through labour and the first weeks of adaptation outside the womb. They also prepare the bodies and minds of the mothers and babies for the profound process of emotional, psychological and physiological relating to each other that must take place in the first weeks after birth.

This suggests that a physiological pregnancy with a spontaneous start of labour is a necessary prerequisite for a physiological labour. However, a physiological labour is often possible even in difficult pregnancies.

Rhythm

Female biology has a cyclic, rhythmic component that moves between hormonal polarities. As noted in Chapter 5, this is also true in labour. The formal approach to labour that most practitioners are used to is based on linear progress that is measured by time, and through clearly defined stages, with the emphasis on speed (Downe & Dykes 2009). Where it is deemed necessary, this is restricted and corrected through regular measurements and an escalating list of interventions. It may seem that we have forgotten the important cyclical law of female physiology. Labour rhythms flow through active and passive phases, peaks and troughs, guided by the needs of the baby and/or the mother, by the physiological constitution of the woman, by her emotional condition, by her sexual energy, by her nutritional reserves, by the dynamic mechanical relationship between the mother's pelvis and the baby's presenting part, and so on. In fact, it seems anecdotally that many practitioners are aware of this through observation of labouring women. However, as this observation is at odds with what is taught, it either seems to be ignored, or to result in dissonance for some practitioners, which potentially causes stress and unease (Festinger 1957; Hunter 2004; Downe *et al.* 2008).

The dilating process

During labour, the woman goes through both physiological and psychological cycles. Her body is physically opening up. She may even feel she is in danger of dying. Her psyche is opening to the baby and to transformation. Some women experience an alteration in their former sense of self once they become a mother. This can be seen as negative and threatening, or as the potential for a positive new identity, with new and unexpected resources. These processes cannot be linear. They move between polar aspects of self-conservation/retraction, and opening to birth/letting go. The physical parallel is that cervical dilation can increase or reduce, and the fetus can descend the birth canal and move up again, or rotate from anterior to posterior position and back again. Woman can cope well, then be in despair, and then cope well again.

It is important not to overreact to the downswing in these cycles, where labour seems to slow and where women lose confidence and faith. An approach that forces the upswing through drugs or other kinds of intervention carries the risk of causing physiological or psychological resistance, and overstimulation of the sympathetic nervous system. This can lead to a domino effect that moves women's physical and hormonal responses, and psychological resources, away from the possibility of the next positive upswing, leading to the need for more external intervention. One of the examples of this effect that is frequently seen in nulliparous women on many labour wards is acceleration of labour in the latent phase; which leads to excessive pain; which leads to loss of confidence and capacity to cope, and a request for an epidural; which leads to lax pelvic muscles; which leads to malrotation of the fetal head and an inability to push; which leads to instrumental birth.

The alternative is to watch and wait, offering support, rest, nutrition, and focusing on the potential for a physiological upswing into the next 'positive wave' of the woman's labour. When this works, the labour progresses.

This approach to labour and birth acknowledges that the optimum psychophysiology of labour balances the hormonal cues produced in situations of fear and anxiety with those produced in situations of euphoria and joy. For example, while the hormonal consequences of fear of pain and of death could be paralysing for a labouring woman, high endorphin levels produced as physiological labour progresses induce a trance-like state, which allows for paradoxical relaxation. Indeed, it is likely that safety is maximised for mother and baby if those attending labouring women can provide an environment that mobilises these physiological resources.

Cycles of labour

This section provides a way of understanding birth as a cyclical phenomenon, rather than as a linear smoothly progressing process. Although it describes a series of cycles, this is not fixed (as in the 'stages of labour' approach). Women do not necessarily experience all of these cycles, and they may spend a longer time in some than in others. The intention is to map out an approach to labour which is much more sensitive to the uniquely normal behaviours, feelings and clinical changes of individual women, than the current population-based standard assumptions about strictly defined labour stages.

The latent cycle (early labour)

This is the most important cycle of labour, because it creates the basic conditions for dilation and descent of the baby, and for physiological adaptation to labour pain. In this phase, contractions tend to be short, irregular and bearable. For the woman, this is an essential time to adapt to the reality of labour, to pain and to the reality of the child that is coming. This can be less or more conflicting for her, and it may demand less or more time, depending on the individual. Indeed, women who have very fast labours, where this phase is contracted, or not present at all, often appear to be stunned and shocked at the end of labour. Despite the strong assumption that shorter labours are better, these women (and, possibly, their babies) may be at a higher risk of being traumatised by labour, and even of post-traumatic stress (Rippin-Sisler 1996).

First transition

The first transition stage is between the latent cycle and active labour. Based on clinical observation and experience, transition stages have different kind of dynamics, depending on the individual woman. Sometimes they are sudden and violent: labour accelerates rapidly, with symptoms of the sympathetic nerve system (vomiting, crying, fear) for a short time, after which the labour moves into a new, stronger rhythm. For other women, labour slows down at this point, giving them the opportunity to restore their energy, to rest, eat and sleep. In this case, the parasympathetic nerve system seems to prevail. In the case of the slow transition, the labour dynamic can change from active labour back to the irregular contractions of the latent phase, and it can take some time until regular contractions with progress are established.

Active cycle, first part

During this time, contractions are regular, grow in intensity and duration and start to push the baby into the lower pelvis. The woman changes states of consciousness between concentrating fully on working with and coping with the sensations of labour during contractions, and recovering control during the pauses between contractions. The activity of the autonomic nerve system is increasing and the signs of the sympathetic and parasympathetic nervous system are both evident. The neocortex is always active during the pause between contractions, and factors that disturb the woman can slow down or stop labour for a while. This process is usually reversible. For example, often, if a woman is transferred from home to hospital in this phase, labour slows down. However, if the woman is properly supported, and if a space is created in which she can feel physically and psychological safe, she can re-engage with the process, and labour will go on again.

A good bond with the baby during pregnancy helps many labouring women to focus on the baby, and to relax in to the work of opening up her body. In contrast, conflicts from the pregnancy and in the woman's life, or concerns about her capacity to parent, can inhibit endorphin production, and prolong this cycle of labour. A key task for the labour attendant at this stage is to minimise external stressors, or, if the labour appears to be blocked, to try to establish if psychological stress might be impeding effective release of the appropriate hormones. If this does seem to be the case, it is important for the caregiver to try to work with the woman to deal with and overcome these factors, if possible. One example of this process in action is given in Walsh's (2006) research on a birth centre when a midwife consoles a teenage girl in early labour by lying on the floor on a mattress and holding her in a lengthy embrace as she sobbed into her shoulder. An authentically caring relationship between the woman and the professional who is with her is essential for this psychologically therapeutic relationship. It is likely that this is at least one of the factors that underpin the effectiveness of one-to-one care in labour.

Second transition

Around this time in labour (usually when the cervix is around 5–6 cm dilated, though this will vary with each individual), there is often another transition. This can be manifest as a sudden increase in intensity of the woman's reaction. She may vomit, swear, have an emotional outburst, demand pain relief, and grasp her partner or anyone else near to her. After this, if she is given the space to recover her equilibrium, she may progress into a trance-like state. If this second transition cycle is slow, labour slows down, or even stops, and the woman can fall asleep. In this case, women appear to need to restore their energies physically. Psychologically, nulliparous women may need to prepare to let their old sense of self go, and open up to the new state of being mother. A gentle massage can help the woman to turn on her parasympathetic nerve system and come back into touch with her hormonal and psychological resources.

Active cycle, second part

Now labour is progressing intensely, and the parasympathetic nervous system prevails, even if the contractions become stronger and stronger. If labour has been allowed to progress physiologically, endorphin levels are very high and dominant (Fettes *et al.* 1984). Many women report that the sensation of pain changes into something that feels more active, even if the expression or reaction to pain is very strong. The woman's body works very instinctively, and, for some women, sexually (see Chapter 12 for an in-depth discussion of this issue). Her breathing is deep. She is completely in her own world, and should not be disturbed. Her body is ready for the process that has been termed the *fetal ejection reflex* (Odent 1987). On an emotional level, this is the most difficult phase for the woman – the moment where she reaches and overcomes her boundaries. This is the point when some women feel that they will die. Many women will cry for help. As Tricia Anderson has noted, women may frame this call in terms of a plea for pain relief, or even for a Caesarean section (Anderson 2000). However, on retrospection, most women in Tricia's study recalled that they wanted support and encouragement, not a scalpel or a needle.

One of the skills of midwives at this point is to know that what seems to be the most vulnerable time for women is actually the moment of empowerment for them. Soon this sense of absolute extremity will be passed over. One of the most important responses at this time is to hear the actual request behind the words spoken by women. For example, do they really want an epidural – or are they in fact asking for someone to help them over this temporary moment, and into the final transition of their labour.

Third transition

When the woman is nearly fully dilated (maybe around 8–9 cm of cervical dilation; though in some women this occurs much sooner) there is a new transition to the cycle where active pushing begins. This has only recently been noted (as 'transition') in midwifery textbooks (Downe 2003, 2004b), though midwives and other labour attendants have known about it for generations. Some women begin to feel pushing urges as the contraction reaches maximum intensity. If the baby's head is in an anterior position and well flexed, this is a sign of progress, and no interference is necessary. The cervix will fully open up under the spontaneous pushing urges of the woman, and she will enter into the second stage. If the transition is slow, contractions will slow down again and the woman will again rest in order to build up enough resources to continue. Sometimes there is an anterior lip, or a small rim of the cervix left. In this circumstance, a slowing down of the labour means that the baby has to rotate and adapt better, and this takes time. However, there is no evidence to date to indicate that spontaneous pushing at the height of the contraction should be stopped, even in this situation, if labour has progressed physiologically up to this point (Downe *et al.* 2008). The practical implications of this are discussed below.

Active pushing

Spontaneous pushing urges will guide the woman through the final cycle of labour. This cycle can also exhibit a latent, active and expulsive phase. If women experience a latent phase, when contractions appear to slow or even stop, it is likely that the fetal head is rotating and descending. In this case, the pushing urges usually only occur at the time of maximum intensity of the contractions, if at all. If women experience this so-called 'rest and be thankful' phase, there is no need to intervene if mother and baby are well. As the baby's head rotates, descends and distends the pelvis muscles, Ferguson's reflex is stimulated, and labour will recommence. Whether women are bearing down early or later, when the presenting part of the baby's head reaches the bulbocavernosus muscles, a sensation of burning and of tearing triggers another oxytocin surge, and the consequent so-called 'fetus ejection reflex' (Odent 1987). This generates an unstoppable bearing down urge, and the baby is born rapidly. While the evidence base is not conclusive (Altman & Lydon-Rochelle 2006), some studies have demonstrated that there is no reason to impose time limits on a second stage of up to at least 4 hours (Hansen *et al.* 2002), if mother and baby are well, and if labour has progressed well up to this point.

Fourth transition

After the expulsion of the baby, there is often a short transition during which the mother realises that the labour is over, and the baby has arrived. Over the next 2 hours or so, the baby adapts to extra uterine life, and the mother adapts to the presence of the baby. While the placenta is attached to the mother's body, it will support transition, even if the cord is collapsed. There is good evidence that the cord should not be cut immediately after the birth (see Chapter 6). Early breastfeeding provides a smooth transition from fetal life, supported by the placenta, to extra uterine life, supported by breast milk and physical and emotional nurturing by the mother. The process of imprinting and bonding on a biological as well as relational basis are basic conditions to start life.

The framework for understanding unusual normal labour described above is based on observation, and on deduction from the known effects and interactions of the neurophysiology of labour and birth. Women will not necessarily exhibit all of the phases described. Every woman has her own rhythm through the birth process, dictated by her physiological, psychological and emotional state, the baby's state, and the environment. Women who experience long but physiologically normal labours can be joyful and satisfied if they undertook the whole process without interventions. As we have noted above, women with very short labours, either spontaneous or after intervention, can be profoundly shocked and traumatised. It is not clear what impact this might have on the baby. It does appear, however, that the cyclic processes of labour permit women to cope with the profound physical, psychological and emotional changes that are taking place, and that interrupting this process should only be undertaken with great caution, and where mother and baby are otherwise truly at risk of adverse outcome. This should certainly not be done just to ensure that women's labours conform to a pre-determined 'norm'.

Midwifery skills for unusual normal labour

This section of this chapter addresses specific situations that are unusual but not necessarily pathological (such as long labours, the early pushing urge (EPU), and breech birth) and situations that are potentially patho-logical, but which can sometimes be facilitated to create an optimal outcome for mother and baby (such as shoulder dystocia). We make reference in these sections to internet sites that provide useful evidence for practice in these areas, both from a clinical perspective, and from a formal research basis. These sites offer dynamic ongoing resources for practitioners to consider, critically assess and use if the practice is judged to be appropriate for the setting and population that is relevant to them. They are not necessarily based on formal evidence, but on empirical observation, usually in specific childbirth settings. They may or may not be appropriate for other types of setting.

Long labour and labour with the baby in the occipito-posterior position

As a longer than normal labour is often associated with a fetus that is in the occipito-posterior position, midwifery skills for correcting malposition are frequently the same as those for prolonged labour in general. For this reason, techniques for fetal positioning are included in this section.

From the point of view of many labouring women, especially where labour is progressing spontaneously, and an epidural is not in operation, time does not have much meaning. In these cases, the woman is much more focused on the immediate sensations and changes in her body. The history of the bodily responses of a particular labouring woman can be an important clue as to what is happening. For example, if a labour appears to be slowing down, the midwife who has paid attention is in a position to discern if this is part of the normal rhythm of that woman, or if there is a block in progression, due to some kind of pathological dystocia. A guide to this distinction is to observe how the woman has responded to the labour cycles described above. If her normal response in early labour has been for a cyclical slowing of progress, alternating with more intense activity, a simple solution could be rest, because an exhausted body will not have the reserves of energy needed for the muscular effort required to create powerful peaks in contractions. Once her body is back to homeostasis, the peaks will come back too. Rest and nutrition can be a very simple and effective alternative to exogenous oxytocics for a labour that is slowing down. If, on the other hand, she is beginning to panic and to move towards a pathological flight reaction, the solution might be calming measures, such as massage, rhythmic movement, or empathetic counselling.

As we have noted above, there is no good evidence to intervene in a long labour if it started spontaneously, is progressing steadily, and if mother and baby are doing well (Hansen *et al.* 2002). As one of us has noted previously, definitions of 'prolonged labour' have changed in official texts over the years. In 1931, Berkeley and colleagues suggested that '(l)abour in primiparae lasts on average about 15 to 20 hours. In multiparae, eight to ten hours can be taken as the average time .... It is foolish to attempt to prophesy more than approximately how long labour will last in any given case.' (Berkeley *et al.* 1931, p. 273). Examination of Myles midwifery indicates that the standard length of normal first stage of labour for a nulliparous woman decreased from 12.5 to 11.75 hours between 1958 and 1975 (Downe 2004b). Presumably this is not long enough for evolution to change women's basic physiology. As Margaret Myles herself suggested, this change was much more likely to be due to the increasingly routine use of oxytocins in labour (Myles 1975). 'Normality' therefore becomes defined by the outcomes of routine intervention. Indeed, an extreme example of this is the statement that:

> Because oxytocin-augmented labor proceeds more slowly than spontaneous labor, 2 hours of active phase arrest ... is not a rigorous criterion for caesarean section ...
>
> (Rouse *et al.* 2001)

In this case, labours that are prolonged as a consequence of the use of oxytocin are seen as uncomplicated, and not needing external help, in contrast to spontaneous labours lasting the same time. The abnormal has become the norm.

This is further compounded by rules of normality that judge labour as if it is a uniformly linear process, like the action line on a partogramme, instead of a process governed by hormonal surges, as we have noted in the first part of this chapter. Officially, normal progress in labour for primigravid women has varied from 1.2 cm per hour (Friedman 1955) to 0.5 cm of cervical dilation per hour (Albers *et al.* 1996). None of these definitions take account of the cyclical nature of labour progress secondary to the fact that endogenous oxytocin is released in pulses, and not in a smooth linear fashion.

Many labours move through active and more passive stages at various points in the process. Some women progress very slowly to around 6 cm of cervical dilation, and then feel a strong pushing urge within an hour or so. Cervical reversal is increasingly recognised as a real phenomenon (instead of a result of misdiagnosis by junior staff) (MANA 1998; Gaskin 2003). The fact that some women need a few hours sleep after some time of active labour and progress is also well documented clinically by midwives working in settings that do not impose strict rules on what labour patterns should be.

Some midwives have noted that women's labour patterns can be like their mothers, or their sisters. This can be a useful clinical rule of thumb if labours seem to be unusual. If she is a nulliparous woman, it is worth asking if this kind of labour is a feature in her family, and what kind of outcomes it has resulted in for other family members. If she is a multigravid woman, comparison can be made to her previous labour, to see if this is normal progress for her. If not, it may be worth considering discussing physiological interventions with her earlier if there are signs that mother or baby are tiring or otherwise adversely affected, or if labour progress ceases.

If a labour does appear to be stalling, but there is no evidence of imminent pathology for mother or baby, a range of solutions have been used by midwives and others. These include the following:

Nutrition: Offering the mother a light diet has not been shown to affect clinical labour outcomes or maternal well-being (O'Sullivan *et al.* 2009). However, it may boost morale, revitalise tired muscles, normalise a situation that may be becoming tense, and provide distraction for the woman and her attendants.

Rest and massage: If the labour is slowing down after a good phase of activity, it may help to find somewhere the woman can lie down comfortably for a few minutes or longer, dim the lights, quieten the atmosphere and allow the woman and her birth companions some time to rest and reflect. If this is acceptable to her, massage can help this process, both in terms of the general sense of relaxation it can engender, and as a technique for allowing women's bodies to retune to the hormonal cues needed to get labour going again.

Counselling: As noted above, if there is a suspicion that emotional blocks are causing muscle tension and/or overstimulation of the parasympathetic nervous system, it can be helpful for the midwife to spend some time quietly talking to the woman about any fears and anxieties she may have about the next phase of the labour and/or about motherhood, or any other issues that might be preventing her capacity to activate her parasympathetic nervous system.

Change of position: Most women will move spontaneously through labour if they are in an environment where they can be subconsciously responsive to the cues given by their baby and their body. For example, women with a baby in the occipito-posterior position will often lean forwards, or rotate their hips, to reduce the pain in their backs. These movements can also shift the fetal head into a more optimal dimension in the pelvis, allowing descent to the pelvic floor muscles, and consequent rotation. As an example of instinctive maternal positioning, Sutton and Scott have observed that, contrary to the regular practice of asking women to abduct their legs up to their chest for pushing when they are on a bed, many women spontaneously throw their arms back and reach behind them when they begin to feel a strong pushing urge (Sutton & Scott 1995). They hypothesise that this reflex acts to straighten the curve of Carus, to facilitate fetal descent. In contrast, the normal management approach accentuates the vaginal curvature, inhibiting rotation and descent.

However, sometimes women need to be guided into positions that may help their labour, especially if they are tired or demoralised. Birth balls have proved to be very helpful in this regard. The change of position offers a change of the dynamic in a birth room. It also helps women to spontaneously widen the diameters of the bony pelvis as they sit astride the ball, and it encourages rocking movements that alter the pelvic diameters. In their seminal work on optimal fetal positioning, Jean Sutton and Pauline Scott also propose the use of positions where one leg is asymmetric with the other (Sutton & Scott 1995). These include standing with one leg on a chair, or walking up and down stairs (forwards or sideways), or marching on the spot. This can again shift the diameters of the pelvis and provide room for a baby that is occipito-posterior or asynclitic. These movements tend to be rhythmic and organised, and they can help to restore a sense of order and control if the labouring woman and/or her attendants are beginning to run out of energy and self-belief. There is an excellent account of how to use these and a range of other positions in Simkin and Ancheta (2005), and on the Home Birth Reference website (http://www.homebirth.org.uk/ofp.htm).

If the expulsive phase of labour is slow, Sutton and Scott also advise kneeling positions, or being on all fours, and they note that asymmetric position at this point, such as kneeling on one knee, can also help with late descent and rotation.

Manual techniques: Less commonly, some practitioners utilise manual techniques, especially when the fetal head is known to be malrotated, and progress is not taking place. Indeed, Reichman *et al.* (2008) report remarkable results using digital rotation of the fetal head in a small case series of 61 women with occiptio-posterior position. They describe digital rotation as ' . . . exerting pressure . . . after placing the tips of the index and middle fingers onto the edge of that part of the anterior parietal bone that overlaps the occipital bone in the area of the posterior fontanelle'. The authors note that this is a technique that provides counter-pressure, permitting the fetal head to rotate spontaneously in response. They contrast this with manual rotation, which is the physical turning of the fetal head by the attendant. In this before and after case series, women who were in the digital rotation group had higher rates of spontaneous vaginal birth than those who were in the group left to continue labour spontaneously (77% vs. 27%). This is, however, a small and relatively uncontrolled study, and so the results would need to be treated with caution until larger studies have been undertaken. Any practice in this area would need to pay careful attention to the position of the fetus, and the biomechanics of the pelvis, if the manoeuvres are to create benefit rather than harm.

Attendants' attitudes: As we have noted above, the mother will sense the way the midwife, or her other attendants, feel about the baby. It is important for the midwife to encourage the positive support of other birth companions, and to pay attention to their needs for rest and nutrition. This will include encouraging them to leave the birth room sometimes for a break from the intense work of supporting the labouring woman. Equally, it is important for midwives to be self aware, and to be able to recognise when their emotional and physical energy levels are too low. Although it is hard to find the space to take care of oneself in many busy labour wards, it is essential for midwives to give themselves space and time away from the labouring woman to rest, eat, drink, and recover their capacity to judge the health of, or danger in, a slow labour.

Hydrotherapy: There is some concern that the use of water in very early labour can slow down progress (Eriksson *et al.* 1997), presumably due to suppression of oxytocin feedback occasioned by deep relaxation. However, the work of Cluett and colleagues offers a possible solution where labour has been progressing, but is now stalling (Cluett *et al.* 2004). In this randomised controlled trial, women with a diagnosis of dystocia who were randomised to the use of water in labour, as opposed to amniotomy and syntocinon, had lower rates of use of epidurals, and of operative birth. The infants of women randomised to water had higher rates of admission to neonatal units, but none of them suffered adverse effects at follow-up.

The Royal College of Midwives Campaign for Normal Birth website has a number of stories about the experience of a long labour, and hints and tips for supporting women who are experiencing this. The site is available at the following url: http://www.rcmnormalbirth.org.uk/

The early pushing urge

For decades, it has been an article of faith in many childbirth settings that women should not actively push unless the cervix is fully dilated. However, this has not always been the assumption. A long-established obstetric textbook, *Obstetrics by Ten Teachers* (1931, the authors of *Midwifery by Ten Teachers*) (Monga & Baker 2006) stated, in its 1931 edition, that 'No good can be done by bearing down before the dilatation of the os is complete *or nearly complete*' (our emphasis) (Berkeley *et al.* 1931, p. 300).

In the 1980s, Jean Roberts began querying the usual practice of assuming that any pushing efforts before diagnosis of full dilation of the cervix were invariably pathological. Based on a range of small observational studies, she and her colleagues concluded that women who experienced the early pushing urge (EPU) at 6 cm or more of cervical dilation were probably experiencing a physiological response, unless there were signs of obstructed or dystocic labour, such as a persistent occipito-posterior position (Roberts & Hanson 2007). In an anonymous incidence survey of four consultant units in Trent Region over a 3-week period in May 1999, a survey carried out by Downe *et al.* (2008) found that, of the 383 women for whom data were returned, about 40% experienced the EPU. The authors note that, if an extreme assumption is made that all those with no returns did not want to push early, the incidence of pushing at or before 9 cm of cervical dilation was around 20% (153/765): approximately one in five of all women labouring over the 3 weeks of the survey. In some cases, the pushing urge was experienced prior to 6 cm dilation, with no apparent ill effects for mothers or babies. While the evidence base in this area is not very comprehensive, there is some indication from the observational studies that women who are prevented from pushing in this circumstance can be highly distressed, and even unable to push once they are finally allowed to do so (McKay *et al.* 1990; Bergstrom *et al.* 1997). Whatever the physiology of the EPU, in all these unusual normal circumstances, the skill of the midwife and the other attendants is to ask, 'what is happening with this woman and this baby at this specific moment, and is this likely to be a salutogenic response for her, even if it is outside of population based norms?'

In the two surveys undertaken in the United Kingdom in this area, it appears that practice varied from complete prevention of pushing unless the cervix was known to be fully dilated, to a complete 'hands-off' approach, leaving the mother to work entirely by instinct (Downe *et al.* 2008). There may be circumstances where each of these approaches may be appropriate. However, in most cases, midwives responding to these surveys would initially passively observe the effect of EPUs for a while, to see if they were productive. If, after half an hour or so there was no sign of the vertex at the introitus, or if the woman or baby exhibited an adverse change in their physical or emotional responses, these midwives would check to see if there were other signs of progress, by abdominal palpation and vaginal examination. This would then either result in more watching and waiting, if progress was evident, or, if not, techniques such as encouraging the woman to breathe through the contraction, lie on her side, or otherwise change position and attempt to work through the bearing-down urge.

Labour with the fetus in the breech position

Following the Term Breech Trial that reported in 2000 (Hannah *et al.* 2000), rates of vaginal breech birth have reduced markedly in many high-resource countries (Hogle *et al.* 2003). However, the 2-year follow-up sub-study published in 2004 showed no difference in combined mortality and morbidity between babies presenting by the breech who were born by Caesarean section, and those born vaginally (Whyte *et al.* 2004). The following anecdote is reported in a study of 'handywomen' midwives who were practising in the United Kingdom in the 1930s:

> 'Oh, I used to love delivering breeches. The breech births were so easy. And we never used to have any problems with them . . . '
> (Leap & Hunter 1993, p. 179)

While one comment from one practitioner cannot be taken as evidence of widespread practice and outcomes, there is a marked contrast between the relaxed approach to breech birth taken by the lay midwife above, and the fear of breech birth experienced by most midwives and other maternity caregivers today. The key issue here is that, even if a diagnosis of breech presentation in late pregnancy leads to a scheduled Caesarean, undiagnosed breech presentation still occurs, and staff need to know how to support women when this happens. Indeed, having weighed the evidence, some women still prefer to birth their breech babies spontaneously, and midwives need to have the skills and experience to support this unusual normal choice.

Mary Cronk is one of the few midwives who has consistently talked and written about this area of practice. Some of her accounts are available at http://www.radmid.demon.co.uk/breech.htm, along with those of other midwives who have been involved in or experienced breech birth (see also www.birthspirit.co.nz). Some of these stories also illustrate the dangers of excessive interference in breech birth, and the fact that some spontaneous labours with undiagnosed breech births can end in tragedy. External Cephalic Version (ECV) is recommended in most cases of breech presentation in late pregnancy, to limit the occurrence of breech birth. However, where the breech does present in labour, some principles seem to be clear from the anecdotal accounts of practitioners with experience in this area:

1. Breech births are likely to maximise optimal maternal and infant physiology, as the body is allowed to descend spontaneously with minimal manipulation, taking the route that brings it optimally through the woman's pelvis. Breech delivery (by active traction and manipulation) may not achieve this end, as it disrupts the processes that might be particular to this mother and this baby.

2. Induction or augmentation of labour, and use of epidural analgesia, also risk disruption of physiological processes. Caesarean section should be considered and discussed with the women early if the labour does not progress spontaneously.

3. Many women with breech presentations spontaneously move to the all-fours position in the active pushing phase of labour. In this case, Mary Cronk says, 'the midwife supports the body once the trunk and arms are born and the head flexes spontaneously (or we can assist it by a finger behind the occiput tipping it forward and a finger in the babies mouth, or two fingers on its cheeks doing the same thing)' (Cronk 2001).

4. Anecdotally, standing breech birth seems to be associated with post-partum haemorrhage (PPH).

5. Women are often observed to begin the active pushing stage kneeling up, then move to a full all-fours position as the head flexes and emerges. This may be a spontaneous response to the mechanisms of a breech birth.

Labouring with twins

Descriptions of skills in normalising twin births are rarely published in the formal literature. Independent midwives, and those working in small non-centralised units or at home are more likely to develop experience in this area than those working in large hospitals. Jane Evans, an independent midwife working in London, published a series of descriptive case studies of spontaneous twin births in 1997 (Evans 1997). Along with additional case studies, these accounts are available on the Association of Radical Midwives website, at http://www.radmid.demon.co.uk/twins.htm.

The general principles underlying the successful stories seem to be the following:

1. The woman herself must be very clear that physiological labour is her goal, but also be prepared to consider intervention if this becomes necessary.

2. The midwife and other caregivers need to have a very clear under-standing of labour physiology, and to be prepared to watch and wait if the labour progresses smoothly, or to make suggestions for change based on this physiological knowledge if progress is not evident, or signs of pathology occur.

3. It helps if all the professional groups involved (midwives, obstetri-cians, paediatricians) have agreed on a plan with the woman and between themselves for a range of eventualities. It is also important for all those involved to accept the benefits of watching and waiting, and, if action is needed, to be willing to act calmly, coherently and with mutual respect for each other and the labouring woman.

4. Twins can be born vaginally in the breech position, or in water. The important elements for successful birth seem to be the positive use of gravity to align the second twin into the pelvic axis, a lack of panic when labour slows between the first and second twin, and a willingness to regularly reconsider what approaches might work for each individual woman/baby triad.

These principles are in line with the approaches that appear to maximise the neurohormonal cycles we have discussed in the first section of this chapter. In each case, seeing the situation through the lens of salutogenesis permits discussion of what is possible, rather than a premature decision about what is impossible. If labour processes are understood using the pillars of health discussed above, more choices become possible for more women.

Labour and birth after Caesarean section

In one of the few published accounts of a salutogenic approach to vagi-nal birth after Caesarean section (VBAC), Hangsleben and colleagues discuss the techniques they used over a 5-year period to support women who were intending to have a VBAC (Hangsleben *et al.* 1989).

Current UK Royal College of Obstetrician and Gynaecologist (RCOG) guidance to women considering a VBAC (based on their Green Top Guideline in this area) cite the risk of uterine rupture after one previous Caesarean section at around 0.5% (RCOG 2007, 2008). The guidance also notes that this risk is higher if labour is induced, if the uterine scar is vertical, or if uterine closure was undertaken in one layer rather than two. These are all factors that need to be established in each woman planning a VBAC.

The RCOG guidelines cite the success of attempted VBAC at 75% after one Caesarean. This indicates that, for most women, the fundamental physiology of a VBAC is the same as for a labour following a previous vaginal birth. Arguably, the only difference lies in the psychological impact on the woman and the caregiver of a fear of uterine rupture, repeat Caesarean, and fetal damage. As we have seen above, the psychology of the situation is a real issue, as such fears have a tangible impact on the physiology of labour and birth. The skills of the midwife in this case are to think salutogenically, to emphasise and encourage normal physiological process, while being quietly vigilant for, and prepared to deal with, the rare but real problems that can arise.

Some practitioners argue that epidural analgesia is contraindicated, as it may mask the pain of uterine dehiscence (Rowbottom *et al.* 1997). This is disputed by others (RCOG 2007). It is possible that the relaxant effect of the epidural agents may reduce the capacity of the pelvic muscles to act as a counterforce to the presenting part, thus limiting fetal rotation, and, consequently, descent, and feedback into Ferguson's reflex and the fetal ejection reflex (Lieberman *et al.* 2005). This outcome, and the inhibiting effects of induction and augmentation of labour on the cyclic processes of labour, would be consistent with our general argument that, if physiological labour processes are disrupted, it is harder for mother and baby to regain the equilibrium and rhythms needed to get the labour back on track. In this case, spontaneous neuro-physiological processes that might help to ease the baby out with minimal disruption to the maternal and fetal 'fit' are overridden by exogenous hormones and pharmacological agents.

This does not mean that VBAC is impossible in the presence of induction, augmentation or epidural analgesia, if the midwife pays attention to some of the techniques and approaches we have suggested above for re-orientating a labour that is veering off track. It is, however, more difficult, and requires more physical effort and more psychological concentration than if a woman undertaking a VBAC is left to enter and progress through labour spontaneously.

In all cases, as for the other unusual labours above, it is crucial to have good relationships with all the maternity team, including with the medical team, so that unexpected pathological events can be quickly identified, and to enable the appropriate response to be taken rapidly, after consultation with the woman. The cardinal sign of imminent or actual uterine rupture is sudden fetal heart rate abnormalities. Suprapubic pain, haemorrhage, or, in extreme cases, maternal shock and collapse may also be present. Given that these events can happen suddenly, optimal birth cannot be achieved for all women without a high level of trust and mutual respect between actual and potential caregivers.

Heidi Rinehart, an American obstetrician, offers the following recommendations to midwives doing home VBACs in the United States (Rinehart 2001). Some of these points are relevant for a UK context, both in and out of hospital:

1. *Learn about the physical and psychological differences in a woman with a previous Caesarean.*

2. *Define the comfort zone of the practitioner to attend VBACs.*
3. *Develop a VBAC practice protocol that reflects the midwife's knowledge or comfort and access to emergency or surgical services in labour.*
4. *Engage in detailed informed consent with the client.*
5. *Perform [or, in the United Kingdom, arrange for] an ultrasound early in the third trimester to rule out a placenta that is overlying the previous scar.*
6. *Know (1) the transport time to the nearest hospital with emergency C-section capabilities, and (2) the time for that hospital to initiate emergency . . . .*
7. *Decide in advance if your VBAC protocol is negotiable or not.*

Shoulder dystocia

True shoulder dystocia is accepted by all practitioners as a situation that carries high risks for the fetus. In this sense, it is not a situation of unusual normality. However, the approach taken by the midwife can significantly reduce the risk of damage to mother and baby, if it is undertaken in line with, and not in opposition to, maternal and fetal physiology. Mismanaged shoulder dystocia can result in mechanical damage (such as Erbs Palsy, or fractures) and acute anoxia, with the ultimate demise of the baby if the situation is not resolved. The issues in this situation are both prevention and management. In terms of prevention, there is no good predictor for a high risk of shoulder dystocia. While fetal weight, maternal obesity, induction and augmentation of labour, slow progress in the first and second stages of labour, and instrumental birth have all been implicated (Gottlieb & Galan 2007; Christie *et al.* 2009), there is still no clear evidence that any or all of these factors are effective predictors of shoulder dystocia. More research work is needed in this area to improve prediction, and, therefore, possibly prevention.

Given that any labour and birth can result in a shoulder dystocia, the key midwifery skills in this situation are recognition and management. The warning signs are widely acknowledged. These include slow advancement of the fetal head in the presence of active pushing, and, specifically, retraction of the head after it is born and prior to restitution. Some midwives refer to this as 'turtle-necking'. This results from a lack of rotation of the fetal shoulders, so that they do not enter the pelvis in the antero-posterior diameter. The shoulders cannot therefore descend from the pelvic brim, and they may become compressed at the brim by further uterine contradictions. The fetal head is retracted back into the vagina as the descent of the shoulders has not occurred.

In a recent clinical review in this area, obstetricians are advised: 'to avoid permanent neuralgic sequelae from shoulder dystocia, clinicians are encouraged to be very mindful of traction applied to the fetal head and neck, to become adept at performance of alternative manoeuvres that instead concentrate on finesse rather than force . . . ' (Gurewitsch 2007, p. 592)

Understanding the physiology of spontaneous labour and birth is critical to the capacity of midwives to use finesse rather than force. With reference to the hormonal cues and actions described above and in Chapter 12, it is crucial that the midwife and all other caregivers continue to work with the labouring woman and her attendants, offering reassurance and support, and enlisting the active help of the woman herself, as a key player in making this birth happen. This will prevent a reversion to a protective fight-or-flight response that might decrease contractions and cause persistent muscular contraction, at a time when the normal mechanisms of labour need to be optimised, and not repressed. Engaging the woman in this way will enable the application of finesse by the midwife in partnership with the woman's efforts, and maximise the chance of a positive birth experience, a healthy baby, and good long-term memories for the mother and her birth attendants.

There are a number of manoeuvres that, if performed properly, do take account of the physiology of the woman and the baby. The McRoberts manoeuvre pays attention to the forces of the uterus and the physiology of the pelvis, and is now well accepted for this situation (Shiers & Coates 2003). It is designed to release the impacted shoulder by helping the mother into a supported supine position, and helping her to hold her legs back in a flexed abducted position to maximise the space in the pelvis. Suprapubic pressure is then applied obliquely to push the impacted shoulder towards the midline and downwards. Shiers and Coates also describe two rotational manoeuvres which are as follows:

Rubins manoeuvre: This is the vaginal identification of the posterior shoulder, which is likely to be further descended into the pelvis than the anterior shoulder, and pushing this anteriorly towards the fetus, to adduct the shoulders and dislodge the posterior shoulder.

Woods screw manoeuvre: This requires rotational force in the opposite direction on the posterior shoulder, causing abduction and rotation, and delivery of the posterior arm to allow more space for rotation of the anterior shoulder.

These manoeuvres are associated with good results in many cases. However, there is an alternative manoeuvre that was developed by the Farm midwives in Tennessee, based on discussion about the possible benefits of using the all-fours position. This discussion was in turn based on observations of indigenous midwives in Latin America, who had learned it from generations of midwives before them. Accounts of using this technique are available at http://www.thefarm.org/midwives/dystocia.html. Bruner and colleagues report that, in a case series of 82 consecutive cases of shoulder dystocia managed with this manoeuvre, 68 (83%) accomplished the birth with no additional intervention. There were no deaths. There was one maternal PPH that did not result in transfusion, two cases of low Apgar scores, and one of a fractured humerous. (Bruner *et al.* 1998). This technique has also been reported in a medical journal more recently (Kovavisarach 2006).

As Meenan and colleagues note:

> The explanation for the success of this maneuver probably lies in movement at the sacroiliac joints at term, which can result in a l-cm to 2-cm increase in the sagittal diameter of the pelvic outlet . . . . . placing the mother on her hands and knees with weight evenly distributed over all four extremities allows rotational movement around a transverse axis through the sacroiliac joints . . . Additional benefit is probably obtained from the movement involved in the actual change of position, which may help to disimpact the shoulders, and the addition of gravity to the forces tending to push the posterior shoulder anteriorly, allowing it to slide over the sacral promontory.
>
> (Meenan *et al.* 1991)

Conclusion

Famously, Nicky Leap has claimed that 'the less we do the more we give' (Leap 2000). In a similar vein, Holly Kennedy has referred to 'the art of *doing nothing* well' (Kennedy 2002). These authors are not describing a passive process of withdrawal and non-engagement, but a sophisticated skill that includes watching, waiting and the kind of active being-with-women that Patricia Benner (borrowing from the phenomenologist philosopher Heidegger) has called 'presencing' (Benner 1984). Kennedy, Anderson and Leap discuss this concept in more detail in Chapter 7. This is a highly focused, concentrated skill that, as Berg and Dahlberg note, can 'support the natural processes, particularly . . . in apparently hopeless cases . . . '. (Berg & Dahlberg 2001). This approach is not just about standing back and letting the woman make blind choices. It involves taking part in a kind of dance in which, according to Lundgren and Dahlberg (2001), expert caregivers 'wait for the woman' when things are going well, but are ready to 'seize' her when she needs the insights, confidence and skills of an expert to refocus the atmosphere and change the conversation, in terms of what is said, what is done and how it is done, and what practical changes might help.

In a systematic review of expert intrapartum care, Downe *et al.* (2007) have hypothesised that the skills required to maximise the best possible outcomes in situations of unusual normal birth are a subtle mixture of wisdom, skilled practice, and enacted vocation. These skills are not acquired overnight by reading up about a list of clinical tricks and methods. Equally, they do not necessarily require years of practice: the expert maternity care practitioner seems to be able to learn quickly and effectively through being constantly curious and open to possibility, while maintaining complete respect for unexpected pathology. This respect includes effective skills to deal with such events if they arise.

The increasingly complex interconnectivity revealed by our growing insights into the science of emotion and physiology provides a way of seeing that can help caregivers to acknowledge and understand the uniquely normal physiological rhythm of most women in labour. It also provides a way of understanding the skills of expert caregivers in these situations, particularly in dealing with uncertainty and complexity. These issues are explored further in Chapter 16. This new scientific paradigm also serves to support a statement made by an obstetrician over 50 years ago:

> ... it is amazing how little of fact is know about the simplest phases of reproduction. The field for research here is widely open.
>
> (Montgomery 1958)

References

Albers LL, Schiff M, Gorwoda JG (1996) The length of active labor in normal pregnancies. *Obstetrics and Gynecology* 87(3): 355–9.

Altman MR, Lydon-Rochelle MT (2006) Prolonged second stage of labor and risk of adverse maternal and perinatal outcomes: a systematic review. *Birth* 33(4): 315–22.

Anderson T (2000) Feeling safe enough to let go: the relationship between the woman and her midwife during the second stage of labour. In Kirkham M (ed) *The Midwife–Mother Relationship*. London, Macmillan Press Ltd, 92.

Andrasik F, Rime C (2007) Can behavioural therapy influence neuromodulation? *Neurological Sciences* 28(Suppl 1): S124–9.

Antonovsky A (1987) *Unravelling the Mystery of Health – How People Manage Stress and Stay Well*. San Francisco, Jossey Bass Publisher.

Beck U (1992) *Risk Society: Towards a New Modernity*. New Delhi, Sage.

Benner P (1984) *From novice to expert: Excellence and Power in Clinical Nursing Practice*. Menlo Park, Addison-Wesley.

Berg M, Dahlberg K (2001) Swedish midwives care of women who are at high obstetric risk, or who have obstetric complications. *Midwifery* 17: 259–66.

Bergstrom L, Seidel J, Skillman-Hull L (1997) 'I gotta push. Please let me push!' Social interactions during the change from first to second stage labor. *Birth* 24: 173–80.

Berkeley C, Fairburn JS, White C (1931) *Midwifery by Ten Teachers*, 4th edition. London, Edward Arnold & Company.

Bruce S, McEwen BS, John C, Wingfield JC (2003) The concept of allostasis in biology and biomedicine. *Hormones and Behavior* 43(1): 2–15.

Bruner JP, Drummond SB, Meenan AL, Gaskin IM (1998) All-fours maneuver for reducing shoulder dystocia during labor. *Journal of Reproductive Medicine* 43(5): 439–43.

Carter CS, Lederhendler II, Kirkpatrick B (eds) (1999) *The Integrative Neurobiology of Affiliation*. Cambridge, MIT Press.

Christie LR, Harriott JA, Mitchell SY, Fletcher HM, Bambury IG (2009) Shoulder dystocia in a Jamaican cohort. *International Journal of Gynaecology and Obstetrics* 104(1): 25–7.

Cluett ER, Pickering RM, Getliffe K, St George Saunders NJ (2004) Randomised controlled trial of labouring in water compared with standard of augmentation for management of dystocia in first stage of labour. *British Medical Journal* 328(7435): 314.

Cronk M (2001) Comment, available from: http://www.radmid.demon.co.uk/breech.htm (accessed 02/02/09).

Downe S (2003) Transition and the second stage of labour. In Fraser D, Cooper M (eds) *Myles Textbook for Midwives*, 14th edition. London, Harcourt Health Sciences.

Downe S (2004a) The concept of normality in the maternity services: application and consequences. In Frith L (ed) *Ethics and Midwifery: Issues in Contemporary Practice*, 2nd edition. Oxford, Butterworth Heinemann.

Downe S (2004b) Transition and the second stage of labour. In Henderson C, MacDonald S (eds) *Mayes Midwifery*, 13th edition. London, Harcourt Health Sciences.

Downe S, Dykes F (2009) Counting time in pregnancy and labour. In McCourt C (ed) *Time and Maternity Care*. Oxford, Elsevier.

Downe S, McCourt C (2004) From being to becoming: reconstructing childbirth knowledges. In S Downe (ed) *Normal Childbirth; Evidence and Debate*. London, Churchill Livingstone.

Downe S, Simpson L, Trafford K (2007) Expert intrapartum maternity care: a meta-synthesis. *Journal of Advanced Nursing* 57(2): 127–40.

Downe S, Young C, Hall-Moran S; Trent Midwifery Research Group (2008) Multiple midwifery discourses: the case of the early pushing urge. In Downe S (ed) *Normal Birth, Evidence and Debate*, 2nd edition. Oxford, Elsevier.

Eriksson M, Mattsson LA, Ladfors L (1997) Early or late bath during the first stage of labour: a randomised study of 200 women. *Midwifery* 13(3): 146–8.

Evans J (1997) Can a twin birth be a positive experience? *Midwifery Matters* 74: 6–11.

Festinger L (1957) *A Theory of Cognitive Dissonance*. Evanston , IL, Row, Peterson.

Fettes I, Fox J, Kuzniak S, Shime J, Gare D (1984) Plasma levels of immunoreactive beta-endorphin and adrenocorticotropic hormone during labor and delivery. *Obstetrics and Gynecology* 64(3): 359–62.

Fleming AS, Corter C, Stallings J, Steiner M (2002) Testosterone and prolactin are associated with emotional responses to infant cries in new fathers. *Hormones and Behavior* 42(4): 399–413.

Friedman EA (1955) Primigravid labor; a graphicostatistical analysis. *Obstetrics and Gynecology* 6(6): 567–89.

Gaskin IM (2003) Sphincter law. In May I (ed) *Guide to Childbirth*. New York, Bantam Books, 167–82.

Gottlieb AG, Galan HL (2007) Shoulder dystocia: an update. *Obstetrics and Gynecology Clinics of North America* 34(3): 501–31.

Grumbach K, Bodenheimer T (2004) Can health care teams improve primary care practice? *The Journal of the American Medical Association* 291(10): 1246–51.

Gurewitsch ED (2007) Optimizing shoulder dystocia management to prevent birth injury. *Clinical Obstetrics and Gynecology* 50(3): 592–606.

Hangsleben KL, Taylor MA, Lynn NM (1989) VBAC program in a nurse-midwifery service. Five years of experience. *Journal of Midwifery and Womens Health* 34(4): 179–84.

Hannah ME, Hannah WJ, Hewson SA, Hodnett ED, Saigal S, Willan AR (2000) Planned caesarean section versus planned vaginal birth for breech presentation at term: a randomised multicentre trial. *Lancet* 356: 1375–83.

Hansen SL, Clark SL, Foster JC (2002) Active pushing versus passive fetal descent in the second stage of labor: a randomized controlled trial. *Obstetrics and Gynecology* 99(1): 29–34.

Health Care Commission (2006) *Investigation into 10 Maternal Deaths at, or Following Delivery at, Northwick Park Hospital, North West London Hospitals NHS Trust*, between April 2002 and April 2005, available from: http://www.healthcarecommission.org.uk/_db/_documents/Northwick_tagged.pdf (Accessed 02/02/09) http://www3.interscience.wiley.com/journal/120829153/abstract?CRETRY=1&SRETRY=0 - c1#c1

Heasman L, Spencer JAD, Symonds ME (1997) Plasma prolactin concentrations after caesarean section or vaginal delivery. *Archives of Disease in Childhood Fetal and Neonatal Edition* 77(3): 237F–8F.

Hodnett ED, Gates S, Hofmeyr GJ, Sakala C (2007) Continuous support for women during childbirth. *Cochrane Database of Systematic Reviews* (3).

Hogle KL, Kilburn L, Hewson S, Gafni A, Wall R, Hannah ME (2003) Impact of the international term breech trial on clinical practice and concerns: a survey of centre collaborators. *Journal of Obstetrics and Gynaecology Canada* 25(1): 14–6.

Hunter B (2004) Conflicting ideologies as a source of emotion work in midwifery. *Midwifery* 20(3): 261–72.

Jordan B (1993) *Birth in Four Cultures*, 4th edition. Prospect Heights, Waveland Press.

Kennedy HP (2002) The midwife as an 'Instrument' of care. *American Journal of Public Health* 92(11): 1759–60.

Kovavisarach E (2006) The "all-fours" maneuver for the management of shoulder dystocia. *International Journal of Gynecology and Obstetrics* 95(2): 153–4.

Kuhn TS (1962) *The Structure of Scientific Revolutions*. Chicago, University of Chicago Press.

Leap N (2000) The less we do, the more we give. In Kirkham MJ (ed) *The Midwife–Mother Relationship*. London, MacMillian Press Ltd.

Leap N, Hunter B (1993) *The Midwife's Tale: An Oral History from Handywoman to Professional Midwife*. London, Scarlet Press.

Lieberman E, Davidson K, Lee-Parritz A, Shearer E (2005) Changes in fetal position during labor and their association with epidural analgesia. *Obstetrics and Gynecology* 105(5, Pt 1): 974–82.

Lundgren I, Dahlberg K (2001) Midwives' experience of the encounter with women and their pain during childbirth. *Midwifery* 18(2): 155–64.

MANA (1998) Report on Cervical Reversal. MANA Newsletter, 16, 2, 16 March 1998.

McKay S, Barrows T, Roberts J (1990) Women's views of second-stage labor as assessed by interviews and videotapes. *Birth* 17: 192–8.

Meenan AL, Gaskin IM, Hunt P, Ball CA (1991) A new (old) maneuver for the management of shoulder dystocia. *Journal of Family Practice* 33(4): 337–8. Also available at: www.thefarm.org/midwives/dystocia.html (accessed 29/01/09).

Monga A Baker P (eds) (2006) *Obstetrics by Ten Teachers.* London, Hodder Arnold.

Montgomery TL (1958) Physiologic considerations in labor and the puerperium. *American Journal of Obstetrics Gynaecology* 76: 706–15.

Myles MF (1975) *A Textbook for Midwives*, 8th edition. Edinburgh, Churchill Livingstone Ltd.

Odent M (1987) The fetus ejection reflex. *Birth* 14(2): 104–5.

Ontario Womens Health Council (2001) *Attaining and Maintaining Best Practices in the Use of Caesarean Sections*, available from: http://www.womens healthcouncil.com/E/index.html (accessed 02/02/09).

O'Sullivan G, Liu B, Hart D, Seed P, Shennan A (2009) A randomised controlled trial to evaluate the effect of food intake during labour on obstetric outcome. *British Medical Journal* 338: b784.

Pedersen CA, Boccia ML (2002) Oxytocin links mothering received, mothering bestowed and adult stress responses. *Stress* 4: 259–67.

Pervanidou P (2008) Biology of post-traumatic stress disorder in childhood and adolescence. *Journal of Neuroendocrinology* 20(5): 632–8.

RCOG (2007) *Green-top Guideline No. 45: Birth after Previous Caesarean Birth*, available from: http://www.rcog.org.uk/resources/Public/pdf/green_top45_birthafter.pdf (accessed 02/02/09).

RCOG (2008) *Birth after Previous Caesarean: Information for You RCOG.* London, available from: http://www.rcog.org.uk/index.asp?pageID=2514 (accessed 02/02/09).

Reichman O, Gdansky E, Latinsky B, Labi S, Samueloff A (2008) Digital rotation from occipito-posterior to occipito-anterior decreases the need for cesarean section. *European Journal of Obstetrics, Gynecology, and Reproductive Biology* 136(1): 25–8.

Rinehart H (2001) *A VBAC Primer: Technical Issues for Midwives Midwifery Today* Issue 57. Also available at: http://www.midwiferytoday.com/articles/vbacprimer.asp (accessed 02/02/09).

Rippin-Sisler CS (1996) The experience of precipitate labor. *Birth* 23(4): 224–8.

Rizzolatti G, Sinigaglia C (2007) *Mirror in the Brain.* Translated by Anderson F. New York, Oxford University Press.

Roberts J, Hanson L (2007) Best practices in second stage labor care: maternal bearing down and positioning. *Journal of Midwifery & Women's Health* 52(3): 238–45.

Rouse DJ, Owen J, Savage KG, Hauth JC (2001) Active phase labor arrest: revisiting the 2-hour minimum. *Obstetrics and Gynecology* 98(4): 550–4.

Rowbottom SJ, Critchley LA, Gin T (1997) Uterine rupture and epidural analgesia during trial of labour. *Anaesthesia* 52: 486–8.

Scaglia HE, Margulies M, Galimberti D *et al.* (1981) Binding of prolactin by fetal human lung cell membrane fractions. *La Ricerca in Clinica e in Laboratorio* 11(3): 279–82.

Schmid V (2007) *Salute e Nascita, la Salutogenesi in Gravidanza*. Milano, Apogeo ed.

Scott LD, Rogers AE, Hwang WT, Zhang Y (2006) Effects of critical care nurses' work hours on vigilance and patients' safety. *American Journal of Critical Care* 15(1): 30–7.

Shiers C, Coates T (2003) Midwifery and obstetric emergencies. In Fraser DF, Cooper MA (eds) *Myles Textbook for Midwives*, 14th edition, 599–619. London, Churchill Livingstone.

Simkin P Ancheta R (2005) *The Labor Progress Handbook*. Oxford, Blackwell Science.

Soloman V (1985) The emerging field of psychoneuroimmunology advances. *Journal of Institute for the Advancement of Health* 2(1): 6–19.

Soltis J, Wegner FH, Newman JD (2005) Urinary prolactin is correlated with mothering and allo-mothering in squirrel monkeys. *Physiology and Behavior* 84(2): 295–301.

Sternberg EM (2000) *The Balance Within: The Science Connecting Health and Emotions*. San Francisco, W. H. Freeman.

Sutton J, Scott P (1995) *Understanding and Teaching Optimal Foetal Positioning*. Birth Concepts. NZ.

Taylor S (2003) *The Tending Instinct, Women, Men and the Biology of Relationships*, Holt Paperbacks.

Taylor A, Fisk NM, Glover V (2000) Mode of delivery and subsequent stress response. *Lancet* 355(9198): 120.

Tolino A, de Conciliis B, Romano L, Graziano E (1983) Fetal prolactin levels and respiratory distress syndrome. *Clinical and Experimental Obstetrics and Gynecology* 10(4): 198–200.

Tyzio R, Cossart R, Khalilov I, *et al.* (2006) Maternal oxytocin triggers a transient inhibitory switch in GABA signaling in the fetal brain during delivery. *Science* 314: 1788–92.

Walsh D (2006) 'Nesting' and 'Matrescence': distinctive features of a free-standing birth centre. *Midwifery* 22(3): 228–39.

Whyte H, Hannah ME, Saigal S; Term Breech Trial Collaborative Group (2004) Outcomes of children at 2 years after planned cesarean birth versus planned vaginal birth for breech presentation at term: the International Randomized Term Breech Trial. *American Journal of Obstetrics and Gynecology* 3: 864–71.

Winberg J (2005) Mother and newborn baby: mutual regulation of physiology and behavior: a selective review. *Developmental Psychobiology* 47(3): 217–29.

Young LJ (2009) Being human: love: neuroscience reveals all. *Nature* 457: 148.

Zadoroznyj M (2001) Birth and the 'reflexive consumer': trust, risk and medical dominance in obstetric encounters. *Journal of Sociology* 37(2): 117–39.

Zak PJ, Kurzban R, Matzner WT (2005) Oxytocin is associated with human trustworthiness. *Hormones and Behavior* 48(5): 522–7.

Chapter 11
Psychology and Labour Experience: Birth as a Peak Experience

Gill Thompson

In this chapter, insights from a doctoral study into women's birth stories are presented. An interpretive phenomenological study was undertaken to explore women's lived experiences and meanings of traumatic and subsequent positive birth experiences. It aimed to gain a greater understanding of how women experience and internalise diverse childbirth accounts and the implications of birth on post-natal well-being.

Whilst this study set out to explore traumatic as well as positive birth experiences, it is the latter experience which is addressed in this chapter. In-depth interviews with 12 women uncovered insights into the nature of a positive birth, and the meanings attached to this experience. Three key themes are presented in this chapter. The first theme of 'the value of connections' explores the relationships formed between women and health professionals during a positive birth. The second theme of 'it was all about me' describes how a joyful birth can represent a unique and embodied experience. Furthermore, by drawing upon the works of a humanist and existentialist psychologist, Abraham Maslow (1962, 1970), the third theme explores how birth can represent a 'peak experience' for some women.

Introduction

Childbirth is considered to be a significant rite of passage in a woman's life, as they move from one social status into another (Hall & Taylor 2004). The experience of childbirth is signified as an emotional as well as a physical experience, which has the potential for permanent or long-term consequences (Simkin 1991) for women, babies and wider social networks. A positive birth is considered to enhance a woman's self-esteem and sense of femininity and move them towards emotional and spiritual growth (Simkin 1991; Raphael-Leff 1991; Callister *et al.* 2003; Brown & Phipps 2004). Moreover, this experience has also been associated with a more successful transition into motherhood through the establishment of maternal bonds and family relationships (Mercer 1985; Simkin 1992). However, empirical insights into the nature of a positive birth and women's perceptions of this experience were difficult to elicit within the literature. An overview of the current research together with its inability to fully explain this phenomenon will now be presented.

The maternity literature identifies a number of factors associated with positive maternal outcomes (such as satisfaction with the birth and emotional well-being). These variables include women's perceptions of pain, expectations, control, social support, number of obstetric interventions performed and quality of care received (Green *et al.* 1990; Brown & Lumley 1994; Waldenstrom *et al.* 1996, 1999). However, one of the key limitations is that the majority of studies utilised quantitative methodologies. Women are presented with a predetermined list of discrete variables, and asked to score their responses using numerical scales. Subsequently, the conclusions from this research are drawn from statistical analysis of the data ('positivist' approach to research). The arguments against this approach are that these methods do not assess the interconnected and multifaceted nature of childbirth, nor do they address women's subjective responses towards these events.

Over the last few decades there has been a surge of interest in the utility of qualitative-based methodologies to elicit the actual meanings of phenomena, as opposed to drawing inferences from quantitative-based data (Sandelowski 1997). In the maternity care literature, qualitative methods such as interviews and observational analysis are increasingly being used to uncover person-centred insights into the childbirth phenomenon. For instance, Halldorsdottir and Karlsdottir (1996a,b) adopted a phenomenological approach to assess women's 'journey' through a natural physiological birth (1996a), as well as women's experiences of caring and uncaring encounters with their caregivers (1996b). A grounded theory approach was adopted by Walker *et al.* (1995) to explore women's experiences of transfer from hospital to home during the second stages of labour. Qualitative research has illuminated insights into women's experiences of types of birth (water, vaginal, Caesarean), birth environments (birth centre, hospital, home), models of care (midwifery or consultant led) as well as specific bio-psychosocial aspects of the birth experience (such as decision-making, control, augmentation, pain and quality of care). However, the main limitation of this research is that they have tended to focus on a specific aspect of birth, rather than women's experiences of childbirth per se. To date, therefore, there appears to be limited qualitative insights into a positive birth event.

A further rationale for the limited insights into positive birth is that a number of authors have highlighted a pathological focus within the childbirth literature (Downe & McCourt 2004). The argument follows that research has been directed towards the identification of potentially negative influences (such as augmentation of labour, obstetric interventions, operative deliveries) and longer term sequelae (such as the development of post-traumatic stress disorder, depression, physical complications) of childbirth. The dominance of this pathological perspective could be argued to perpetuate and magnify the fear and permeation of a 'risk surveillance' (Walsh *et al.* 2004) culture within maternity care. Furthermore, searching for negatives and dissatisfaction in maternity care is unlikely to uncover positive aspects of birth.

Limitations with current research and rationale for study

The profound and transformative nature of childbirth is frequently cited in the literature (Mauger 1996; Callister *et al.* 2003; Beech & Phipps 2008). Empirical research into the positive birth phenomenon is however, somewhat limited. Whilst research has identified predictors of positive childbirth, these findings tend to be generated through inferential statistics, rather than a person-centred perspective. The danger of this approach is that meanings are objectively constructed rather than subjectively generated. Whilst qualitative- and interpretive-based accounts have been undertaken, they have largely focused on specific aspects of the birth, rather than the nature and meanings of a positive birth experience.

The research discussed here embraced a more 'appreciative focus' towards childbirth, by uncovering insights into what was good, positive and working well in maternity services. This chapter presents a number of the themes into women's experiences of a positive birth. The findings presented illuminate how a positive birth was achieved, experienced and internalised.

Study method

Recruitment methods

A purposive sampling method was adopted to identify participants who had experienced a traumatic and subsequent positive birth to take part in the research. All participants were recruited through the local consultant midwife from a North-West Maternity Unit in England.

Within the selected National Health Service (NHS) trust, all women who have experienced a self-defined difficult and distressing childbirth are referred through to the consultant midwife for after-birth services. The sample of women engaged in this study related to those who had recently completed or were receiving ongoing support through this service. All, bar one of the women approached, agreed to participate in this study; the remaining women provided no response.

There were two recruitment phases within the research. Phase one consisted of recruiting women who had already experienced a self-defined traumatic and positive birth. Eight women were recruited during phase one; and these women presented at various post-natal periods. Phase two adopted a longitudinal design. Four women were interviewed who had previously experienced a traumatic birth, and were currently pregnant with a subsequent baby (interview 1). A further interview (interview 2) was conducted at 3 months post-natally. All women (across both phases) were also engaged in a final interpretation meeting to discuss the key themes generated from the findings. A total of 28 interviews were conducted.

Procedure

In-depth interviews were undertaken during August (2005) to November (2006). At the start of the interview, women were presented with a broad open-ended question designed to elicit their birth story, and their emotional responses towards their experiences: 'Please can you tell me about your childbirth experience(s) and your feelings and perceptions regarding this/these experience(s)?' Once the women's story had been recounted, open prompt questions were used to obtain clarification and description of the key issues which had emerged.

During the final interpretation meeting, a more conversational approach was adopted. During this meeting, I discussed each of the thematic areas with women, collecting additional information and exploration of the issues identified.

Participants

The participants were aged between 27 and 40 years. One of the participants was of Indian ethnic background, and the remaining women were of white-British descent. Ten of the women were married, and two were currently residing with partners who were not the biological father of their first child.

Nine of the twelve self-defined traumatic births involved an assisted vaginal or operative delivery, and the remaining three were officially recorded as uncomplicated vaginal deliveries. With regard to the positive birth experiences, eight were recorded as uncomplicated vaginal deliveries and four were Caesarean sections (two elective and two unplanned).

In the subsequent birth, four of the women changed NHS Trusts. Six of the women were allocated to a caseload team and the rest received care under a 'traditional' model. A definition of a 'traditional' model in the context of this research is where the woman received care from different midwives across pre, intra- and post-partum periods. The midwife who attends the birth was allocated on the woman's arrival at the delivery suite. Apart from one woman who opted for a home birth for her second parturition, the remaining birth experiences took place in a large maternity unit.

Ethical issues

Ethics approval was obtained through the local NHS Research Ethics Committee, and the sponsoring University Ethics' Committee.

Data analysis

An interpretive phenomenological approach was adopted for this research, based on Gadamer (2004) philosophical hermeneutics. Hermeneutics is a contemporary philosophy that emphasises the human experiences of understanding and interpretation (Thompson 1990). It offers a person-centred approach in exploring the meanings and lived experienced of phenomena.

All interviews were audio-taped and transcribed, and data analysis was supported by MaxQDA qualitative data-analysis software.

The stages adopted for analysis are listed below. For further information on their detail, please email the author (see Credits Page).

1. Explication of pre-understandings
2. Submersion within phenomena
3. Fusion of horizons (exposition of themes)
4. Rich descriptions of phenomenon

Study findings

Three themes have been presented in this section to illuminate the meanings and lived experiences of positive birth experiences. The theme 'the value of connections' portrays the significance of the woman–caregiver relationship. The second theme 'it was all about me' explores how a positive birth is a unique woman-led affair. An experience of mind–body connection as women felt that they birthed their babies irrespective of the mode of birth. The final theme draws upon the work of Abraham Maslow to explore 'birth as a peak experience'. The resonances between Maslow descriptions of a peak experience and positive birth reflect how birth can be a euphoric and transformative experience for some women.

The value of connections

The women's narratives suggested that social, emotional, physiological and intuitive connections were forged between women and caregivers (midwifery as well as medical professionals) during a positive birth. This is not to say that all of the interactions with clinical staff during a positive birth were happy ones; rather that the ethos and dominant philosophy overarching a positive birth experience was one of connectivity, reciprocity and mutuality.

All of the women in this study received continuity of carer during their positive birth in that the same caregivers attended throughout their labour and delivery.

> She [midwife] was great, she was wonderful, there was just me, X [husband] and her right the way through to the end (Kate)

Ultimately, however, it was not due to continuity per se which created a meaningful and valued relationship; rather it was the women's trust in their caregivers.

> I just felt like, because I had so much trust in her [midwife] I knew that whatever happened it would be OK, it would be OK (Diane)

Through trust, a number of these women considered that their intrinsic needs would be met. Furthermore, it was the personal and professional qualities of the clinical staff which appeared to determine whether trust was formed. Women spoke of the 'support', 'kindness', 'reassurance' and 'encouragement' provided by the health professionals. Caregivers in a positive birth were characterised by a 'natural', 'calm', 'relaxed' and 'professional' manner, as well as an ability to find humour to 'break the tension'.

These health professionals were considered to be an essential part of a woman's positive birth journey.

> Just the feeling that they really are there for you, they really get you through it and they want the best for you, and just got real bonding and understanding (Janet)

The women believed that their birth was important to caregivers, and that they 'really mattered' as a unique person, woman and expectant mother. This depth of connection was considered to make the experience 'so special' for women.

Women also made reference to the 'presence' of their caregivers. The term 'presence' in the nursing and midwifery literature is used to describe care which operates from a humanistic paradigm.

> embodiment of mind, body and spirit, that is a conscious ability of the nurse to value presence within nurse-patient encounters as essential to understanding patients' experiences
>
> (Welch & Wellard 2005, p. 5)

In a positive birth experience, women frequently viewed the midwife's presence as being 'there when I needed her'.

> X [husband] and I were left on our own a lot of the time really, we just got on with it and then X [midwife] just popped back in and out and do bits of monitoring and go back out again and it was nice just the two of us, that's how it started, just the two of us (Kate)

As highlighted within Kate's birth narrative, her caregiver intuitively knew when her physical presence was warranted, and when she wanted to labour on her own with her birth partner. These perceptive connections between health professionals and women enabled women to labour the way they had envisioned.

A selection of the women in this research described their caregivers as 'friends'. The women allocated to the caseload team were able to forge these 'friendships' during the prenatal period. However, the other women like Sonia who received care under a traditional model described a bond which was formed instantaneously.

> it was almost like a best friend was there (Sonia)

Whilst the concept of 'friend' has been alluded to within the literature (Leap 2000; Pairman 2000), the insights from this research suggested that women viewed caregivers as a 'professional friend' (Pairman 2000). Women valued their caregivers' professional expertise over the physiological processes of childbirth, as well as the personal consideration of what they wanted to achieve.

> she [midwife] showed me how to maybe go into a different position where it might be easier because of the way you know my cervix was and everything to deliver and she was just so nice ... she really was ... so glad to have met her (Holly)

The women in this study appeared to treasure the specialist as well as the emotional basis of care provided by their health professionals. They viewed their engagement with health professionals as a partnership; a shared relationship in which both parties worked towards an optimum birth experience.

As the woman in this research received care from either a caseload team or a traditional model, a significant difference to emerge amongst the narratives related to 'being known'.

All the women who received midwifery-led care spoke of the reassurance, trust, encouragement and empathic understanding they received prenatally. Through 'being known', their caregivers were considered to understand where they were 'coming from' and what they ultimately wanted to achieve. Women felt safe in the knowledge that their midwives wanted 'the best experience' for them. In turn, this enhanced their confidence and reduced their stress levels prior to and during the labour and birth.

Within this research, however, mothers allocated under both models of care (traditional and midwifery) described the same value-based humanistic model of care provision. All women trusted their caregivers, and highlighted respect, support, value, encouragement as well as professional expertise in the care they received. Therefore, the women in this research may register 'being known' as a facet of care which 'really mattered' because they were provided with this option, rather than this demonstrate some 'gold standard' of care.

It was all about me

> I was centre stage. I took the lead and they were there as the supporting cast (Kate)

The narratives revealed that a positive birth was a unique, individually determined, woman-led affair. It represented an embodied experience: an integration of mind, body and spirit, as women were active, engaged, informed and 'in control' over the birth.

In Clare's birth story she had originally planned for a home birth. Whilst a forceps delivery (due to breech presentation) was performed in the hospital delivery suite, she still considered the birth to be a fulfilling, joyful experience.

> he [doctor] asked me, and it was amazing really I was asked, so it was my choice and I'm in control and even though she [daughter] was breech and needed forceps with the head and stuff it was me, it was still me, I was in control and I gave birth to her vaginally (Clare)

Within the positive birth scenarios, clinical practices and procedures (such as fetal monitoring) were undertaken to suit the labouring woman. Sonia talked about her 'space' within the delivery suite as she tried various positions and labouring aids (such as the birthing ball). Fetal monitoring was undertaken in whatever position she was in, rather than determined by the needs of her caregivers.

Previous research has suggested that 'being informed' is central to a woman's perception of control (Lundgren & Dahlberg 1998; Lavender *et al.* 1999; Kennedy *et al.* 2004; Edwards 2005). In Kate's story, her midwife showed and explained all the equipment in the delivery suite, 'just in case'.

> if you've got that information knowledge, like she [midwife] said I'm gonna have to apply a bit of pressure, I'm gonna have to pull, do a bit of tinkering. It's like right fine, tinker away (Kate)

The information and concern taken to explain these obstetric tools enabled Kate to feel informed and in control over what happened to her. Furthermore, Kate was happy for the midwife to take unilateral decisions, safe in the knowledge as to why these procedures were required. Indeed, across a number of the women's narratives it was generally only when their birth deviated from an anticipated outcome (such as the decision for Caesarean) did they become engaged in decision-making. These insights thereby suggested that it is not necessarily the procedures or interventions which women object to during childbirth. It is whether the women felt fully informed as to the justification for procedures, mediated by the mutual respect and feeling valued by caregivers.

A joyful birth was characterised by a calm, quiet and relaxed sense of normality for women.

> it was dead peaceful, you read about books in natural birth having candles and soft music and this environment was great, it was like that even though I was in an operating theatre, it was calm and happy (Kathy)

Furthermore, these descriptions were provided irrespective of how and where the baby was delivered (vaginal (delivery room) or Caesarean (operating theatre)).

A positive birth was also facilitated by natural, cyclical and embodied time.

> didn't feel rushed about anything or pushed into any decisions, plenty of time to make choices, there was no urgency even when we went to hospital there was no urgency because we were both fine and that's way I wanted it really I didn't want us to get distressed (Jill)

There was no 'urgency' or 'rush' during a positive birth. Time was available for women to labour at their own pace, and they were afforded sufficient time to make decisions. In Jill's birth story, this represented her eventual request for an elective Caesarean.

A spiritual perspective of childbirth is that when women give birth they have to face the unknown – a dark, anxiety-provoking situation through which they become transformed into mothers (Burkhardt & Nagai-Jacobson 2002). The interpretive insights of Anderson (2000) have suggested that women enter the liminal phase of childbirth by 'letting go' (2000). 'Letting go' characterises a state in which women are free from psychological interruptions or concerns as they submit to the will (physiological processes) of childbirth (Anderson 2000). This concept reflects a paradoxical situation in that as women felt 'in control' of their labour, they were able to be 'out of control' to give birth; to surrender to the transformational process of childbirth.

The paradox of 'letting go' was evident within a number of the women's birth stories; and is reflected in Janet's narrative as follows.

> With X's [son] birth I was just able to get on with what my body was doing and I didn't think about anything (Janet)

In the literature, 'letting go' is associated with a natural physiological birth (Anderson 2000; Parratt & Fahy 2003; Edwards 2005; Lundgren 2005). In the current study, 'letting go' also appeared to happen for women who underwent a Caesarean or instrumental delivery. Although these women were not necessarily succumbing to physiological impulses, the women's bodies still experienced sensations outside of their normal boundaries of personal control. To be an integral part of the birth experience and retain control over what was happening to them, women still needed to let go of their fears and surrender to the birth. Lowe (2000) suggested that the ultimate control relates to a woman's ability to relinquish control, to be one with her body and actively participate in the experience of childbirth. During a positive birth, it would appear that the release of control to be in control occurred irrespective of the mode of birth. This is revealed by Kathy who described her Caesarean section as:

> I still feel that my body did it (Kathy)

The descriptions offered by women portray an embodied experience of birth. This represents mind–body connectedness, as psychological and physiological responses operate in harmony to create a transcendental experience. Subsequently, the majority of women in this study felt that they had given birth to their babies, regardless of whether the baby was a vaginal, instrumental or operative birth.

Birth as a peak experience

> Straight after X's [son] birth I felt elated, exhausted, erm, amazed,
> exhilarated, like I'd just .. conquered the world . . . . I felt fantastic
> (Diane)

The findings from this research have revealed that women's experiences of a positive birth resonate with Maslow's (1962, 1970) insights into 'peak experience'. To illuminate these similarities, Maslow's description of a peak experience has been elaborated on below, interleaved with extracts from the women's narratives.

Whilst Maslow was studying the psychology of health, he identified frequent reports of transcendental mystical experiences. These were referred to as *peak experiences* to reflect a naturally occurring phenomenon rather than denoting a religious context (Maslow 1970). Maslow believed these experiences, which occur in any culture at any time, to be universal (Maslow 1970). Whilst these experiences may only last from a few seconds to a few minutes, he considered that they represent our 'healthiest moments' (Maslow 1962).

Maslow uncovered that whilst there was no conformity in the nature or form of peak experiences, there were strong parallels in the emotional responses they induced. He also conceived that these occurrences are not created through will, but occur as a by-product of an experience.

> We cannot command the peak experience, it happens to us.
> (Maslow 1962, p. 87)

In drawing comparisons with positive birth experiences, the element of 'surprise' was evident in the narratives. A number of women I interviewed expressed surprise that birth could be an enjoyable event. For women to be able to 'enjoy', 'love' and even 'relish' childbirth was often met with amazement.

> I could go as far as saying ... I know it sounds a bit bizarre but
> I actually enjoyed the experience. (Clare)

Maslow considered peak experiences to be eureka moments; transcendental ecstatic states through which we can find enlightenment ('defining moments of being', Maslow 1959). Similarly, the majority of women in this research had euphoric reactions to their positive birth. Metaphors such as 'conquering' and on 'top' of the world were used to express their ecstatic reactions. The intense and overwhelming nature of emotions was described by Jules following her planned Caesarean section.

> Oooh you couldn't get that feeling with anything on earth, drugs, alcohol, anything, I just wanted to bottle it and keep it forever that feeling, and I still get it (Jules)

Peak experiences are described by Maslow (1962) as self-validating events, in that they carried intrinsic values to the individual (1962, p. 79). This depiction was evident in the positive birth scenarios through the enhanced self-worth and new-found capabilities that ensued. A fulfilling, joyful birth left women feeling 'strong', 'powerful' and 'capable of anything'.

> I thought yeah I've done that (given birth) and I just felt that I could achieve anything it was a real, you know, sort of really boosted my self-esteem, it was amazing, I just felt wow, I am incredible (Jackie)

A further point of convergence between these descriptions is that like peak experiences, a selection of these women made reference to the 'overflow of energy' (Maslow 1970) which accompanied a positive birth. This uplifted them into a transformed metaphysical state: an incredible adrenaline burst which led them to define themselves as 'amazing', 'tremendous' and 'fantastic' beings. For Ann, the unending source of positive energy she experienced following the birth made her feel 'good to be alive'.

> you know my energy had no boundaries . . . . I was bouncing around the house, and I was really erm, erm, full of the .. joys you know, I was just really . . . it was good to be alive . . . (Ann)

The disorientation of time and space associated with peak experiences (Maslow 1970) was also evident in the birth stories. Clock time appeared to be irrelevant in a positive birth experience.

> it all becomes a blur doesn't it? (Janet)

Moreover, during antenatal planning, a number of women had placed significant value on their birthing environment. However, during second stages of labour, the spatial context became unimportant, as their focus turned inwards.

> X [midwife] asked me which room I would like to go in as when we'd talked the environment had been really important but when it came to it, it wasn't. I said anywhere (Diane)

A positive birth, like a peak experience, was therefore associated with disorientations to the temporal and spatial nature of everyday awareness.

Maslow (1962) explained that there are two opposite physical reactions to peak experiences. One represented high tension and excitement, the other a relaxed peaceful calm (1962, p. 87). These bitter–sweet moments were described in Diane's birth story.

> I felt fantastic, I was sore, but then I'd just passed an 8 lb 10 baby so I was bound to be sore ... and I was tired, but such a happy tiredness, such a lovely tiredness, it was like being in a dream .. felt really quite serene and .. very calm, very relaxed ... and also very excited and exhilarated and I just wanted to shout, I've just delivered a baby normally (Diane)

A further characteristic of peak experiences was that they were often accompanied by a total loss of fear and control. The participants succumbed with total abandonment to pure and absolute pleasure (Maslow 1970). During childbirth, a selection of women identified the pain of birth to be an intensely painful but also pleasurable, almost sexual experience. During the height of labour, the peaks of pain were described as 'exhilarating'.

> It was like orgasmic and even feeling in between my legs that incredible burn, that burn, sting, just like your legs are just going to fly off each side. It is a wonder you go back to being a normal person afterwards (Kate)

Furthermore, similar to peak experiences, a positive birth was considered to be ineffable.

> it was just so incredible ... beyond words it was just so lovely (Ann)

It represented an indescribable experience that operated outside of conscious awareness or comprehension. Any attempts to define these experiences by mere words were considered to lead to altered and inaccurate representations (Maslow 1962).

A number of the women described themselves as 'special' and 'lucky' to have experienced a positive birth.

> I can't even describe how lucky I felt with X's birth (Janet)

Notions of luck, good fortune and grace are all characteristic of peak experiences (Maslow 1970). Furthermore, the notion of completeness and wholeness the women experienced through a fulfilling birth characterised the totality, the 'gestalt closure of peak experiences' (Maslow 1962, p. 111).

> I can remember when they were in theatre, X (consultant) lifting X (daughter) up and I can remember it for the rest of my life and just thinking, it just made me complete, just seeing her, as soon as she was here (Jules)

A final analogy was identified in that the transformational nature of a peak experience was suggested to create benevolent behaviours. Maslow believed that those who had experienced a peak event were fuelled by desires and even a sense of obligation to do some good for the world (Maslow 1962: 113). These acts of benevolence were witnessed in the women's birth stories. Some of these women expressed how they wanted to use their experience to change their life-world. This was initiated through public storytelling; to encourage and empower other women to achieve fulfilment through childbirth.

> I rang one of the X [work colleagues] who's pregnant and said how are you feeling and she said oh gosh I'm due such and such a date and I said don't worry about the birth, just get your head around it, it is a most fantastic experience you will ever have, you've got to go in there positive and you've got to believe that your body can do it, we're women we can do it, you've got to believe it and I said it's absolutely fantastic, it's brilliant, I can't find the words to tell you how amazing it is. She said you're the first person who's said that to me all this lot are telling me horror stories, oh I did this and I did that, and I said well don't listen to them because it is amazing (Diane)

Discussion

In this chapter, insights into women's experiences and internalisations of a positive birth have been presented. The three themes described and discussed have uncovered how a positive birth can be achieved (through women–caregiver relationships), experienced (on a unique and individual basis) and internalised (through enhanced self-perceptions) by women.

The findings suggest that a positive birth can transcend the mode of birth, birth environment and model of care. First, the women in this research described positive vaginal, instrumental and Caesarean birth experiences. Therefore these insights do not confirm with previous research which has associated obstetric interventions with maternal dissatisfaction (Waldenstrom 1996, 1999). In the current research, the mind–body harmony that women experienced during childbirth led them to feel they had given birth, irrespective of how the baby was born. A woman's belief that she has not given birth has previously been associated with instrumental or operative childbirth (Berg & Dahlberg 1998; Kitzinger 2006). The findings of this study thereby extend these reports to suggest that it is an embodied experience of birth, rather than the actual method of delivery that makes an essential difference for women. An embodied experience appeared to represent a peak event (Maslow 1962, 1970) for women: an experience in which women felt totally connected; a state of unity and wholeness during the childbirth process; when women are transformed into mothers through joy, love and new-found self-worth.

In respect to the birth environment, previous research, highlighted in this book, has stressed the importance of the physical aspects of labour and delivery rooms for labouring women (Walsh 1999; Newburn 2003). The findings from this study revealed that for a number of women in this research, the birth environment 'didn't matter'. A joyful birth was characterised by a calm, quiet and relaxed sense of normality irrespective of where the baby was delivered (home, delivery ward or operating theatre).

In regard to the model of care, this research uncovered that positive experiences of childbirth were associated with medical as well as midwifery models of care. Previous research in this area has compared different ideologies of maternity care with maternal outcomes (for examples, refer to Morgan *et al.* 1998; Tinkler & Quinney 1998; Farquhar *et al.* 2000; Homer *et al.* 2002; Borquez & Wiegers 2006). In this research, comparisons have been made between standard hospital (obstetrician units) care and midwifery-led care, or between different models of midwifery-based practice. Whilst there have been some inconsistencies in the findings, women who accessed midwifery-led services were found to be more satisfied with their care and their childbirth experiences. In the current research, however, it was particular professionals from a range of disciplines that shared and engaged in childbirth. These findings thereby extend the 'with woman' paradigm (Coyle *et al.* 2001; Hunter 2004) in the literature that tends to be focused on the value of the midwife–woman relationship.

The continuous presence of a supportive birth companion is believed to be one of the most effective forms of intervention in childbirth (Kirkham 2000; Hodnett *et al.* 2003). However, as the current findings revealed that positive connections were formed with health professionals from midwifery-led and traditional models of care, these findings are consistent with previous accounts in that 'being known' is less important than the qualities of care received (Lee 1997; Morgan *et al.* 1998; Rennie *et al.* 1998; Waldenstrom 1998; Green *et al.* 1999; Hodnett *et al.* 2003).

The finding that a positive birth surpasses the mode, environment or model of care would reflect that the relationships forged between women and caregivers play an important role in facilitating a positive birth experience. Furthermore, as this study has uncovered the processes and characteristics of sensitive, empowering and effective care, the findings offer important insights for clinical practice. In this study, women highlighted the connections formed with health professionals during a joyful birth event. These connections were evident on an emotional, social, physiological and intuitive level. During a positive birth, women and health professionals appeared to operate on a symbiotic and co-dependent basis. The care they received symbolised the value and agency of women. Women felt informed, engaged and in 'control' of what was happening to them during the birth. Power was retained by women as their unique needs and expectations of birth were acknowledged and considered. The findings indicate that during a positive birth, caregivers operated as partners, 'professional friends' (Pairman 2000) to facilitate an optimal birth experience for women. Furthermore, these relationships resonate with the partnership model proposed by Guilliland and Pairman (1995). That model views trust, shared control and responsibility, and shared meaning through mutual understanding as the basis of an effective midwife–mother relationship (Guilliland & Pairman 1995: 7).

As indicated in previous research, trust emerged as key characteristic of the women–caregiver relationships (Berg & Dahlberg 1998; Anderson 2000; Parratt & Fahy 2003; Lundgren 2004; Reibel 2004; Edwards 2005; Lundgren 2005). Through trust, women felt safe, cared for, valued, supported and that their intrinsic needs were being addressed. Women described themselves as active and integral members of a positive birth team. However, in a number of occasions, women spoke of how they were happy for their caregivers to make unilateral decisions, such as the need for obstetric procedures. These women considered that they were offered the 'right choice', due to the belief that it represented their best interests. These insights thereby reflect that it is not necessarily the procedures that women object to during childbirth. It is whether the women felt fully informed as to the justification for procedures, mediated by the mutual respect and feeling valued by caregivers.

In contemporary maternity care, the influence of the culture and environment on the health professional's ability to support expectant women is well reported across the literature (Salariya 1991; Kirkham 2000; Edwards 2005; Dykes 2006). Culture and environment are considered to operate as a pervasive and significant influence on organisational practice. Culture refers to the accepted ideas and codes of behaviour, written rules, organisational standards, beliefs, assumptions, rituals and 'personality of the organisation' (Ranade 1998).

> If care is to improve - the culture within the NHS must be addressed.
> (Kirkham 2000, p. 241)

One of the ways the culture could be addressed is through multi-disciplinary training and seminar events. These events would aim for professionals to recognise and value the implications of care on women's experiences of birth, as well as the influence of childbirth on maternal well-being. A 'Being with Patients' project' has been developed by Cumbria and Lancashire Workforce Development Confederation (Reid 2004). The programme was developed from interpretive research which focused on patients' experiences of nursing care. Delivery of the project has been through a 1-day seminar programme. This seminar uses role play and performances of patient's experiences structured around the key themes generated by the research. The aims of this training are to positively influence staff's understanding of what it means to be a patient, and to promote the acquisition of practical strategies to enhance patient's care. The project could well serve as a model to create a similar programme of support for maternal-care professionals, based on the findings generated by this research.

Limitations of, and suggestions for future research

There are a number of limitations in the interpretation of these findings. First, the findings are based on a small sample of participants from a limited geographical area. These accounts have also been generated by women who had previously experienced a traumatic birth. The reason as to why this experience was such a joyful event may be because it followed adversity. These insights may therefore reflect a 'much better' experience through comparisons with their former distress, rather than a positive experience per se. Further research is warranted to explore positive birth experiences in primiparous women. These additional insights would help to elucidate and authenticate the positive birth phenomenon.

All the women recruited for this research were in receipt of, or had previously received support through the consultant midwife. These women may well have agreed to take part in this research through a sense of indebtedness, or concern as to how a refusal may impact upon future access to services. Future research in this area should therefore seek alternative methods to access participants, such as via antenatal clinics.

A further limitation inherent within qualitative-based research is that interpretations are ultimately constructed by the interpreter. From a hermeneutic perspective, it is only through our pre-understandings that we are able to interpret our life-world. The fact that my pre-conceptions may have introduced limitations in the interpretations cannot be excluded. Supplementary research will help to minimise any confounding influences in how women's voices are represented.

In general, stories are presented as 'snap shots' in time. They offer representations of life at a given moment rather than a representation of life itself (Sandelowski 1991). Furthermore, according to Gadamer, once we understand, this changes our perceptions of how we view our life-world which in turn alters our understanding (Gadamer 2004); interpretation is therefore circular, and never ending. These findings thereby offer insights at one moment in time. Future research in this area will go some way to substantiate the interpretations generated.

Conclusions

This interpretive phenomenological study has offered insights into the women's lived experiences and meanings of a positive birth experience. The findings have illuminated the connections forged between women and caregivers during a positive birth. They have also revealed how a positive birth is linked with the value and agency of women. Furthermore, the resonances between Maslow's descriptions and women's birth experiences reveal that a joyful birth can be an intense, powerful and transformative event for women. These findings signify that a positive birth was not just related to the birth of a healthy baby, but also to maternal well-being through the birth of a happy, confident and empowered mother.

The findings have suggested that a positive birth can transcend the mode of birth, birth environment or model of care. In turn, these insights magnify the importance of the relationships forged between women and health professionals to facilitate a positive experience. Through an 'appreciative focus' into positive birth, this study has uncovered what is positive and working well within maternity services. These messages should underpin the delivery of multidisciplinary training or seminar events, and should be built upon for the sake of future service provision.

References

Anderson T (2000) Feeling safe enough to let go: the relationship between a woman and her midwife during the second stage of labour. In Kirkham M (ed) *The Midwife–Mother Relationship*. Basingstoke, MacMillan Press Limited, 92–118.

Beech BA, Phipps B (2008) Normal birth: women's stories: In Downe S (ed) *Normal Childbirth: Evidence and Debate.* Churchill Livingstone, Edinburgh, 67–79.

Berg M, Dahlberg K (1998) A phenomenological study of women's experiences of complicated childbirth. *Midwifery* 14: 23–9.

Borquez HA, Wiegers TA (2006) A comparison of labor and birth experiences of women delivering in a birthing centre and at home in the Netherlands. *Midwifery* 22: 339–47.

Brown S, Lumley J (1994) Satisfaction with care in labor and birth: a survey of 790 Australian women. *Birth* 21(1): 4–13.

Brown BL, Phipps B (2004) Normal birth: women's stories. In Downe S (ed) *Normal Childbirth: Evidence and debate.* London, Churchill Livingstone, 59–70.

Burkhardt MA, Nagai-Jacobson MG (2002) *Spirituality: Living our Connectedness.* New York, Delmar Thomson Learning.

Callister LC, Khalaf I, Semenic S, Kartchner R, Vehvilainen-Julkunen K (2003) The pain of childbirth: perceptions of culturally diverse women. *Pain Management Nursing* 4(4): 145–54.

Coyle K, Hauck Y, Percival P, Kristjanson L (2001) Ongoing relationships with a personal focus: mothers' perceptions of birth centre versus hospital care. *Midwifery* 17(3): 171–81.

Downe S, McCourt C (2004). From being to becoming: reconstructing childbirth knowledge. In Downe S (ed) *Normal Childbirth: Evidence and Debate.* London, Churchill Livingstone, 3–24.

Dykes F (2006) *Breastfeeding in Hospital: Midwives, Mothers and the Production Line.* Oxon, Routledge Press.

Edwards NP (2005) *Birthing Autonomy: Women's Experiences of Planning Home Births.* New York, Routledge Press.

Farquhar M, Camilleri-Ferrante C, Todd C (2000) Continuity of care in maternity services: women's views of one team midwifery scheme. *Midwifery* 16: 35–47.

Gadamer HG (2004) *Truth and Method.* London, Continuum Press.

Green JM, Coupland VA, Kitzinger JV (1990) Expectations, experiences and psychological outcomes of childbirth: a prospective study of 825 women. *Birth* 17(1): 15–24.

Green JM, Renfrew MJ, Curtis PA (1999) Continuity of carer: what matters to women? A review of the evidence. *Midwifery* 16: 186–96.

Guilliland K, Pairman S (1995) *The Midwifery Partnership: A Model for Practice.* New Zealand, Victoria University of Wellington.

Hall H, Taylor M (2004) Birth and spirituality. In Downe S (ed) *Normal Childbirth: Evidence and Debate.* Sydney, Churchill Livingstone, 41–56.

Halldorsdottir S, Karlsdottir SI (1996a) Journeying through labour and delivery: perceptions of women who have given birth. *Midwifery* 12: 48–61.

Halldorsdottir S, Karlsdottir SI (1996b) Empowerment or discouragement: women's experience of caring and uncaring encounters during childbirth. *Health Care for Women International* 17: 361–79.

Hodnett E, Gates S, Hofmeyr G, Sakala C (2003) Continuous support for woman during childbirth (Cochrane Review). *The Cochrane Library*, Issue 3, Chichester, John Wiley & Sons, Ltd.

Homer CS, Davis GK, Cooke M, Barclay LM (2002) Women's experiences of continuity of midwifery care in a randomised controlled trial in Australia. *Midwifery* 18(2): 102–12.

Hunter B (2004) Conflicting ideologies as a source of emotion work in midwifery. *Midwifery* 20: 261–72.

Kennedy HP, Shannon MT, Chuahorn U, Kravetz MK (2004) The landscape of caring for women: a narrative study of midwifery practice. *American College of Nurse-Midwives* 49(1): 14–23.

Kirkham M (2000) How can we relate? In Kirkham M (ed) *The Midwife–Mother Relationship*. London, Macmillan Press Limited, 227–50.

Kitzinger S (2006) *Birth Crisis*. London, Routledge Press.

Lavender T, Walkinshaw SA, Walton I (1999) A prospective study of women's views of factors contributing to a positive birth experience. *Midwifery*, 15: 40–6.

Leap N (2000) The less we do, the more we give In Kirkham M (ed) *The Midwife–Mother Relationship*. London, Macmillan, 1.

Lee G (1997) The concept of 'continuity' – what does it mean? In Kirkham M, Perkins E R (eds) *Reflections on Midwifery*. London, Balliere Tindall, 1–25.

Lowe NK (2000). Self-efficacy for labor and childbirth fears in nulliparous women. *Journal of Psychosomatic Obstetrics and Gynecology* 21: 219–24.

Lundgren I (2004) Releasing and relieving encounters: experiences of pregnancy and childbirth. *Scandinavian Journal of Caring Sciences* 18(4): 368–75.

Lundgren I (2005) Swedish women's experience of childbirth 2 years after birth. *Midwifery* 21: 346–54.

Lundgren I, Dahlberg K (1998) Women's experience of pain during childbirth. *Midwifery* 14(2): 105–10.

Maslow A (1959) Cognition of being in peak experiences. *Journal of Genetic Psychology* 4: 43–66.

Maslow AH (1962) *Toward a Psychology of Being*, 2nd edition. New York, Litton Educational Publishing.

Maslow, AH (1970) *Religions, Values and Peak Experiences*. New York, Penguin Books.

Mauger B (1996) Childbirth as initiation and transformation: the wounded mother. *Pre and Peri-natal Psychology Journal* 11(1): 17–30.

Mercer RT (1985) Relationship of the birth experience to later mothering behaviours. *Journal of Nurse-Midwifery* 30(4): 204–11.

Morgan M, Fenwick N, McKenzie V, Wolfe CDA (1998) Quality of midwifery led care: assessing the effects of different models of continuity for women's satisfaction. *Quality and Safety in Health Care* 7: 77–82.

Newburn M (2003) Culture, control and the birth environment. *The Practising Midwife* 6(8): 20–5.

Pairman S (2000) Women-centred midwifery partnerships or professional friendships. In Kirkham M (ed) *The Midwife–Mother Relationship*. Basingstoke, Macmillan Press Limited, 207–25.

Parratt J, Fahy K (2003) Trusting enough to be out of control: a pilot study of women's sense of self during childbirth. *Australian Journal of Midwifery* 16(1): 15–22.

Ranade W (1998) *Making Sense of Multi-agency Groups*. Northumbria, Sustainable Cities Research Institute.

Raphael-Leff J (1991) *Psychological Processes of Childbearing*. London, Chapman & Hall.

Reibel T (2004) The language of birth: how words colour women's experiences. *Birth Issues* 13(1): 18–23.

Reid B (2004) The "Being With Patients" Project – developing nurse's caring behaviour and attitudes: an experiential approach to learn from patients' experiences of care. In Shaw T, Sanders K (eds) *Foundation of Nursing Studies Dissemination Series*. Vol. 2 (9) London, Kings Fund.

Rennie AM, Hundley V, Gurney E, Graham W (1998) Women's priorities for care before and after delivery. *British Journal of Midwifery* 6(7): 434–8.

Salariya E (1991) Parent-infant attachment. In Alexander J, Levy V, Roch S (eds) *Postnatal Care: A Research Based Approach*. London, Macmillan Press.

Sandelowski M (1991) Telling stories: narrative approaches in qualitative research. *Image* 23(3): 161–6.

Sandelowski M (1997) To be of use: enhancing the utility of qualitative research. *Nursing Outlook* 45: 125–32.

Simkin P (1991) Just another day in a woman's life. I. Women's long-term perceptions of their first birth experience. *Birth* 18(3): 203–10.

Simkin P (1992) Just another day in a woman's life. Part II: nature and consistency of women's long-term memories of their first birth experience. *Birth* 19(3): 64–81.

Thompson JL (1990) Hermeneutic inquiry. In Moody LE (ed) *Advancing Nursing Science through Research*, Vol. 2. Newbury Park, Sage Publications, 224–67.

Tinkler A and Quinney D (1998) Team midwifery: the influence of the midwife-woman relationship on women's experiences and perceptions of maternity care. *Journal of Advanced Nursing* 28(1): 30–5.

Waldenstrom U (1996) Modern maternity care: does safety have to take the meaning out of birth. *Midwifery* 12: 165–73.

Waldenstrom U (1998) Continuity of carer and satisfaction. *Midwifery* 14: 207–13.

Waldenstrom U (1999) Experience of labour and birth in 1111 women. *Journal of Psychosomatic Research* 47(5): 471–82.

Walker JM, Hall S, Thomas M (1995) The experience of labour: a perspective from those receiving care in a midwife-led unit. *Midwifery* 11: 120–9.

Walsh D (1999) An ethnographic study of women's experience of partnership caseload midwifery practice: the professional as a friend. *Midwifery* 15(3): 165–76.

Walsh D, El-Nemer A, Downe S (2004) Risk, safety and the study of physiological birth. In Downe S (ed) *Normal Childbirth: Evidence and Debate*. Edinburgh, Churchill Livingstone, 103–19.

Welch D, Wellard S (2005) The phenomenon of presence within contemporary nursing practice: A literature review. *Australian Journal of Holistic Nursing* 12(1): 4–10.

Chapter 12
Sexuality in Labour and Birth:
An Intimate Perspective

Sarah Buckley

Introduction

Labour and childbirth are intrinsically sexual events. This may not be obvious in modern, patriarchal settings, where female sexuality is recognised only in context of, or as equivalent to, male coitally directed sexuality. However, childbearing, from menstruation through to breastfeeding, forms part of a woman's wider sexual and reproductive cycle. This cycle encompasses menstruation, ovulation, conception, pregnancy, labour, birth and breastfeeding, eventually cycling back to menstruation and the possibility of another reproductive cycle.

This female sexual cycle is the foundation of human existence, and was likely the focus of awe and ceremony for our ancestors. Some of these events – for example, the onset of fertility with first menstruation – are still celebrated in other cultures today. However, the sexuality of childbirth, the central event in the fertile cycle, has been almost completely dismantled in westernised cultures. The advent of male birth attendants, beginning in Europe in the 17th century, substantially changed the intimate, female-focused birth atmosphere that had existed for most of human history (Tew 1998). The opportunity for intimacy and privacy during labour and birth lessened again as the majority of Western women, over the course of the 20th century, moved from homes to institutions to give birth (Tew 1998) as noted in earlier chapters. Our current emphasis on medical and time-based views of birth, both inimical to sexual expression, has further reduced the opportunity to perceive and protect the sexual elements of labour and birth.

This chapter focuses on both women's experiences and perspectives, and the physiological data that connect birth and sexual experiences. The underlying premise is that recognition of the sexuality of birth is helpful, and may in some cases be transformative for the labouring mother, her partner and carers. An increased awareness of the sexuality of birth also offers new perspectives that can be incorporated into birth care in any 21st century setting.

Rediscovering the parallels

Perhaps the first modern, scientific exploration of the sexuality of birth was published by psychologist Niles Newton in 1955 as *Maternal emotions: A Study of Women's Feelings Toward Menstruation, Pregnancy, Childbirth, Breastfeeding and Other Aspects of Their Femininity* (Newton 1955). In *Maternal emotions*, Niles Newton discusses the observable similarities between women experiencing 'uninhibited, undrugged childbirth' as described by UK doctor Grantly Dick Read among his home-birth clientele (Read 1949) and female sexual excitement, as described in Kinsey's report on female sexual behaviour (Kinsey 1953).

Newton notes 15 parallels between women's behaviour during natural birth and sexual activity, including similarities in: breathing patterns and vocalisations; facial expressions; uterine contractions; choice of bodily position; loosening of the mucus plug; loss of social inhibitions; unusual strength and agility at delivery and orgasm; sudden return of awareness afterwards; and feelings of elation, joy and well-being following both experiences. Elaborating on this material in Psychology Today in 1971 (Newton 1971), Newton also notes parallels between female physiological responses to sexual arousal and to breastfeeding, including the occurrence of nipple erection and uterine contractions. She concludes, 'sexual arousal, lactation and birth share a common neurohormonal level . . . oxytocin is so much involved that I am prompted to call it "the hormone of love"' (Newton 1971).

Newton further discusses the effects of disturbance in birth from her experiments with mice (mentioned in more detail below) and notes that sexual activity, birth and breastfeeding all require a subjective sense of safety because of the relative incapacity for fight or flight during all three engrossing events.

Sexual liberation and birth

Exploring this sexual perspective for women rather than professionals, Sheila Kitzinger's (1984) book *The Experience of Childbirth* defined birth as a psychosexual event, and part of a woman's wider sexual nature. Kitzinger describes ' . . . the intense and thrilling sensations of the descent of the baby's head . . . the keen sensuous pleasure . . . even when it involves some pain' (Kitzinger 1984, p. 23).

In the United States, the sexual nature of birth was recognised in a more alternative context by Ina May Gaskin in her classic book *Spiritual Midwifery*, first published in 1977 (Gaskin 2002). Gaskin gained her midwifery skills by attending births in her alternative community, and was later mentored by a local doctor, but her un-medicalised beginning allowed her to see birth freshly and, like the best of scientists, to observe, reflect and experiment with different variables in labour and birth.

In the context of several difficult births, where she felt that the 'energy' between the labouring mother and father was stalling labour, Gaskin discovered that sexual contact – for example, deep kissing – could remedy the situation (Gaskin 2002). She concluded, 'The energy that gets the baby in, can help to get the baby out' and subsequently encouraged sexual interactions in labour, most often by leaving the prospective parents alone to enjoy intimate time.

The sexuality of birth was brought into the public eye in the United Kingdom in 1982, with the screening of the BBC documentary *Birth Reborn*, filmed in Michel Odent's birth clinic in Pithiviers, France. In one scene, a naked woman holding her newly born baby is asked how she felt as she pushed out her footling breech baby: she replies unhesitatingly to the camera 'It was like an orgasm.' *Birth Reborn* captured the intimate, quiet and low-lit atmosphere of the birthing rooms at Pithiviers, and linked the exceptional outcomes among Odent's clientele with his emphasis on the need for privacy in labour (Mills 1982).

Others have also noticed that sexual activity and orgasm, including masturbation, can help with pain as well as the progress of labour (Shanley 1994; Ariel Drori 2005). These effects may relate to the increases in oxytocin and endorphins associated with sexual activity, both of which have pain-relieving properties, as mentioned later.

Sexual birth in the 21st century

Unfortunately, these useful perspectives have not translated into readily available maternity-care options. This may reflect birth attendants' discomfort with recommending or witnessing overtly sexual behaviour in labour, especially within institutional settings. Opportunities to allow a labouring couple time alone may also be limited in many circumstances.

However, many women have recognised the importance and perhaps practical applications of sexual expression in labour, and made choices that allow themselves this freedom. This includes choosing unassisted or free birth, and much of the subjective writing on the sexual experience of birth comes from women who have made this choice (Moran 1981; Shanley 1994; Moran 1997; Griesemer 1998; McCracken 2000; Seaman 2000; Baker 2001; Morgan 2003).

In particular, Laura Shanley in her 1994 book *Unassisted Childbirth* (Shanley 1994) explores the sexual nature of birth and suggests that feelings of shame, perhaps stemming from cultural or religious beliefs and attitudes to female sexuality, may be a hindrance during labour and birth. Shanley states, 'If a woman believes her sexuality is shameful, she will find it difficult to spread her legs and give birth to a child who is the result of sex' (Shanley 1994, p. 69). Her associated website is also an enlightening look at the sexuality of birth (Shanley 2008c).

What is perhaps most radical amongst this literature, and probably a new development for childbirth in any context, is the idea of sharing the sexual nature of birth with the male partner, in the context of unassisted birth. Helen Wessel first wrote about this from a Christian perspective (Wessel 1963) and the theme was continued by Marilyn Moran (1981) whose 1997 title, *Pleasurable Husband/Wife Childbirth: The Real Consummation of Married Love*, (Moran 1997) sums up this philosophy.

Similarly, there are reports from men who have also experienced and appreciated the sexual dimensions of birth. For example Lewis Mehl, now a US Professor of Family Medicine and Psychiatry, reports, 'My feelings throughout my wife's labors I can describe only as those of a very close, physical-emotional, sexual union with her and what I felt to be the transcendent force flowing through her. The sensation was warm and soft, like making love, but was also strong, forceful and awesome' (Mehl 1980).

Note that providing the conditions necessary for sexual expression may have major advantages for a woman's birth physiology. As Newton observes, both labour and sexual activity require a subjective sense of safety and privacy, without which both processes are more difficult. In choosing such conditions – which are necessary for every other birthing mammal – there may be a higher likelihood of a normal labour and birth. Some intrinsic hormonal safety factors may also be enhanced (Buckley 2009).

Orgasmic birth

Gaskin and others have noticed that woman in the throes of intense labour, and/or at the moment of birth, can look or behave as though they are experiencing orgasm (Gaskin 2003; Pascali-Bonaro 2007). Many women have described their child's birth in orgasmic language, or actually described having an orgasm at the moment of delivery (Baker 2001; Gaskin 2002, 2003; Shanley, 2008a, 2008b). Conducting her own casual survey, Gaskin found that 32 out of 151 interviewees reported having an orgasm at the moment of birth (Gaskin 2003). Similarities in the hormonal physiology of birth and orgasm, detailed below, underline this possibility.

Although most stories of orgasmic birth come from women in relaxed, private settings such as home birth and birth centres, some women also have reported orgasmic birth in hospital in the presence of oblivious (or shocked) nurses and doctors. However Gaskin comments, '... orgasm during labor and birth doesn't seem to happen very much in women whose labors are medicated with narcotics, epidurals or barbiturates ... this may be a significant reason why this phenomenon is so under-recognized by birth professionals and the general public' (Gaskin 2003, p. 161).

These powerful sexual experiences during an unmedicated labour and birth can obviously occur in many settings, and it may be useful for all birth attendants to be aware of and sensitive to this possibility.

Israeli birth coach Shiraz Ariel Drori promotes the deliberate use of orgasm in early labour, and reports her own experiences of progressing from 2 cm to delivery in 30–60 minutes following orgasm. Her story also highlights the possibility of achieving sufficient privacy for sexual activity, even in a hospital setting (Ariel Drori 2005).

Sexuality in the labour ward

These authors are surely not the only observers to wonder about the sexuality of labour and birth. Many birth attendants have (or could) recognise the sexual sounds, looks and behaviour of labouring women in their care. For example, in *The Secret Life of the Expectant Mother*, a US maternity nurse comments, 'The first time I heard a woman giving birth naturally in a childbearing center, I was stunned! I felt like I was intruding on someone making love' (Jones 1997). Newton describes an 'intense strained look' that woman may have close to delivery, and which may be misinterpreted as indicating great pain, but which may be equivalent to the 'tortured expression' described by Kinsey (Kinsey 1953) just before sexual climax (Newton 1955).

Carers may also recognise disinhibited behaviour that may lead a woman to 'do what she would never dare' in labour (Odent 2001) including taking her clothes off in the presence of strangers. The labouring woman will also often choose movements and positions that are uninhibited and out of the range of social norms.

Even when conditions do not accommodate a labouring woman's spontaneous sexual sounds and behaviours, the sexual nature of childbirth is difficult to overlook. For example, it is obvious (but nowadays not inevitable) that the baby is destined to emerge from the sexual parts of a woman's body, which are also the focus of caregiving and monitoring behaviour in labour. A woman's vagina further becomes the focus during the birth, and various vaginal manipulations and procedures such as perineal support, manipulations of the baby, episiotomy and repair, and cord traction may be performed during and after she births her baby and placenta.

Sexual expression and its control during labour

If the sexuality of labour and birth is so obvious, why is it unacknowledged by most women and their carers? Why would most women deny, perhaps vehemently, that their birth experience has sexual dimensions? A full discussion of current social, anthropological and/or feminist perspectives on female sexual expression is beyond the scope of this chapter, but it is likely that patriarchal 'ownership' of female sexuality, and specifically male ownership of the sexual expression of their female partner, contributes to strict cultural boundaries for female sexual behaviour, including behaviour during labour.

Many obstetric procedures, past and current, (hospital clothing, shaving of the pubic hair, use of drapes and gloves, hands-off care such as electronic monitors) could be interpreted as rituals that de-sexualise the processes of labour and birth in order to allow procedures that would otherwise be taboo, such as vaginal examinations. These rituals also create a power imbalance, and create a disembodied, technocratic (and therefore asexual) experience at this powerful time (Davis-Floyd 2003).

The custom in many countries for a labouring woman to be under the care of, and often in the presence of, an unrelated male is likely to further restrict a woman's comfort with sexual expression in labour. Care by a socially unrelated female may be less inhibiting, depending on the woman, her carer and their relationship.

Drugs and procedures, as Gaskin notes, may also interfere with sexual expression. In relation to her comparison of sexual and labour behaviour, Newton remarks: 'Since in this country [US] it is customary to move, strap down and otherwise disturb even undrugged woman as they approach [birth] climax, the behaviour noted by Read [among UK women labouring at home] may be not so frequent nor so pronounced here' (Newton 1955, p. 89). Kitzinger notes that interventions, especially epidurals, negate the sexual aspects of childbirth, leaving the woman '. . . perfectly controlled and rational, and in no way overpowered by the emotions or by the intensity of the labour experience . . . ' which, she observes, is more acceptable to obstetricians and other carers in a busy hospital setting (Kitzinger 1984, p. 22).

The physical environment for labour and birth is also likely to markedly influence a woman's sexual expression. As Buckley (2004) laments elsewhere: '. . . the passion of birth is neither recognised nor accommodated. Birth has become a dispassionate medical event, usually occurring in a setting that discourages emotional expression.'

Birth as rape

The sexual nature of birth may also become obvious when birth has been a bad experience. In extreme (but not uncommon) circumstances, women can feel a violation that is akin to rape (McCracken 2000; Kitzinger 2006) or their experiences as birth rape (Fraser 2008; Freeze 2008). Midwife Barb Herrera, interviewed in Rixa Freeze's PhD thesis on unassisted childbirth, describes birth rape as, 'The experience of having fingers, scissors, and/or tools put/pushed/shoved inside a woman's vagina or rectum without her direct (or indirect) permission . . . ' (Freeze 2008). Such procedures would in fact be defined as rape if they occurred in a different setting.

For a woman who has experienced sexual abuse in the past, the sexuality of birth, and especially the need to use parts of her body that have previously been traumatised, can be extremely challenging, even in ideal circumstances. Skilled care is especially necessary for survivors of sexual abuse, with great awareness of, and sensitivity to, the sexuality of birth. Authors Penny Simkin and Phyllis Klaus note that, according to numerous surveys, between 25 and 40% of women have experienced significant sexual abuse over their lifetimes (Simkin & Klaus 2004).

It is interesting to observe that Caesarean rates have been increasing worldwide under current medicalised models of maternity care. One might wonder whether our discomfort with the sexuality of birth might lead both carers and women to accept the 'vaginal bypass', which removes sexuality (and the chance of feeling sexually violated during birth) even further. This perspective is supported by evidence that women who have had a previous negative birth experience may prefer a subsequent Caesarean (Gamble & Creedy 2001). The sole remaining (but flawed) (Press *et al.* 2007) justification for Caesarean – that it protects the woman's pelvic floor – also hints at sexual protection, as well as sexual ownership by the male partner.

These women's experiences and comments underline the need for extreme sensitivity from carers.

Birth as agony and ecstasy

Birth obviously has the potential to bring suffering and pain – our usual social view of birth – or reward and pleasure, including sexual pleasure. These two perspectives, as Kitzinger reminds us, are not mutually exclusive. When we examine the hormones associated with childbirth, this pleasure–pain continuum becomes clearer. Stress and pain lead to the release of high levels of stress hormones including endorphins, adrenaline-noradrenaline (A/NA) and cortisol. These naturally produced chemicals are designed to bring the body back into physiological balance. When the stress and pain continue for some time, as in labour, high levels can not only aid with stress-reduction, but may also induce euphoria, excitement and even pleasure. Such states are well known to occur when these substances are used therapeutically or recreationally.

The ecstatic hormones

Four of the major hormones of mammalian parturition – oxytocin; beta-endorphin (BE); A/NA; and prolactin – have been called the 'ecstatic hormones' because of their powerful psycho-emotional effects during pregnancy, labour, birth and post-partum (Buckley 2004, 2009). These hormones are produced predominantly in the limbic system – the middle layer of the human brain – and released into the blood stream, where they have systemic or bodily effects during labour and birth.

The ecstatic hormones are also released locally into brain areas close to production (Gimpl & Fahrenholz 2001). This dual release ensures that the hormone's systemic (bodily) effects are coordinated with emotional and behavioural influences. This is especially important during labour and birth, when the unfolding of appropriate post-partum maternal behaviour is critical for infant and, therefore, species survival.

These hormones are not only released during labour, birth and other reproductive acts, but comprise important physiological and psycho-behavioural systems that operate lifelong. For example, oxytocin is also a hormone of 'relaxation and growth', (Uvnas-Moberg 2003) influencing digestion, insulin release, (Uvnas-Moberg 1989) and cardiovascular function (Gutkowska *et al.* 2000). Prolactin has important effects on metabolism (Ben-Jonathan *et al.* 2006) and immune function (Goffin *et al.* 1998). BE has widespread influences on bodily processes and behaviours including eating and drinking, seizures and neurological disorders, and cardiovascular and immunological responses, among many others (Bodnar 2007). Finally, A/NA are prime influences on autonomic function and bodily homeostasis (Nestler *et al.* 2001).

The widespread influence of these hormonal systems raises questions about the possible long-term effects when these systems are disrupted or mis-set during labour and birth. This disturbance has been called *hormonal imprinting*; see Csaba and Tekes (2005) for further discussion.

Oxytocin

Oxytocin is a classical mammalian hormone of reproduction, earning, as mentioned earlier, the title of 'hormone of love' because of its release during activities including sexual behaviour, parturition and lactation (Newton 1971). Oxytocin is produced by cells in the hypothalamus and released in pulses from the posterior pituitary during labour, when it catalyses rhythmic contractions of the labouring mother's uterus. Oxytocin activity increases as labour progresses, with more frequent pulses creating more closely spaced contractions (Fuchs *et al.* 1991). At the same time, oxytocin released in the limbic system and the central nervous system (CNS) has an analgesic effect (Lundeberg *et al.* 1994) (Gimpl & Fahrenholz 2001).

Close to the time of birth, the baby's head (or presenting part), impelled by the oxytocin-mediated uterine activity, begins to stretch the mother's lower vagina. This activates stretch receptors in her vagina and cervix that send a signal to her pituitary to increase oxytocin release. This leads to stronger contractions that produce more descent and stretch, creating a positive feedback loop that ensures an efficient second stage (Blanks & Thornton 2003). This late-labour outpouring of oxytocin and its powerful effects on uterine contractions was first validated in animal experiments by Ferguson, after whom this reflex is named (Ferguson 1941).

High levels of oxytocin produced at this time ensure that the new mother is primed with this hormone of love, inducing relaxation and reward at first meeting with her baby. She will experience ongoing oxytocin release during the first hour after birth through skin-to-skin contact with her newborn, augmented by the baby's pre-breastfeeding and breastfeeding behaviour (Matthiesen *et al.* 2001). The new mother's oxytocin levels peak around the time she births her baby's placenta (Nissen *et al.* 1995).

There is evidence that these peaks of oxytocin activate the 'maternal circuit' – brain areas involved with early instinctive mothering behaviours – in other mammals (Lin *et al.* 2003; Kinsley & Lambert 2006). Ongoing positive maternal motivations may also be mediated through activation of oxytocin-related brain areas, including the powerful mesocorticolimbic dopamine reward system (Insel 2003; Ferris *et al.* 2005; Numan 2006).

Oxytocin in sexual behaviour

A large number of animal studies have confirmed the important role of oxytocin in sexual behaviour. Stimulation of the genitals (whether through mating, birth or manually) results in oxytocin release from the brain, and similarly, oxytocin administration into the brain of steroid-primed animals increases sexual receptiveness in females and hastens ejaculation in males (McCarthy & Altemus 1997).

Human studies have also shown a rise in oxytocin levels during sexual activity for men and women (Carmichael *et al.* 1987; Thackare *et al.* 2006) with an oxytocin peak at orgasm (Exton *et al.* 1999; Kruger *et al.* 2003). In one study, the intensity of muscular contractions during orgasm correlated with blood levels of oxytocin (Murphy *et al.* 1987). These studies show that, as predicted by Newton, the release of oxytocin during sexual activity is almost identical to its release during labour and birth, with a peak at orgasm paralleling the oxytocin surge at birth.

Beta-endorphin

Beta-endorphin (BE) is one of a group of opiate-like compounds that are naturally produced within the body ('endogenous opioids') and has properties in common with 'exogenous' (from outside the body) opiates, originally derived from the opium poppy. Exogenous opiates include morphine, pethidine and heroin as well as synthetic opiates and opiate derivatives such as fentanyl, sufentanil and codeine.

BE is released from the pituitary into the blood stream as part of the general stress response, triggered by the hypothalamic release of the executive stress hormone corticotrophin releasing hormone (CRH). The pituitary releases adrenocoticotrophic hormone (ACTH), which activates cortisol release from the adrenal, at the same time as BE and usually in equal parts, thus helping to co-ordinate the body's responses to stress.

Like the exogenous opiates, endorphins also have analgesic and euphoric effects, as well as a myriad of influences on many other bodily processes including: addiction and tolerance, learning and memory, food and water intake, alcohol abuse, sexual and reproductive functions (including maternal behaviour), and cardiovascular, respiratory, kidney, liver and gut functions (Bodnar 2007).

High levels of endorphins are also associated with altered states of consciousness, including euphoria, intense pleasure, ecstatic experiences, and excitation. These effects may reflect activation of the powerful mesocorticolimbic dopamine reward system (Ribeiro *et al.* 2005). An alteration in consciousness may be important for the labouring female, helping her to behave instinctively and to use the bodily movements that will help her baby to descend most efficiently (Buckley 2009).

BE levels rise as labour progresses, (Newnham *et al.* 1984; Brinsmead *et al.* 1985; Bacigalupo *et al.* 1990; Laatikainen 1991) increasing particularly during active labour when pain is reported as severe (Raisanen *et al.* 1984; Bacigalupo *et al.* 1990) and/or when the membranes have ruptured (Hofmeyr *et al.* 1995).

Levels of BE peak around the time of birth and gradually subside over the following hours (Pancheri *et al.* 1985; Bacigalupo *et al.* 1990). However, BE psychoneurological effects may persist for some hours, as the half-life of BE in the brain and cerebrospinal fluid (CSF) is estimated at 21 hours (Foley *et al.* 1979). BE will continue to be released with maternal–infant contact and breastfeeding (Franceschini *et al.* 1989).

BE elevation in the post-partum period may contribute to maternal euphoria as well as analgesia, and may also reward pleasurable interactions between mother and baby, helping to establish a positive mutual dependency that will enhance attachment for both partners (Panksepp *et al.* 1994; Buckley 2009).

Beta-endorphin in sexual behaviour

The role of BE in sexual arousal, mating and the post-coital phase is not well understood. As with other areas of BE research, there seem to be different effects on sexual behaviour according to the level of opiate exposure or release (Panksepp *et al.* 1994; Argiolas 1999).

While higher doses of administered exogenous opiates are well known to inhibit, some researchers have found that low doses can enhance sexual behaviour. This may fit with a natural increase in endogenous opiates with sexual arousal, which increases motivation and reward. High levels of exogenous (or endogenous) opiates may saturate the reward system, reducing sexual motivation (Argiolas 1999). This is supported by studies suggesting that opiates promote sexual satiety (Hull & Dominguez 2007).

However studies measuring blood beta-endorphin levels during and following sexual behaviour in humans have not found hormone elevations (Kruger *et al.* 1998; Exton *et al.* 1999; Argiolas & Melis 2003). Human studies using opiate antagonists, which would inhibit brain opiate effects, have also not found measurable inhibition of sexual function (Goldstein & Hansteen 1977).

Note however that all of these studies have used masturbation as a human model. This model may not reflect dyadic sexual activities, which are likely to involve skin-to-skin contact and other affiliative interactions that are known to increase endorphins (Young *et al.* 2001). This perspective is supported by one study which showed positive medium-term psychological benefits in woman following dyadic sex but not masturbation (Burleson *et al.* 2007).

In summary, the involvement of BE in human sexual behaviour is still poorly understood, but may parallel its release during labour and birth. Post-orgasmic opiate peaks may promote reward, satiety and bonding between sexual partners, similar to its pro-attachment effects on mother and baby.

Adrenaline and noradrenaline

Adrenaline and noradrenaline (A/NA), also known as epinephrine (E) and norepinephrine (NE), are the major chemicals mediating the short-term stress response, also called 'fight or flight', under the influence of the sympathetic nervous system (SNS).

Activation of the SNS in response to perceived danger produces widespread effects on brain and body aimed at enhancing the chances of survival by fight or flight. Physiological effects include a shift in blood supply from the skin and viscera (internal organs, including the uterus) to major muscle groups, increased heart rate and force of contractions, increased blood pressure, mobilisation of fuels including an increase in blood glucose and fats, dilation of pupils for keen vision, dilation of airways for efficient respiration, inhibition of secretions (leading to dryness) in the nose and mouth, decrease in gut activity and increased alertness and vigilance (Nestler *et al.* 2001).

The appropriate release of A/NA is very important during labour and birth. Researchers have shown that markedly elevated levels of A/NA early in labour (as measured in the labouring woman's blood) are associated with longer labour and more fetal heart rate abnormalities, indicative of insufficient fetal blood and oxygen supply (Lederman *et al.* 1985). This is not surprising, given that these hormones divert blood away from the baby to the fight-or-flight pathways, as above. Adrenaline also has directly inhibiting effects on uterine contractions (Carter & Olin 1972; Rosenfeld *et al.* 1976; Roman-Ponce *et al.* 1978).

These A/NA effects make sense when we consider that a labouring female of any species is extremely vulnerable to predators in the wild. If she senses danger, she needs an active fight-or-flight reflex to give her a respite from labour, and the muscular energy for fight (or more likely flight). Mother Nature designs this as a short-term strategy, with stress or danger during labour provoking high A/NA levels that will subside once the female reaches a safe situation.

However, this fight-or-flight reflex persists in modern women, who are just as alert to danger in modern maternity settings as were our ancestors giving birth in the wild. Being in, or moving to, an unfamiliar environment (e.g. from home to hospital) may bring a subjective sense of unease, with elevations in A/NA that will and slow or stall labour, at least in the short term.

Feeling observed by strangers, which would also have been a signal of potential danger in the wild, may also activate the SNS and hinder the progress of labour for modern woman. Ironically, if labour stalls because the labouring woman feels unsafe and observed, the usual obstetric reaction is to redouble observations, including various intrusive forms of monitoring, which is likely to further increase anxiety and SNS activation.

In contrast, surgeon and birth attendant Michel Odent believes that a stalled labour is a signal for him to withdraw and allow the labouring woman some privacy. This response is more physiologically likely to reduce her SNS hormones and normalise labour.

Other researchers have measured urinary hormone levels in women through normal labour and found a slow and gradual rise, with a significant increase from mid to late labour. In this study, peak levels of A and NA were around nine and two times (respectively) those of late pregnancy, as measured in the same individual at the same time of the day (Alehagen *et al*. 2005). In contrast to large A/NA elevations associated with the fight-or-flight reflex, this gradual rise in A/NA may help with alertness and energy as labour progresses. The late-labour A/NA peaks may reflect, in some women, activation of the fetus ejection reflex (FER).

The FER refers to the large pre-birth surge in A/NA that will paradoxically stimulate contractions and so ensure a quick and easy birth. This reflex also benefits the female giving birth in the wild who, near the time of birth, would be more advantaged by a rapid birth than by the cessation of labour for fight-or-flight. According to Odent, a genuine FER is unlikely if the labouring female has been disturbed earlier in labour, and is rarely seen in women giving birth in hospital settings (Odent 1987).

The FER model is supported by studies showing a very wide range of A/NA blood levels among individual women (Lederman *et al*. 1978; Lederman *et al*. 1985; Mahomed *et al*. 1995; Alehagen *et al*. 2005) and by one *in vitro* study that documented the paradoxically stimulating effects of high doses of mixed A and NA (Segal *et al*. 1998).

Overall, these studies reflect the effects of maternal anxiety and fear during labour, with activation of the fight-or-flight reflex leading to possible compromise in fetal blood supply. This mechanism underlines the importance of subjective feelings of safety and privacy during human labour.

Animal studies also highlight the requirement for the labouring female to feel safe and private during labour and parturition. Researchers applying stress during labour to mammalian females of various species have shown reduced uterine blood flow in stressed sheep (Shnider *et al*. 1979), reduced uterine blood flow, abnormal fetal heart rate (FHR) and compromised fetal oxygenation in stressed baboons (Morishima *et al*. 1979), fetal hypoxia in rhesus monkeys (Morishima *et al*. 1978), increased maternal blood pressure and heart rate along with fetal bradycardia in stressed monkeys (Myers *et al*. 1972; Myers 1975), slowing of labour by 65–72% in stressed mice (Newton *et al*. 1966a), and prolonged atypical labour with up to several hours between pup births among stressed mice (Newton *et al*. 1966b).

Dutch biologist Naaktgeboren summarises, 'In all mammalian species, the course of delivery can be influenced by environmental disturbances ... Anxiety and fright inevitably lead to prolongation of the duration of labour ... For many animals, the mere presence of an observer acts as a stress-stimulus' (Naaktgeboren 1989).

Interestingly, the need for privacy in labour is familiar to most farmers and animal breeders, who go to some effort to leave a labouring female alone, unless assistance is really necessary (Andrews 1999; Florence 2002; Miller 2003).

Adrenaline/Noradrenaline in sexual behaviour

These hormones are also involved in sexual activity in mammalian species. Adrenaline and noradrenaline levels both rise with sexual arousal, increase as arousal increases and peak at orgasm in masturbating men and women (Exton *et al.* 1999; Kruger *et al.* 2003). Levels of E and NE at orgasm are around three times those of controls for men (Kruger *et al.* 2003) and increase half to one and one half times for women (Exton *et al.* 1999).

The physiological disturbances that ensue with environmental disturbances during labour, including disturbance by the presence of an observer, are likely to have parallels with sexual behaviour, although this does not seem to have been studied in humans or other mammals. Perhaps the need to feel private, safe and unobserved during sexual activity is so obvious and universal that it has not warranted study. Note however that the physiological monitoring and blood sampling performed during the studies of solitary human sexual behaviour was done using an elaborate system that was hidden behind a wall, therefore ensuring privacy.

In summary, both sexual activity and labour and birth involve relative immobility and vulnerability to predators. Therefore, both require participant vigilance and a subjective sense of safety. Because both are essential reproductive acts, it is likely that there has been intense evolutionary investment in a system to ensure that both sex and birth take place only under the safest of conditions.

The above evidence supports the A/NA SNS as the system that regulates these activities in terms of safety, and implies that a subjective sense of safety and privacy is as important during labour and birth as during sexual activities.

Prolactin

Originally named for its powerful pro-lactation effects, prolactin is the major hormone of breast-milk synthesis among all mammals. However research has uncovered over 300 other physiological effects on the body (Freeman *et al.* 2000). These include effects on immune function, metabolism (Ben-Jonathan *et al.* 2006), growth and other crucial aspects of homeostasis (Freeman *et al.* 2000).

Prolactin is also important in other facets of reproduction. Mice bred to be deficient in prolactin have major reproductive dysfunctions including low fertility, deficits in implantation and deficient maternal behaviour (Harris *et al.* 2004).

Prolactin has been called the 'mothering hormone', because of the ability of exogenous prolactin to promote maternal behaviours and its involvement with instinctive mothering behaviours post-partum (Freeman *et al.* 2000; Torner & Neumann 2002). Prolactin has also been implicated in nurturing paternal behaviours (Ziegler 2000).

Psychologically, high levels of prolactin in post-partum women have been associated with anxiety and aggression, which benefit offspring by increasing maternal vigilance and aggressive–defensive behaviour. Prolactin also benefits human mothers by increasing social desirability, making them more able to submit their own desires to the care of the baby (Uvnas-Moberg 1989).

During labour, maternal prolactin has a multiphasic pattern of release. In some species, a rise in prolactin has been documented in the nocturnal period before labour begins (Andrews 2005). This pre-birth surge is thought to be an essential preparation for post-natal lactation and maternal behaviour, at least in rats (Grattan 2001; Andrews 2005) but has not been studied in humans.

Subsequently, prolactin levels decline from early labour, reaching the lowest point close to the time of full dilation. Prolactin levels then rise dramatically, peaking 1–2 hours following birth and declining over the next 4–6 hours (Rigg & Yen 1977; Volpe *et al.* 1982; Fernandes *et al.* 1995; Stefos *et al.* 2001). A second nadir at 9 hours or so is maintained up to 24 hours after delivery (Buhimschi 2004).

This post-partum maternal surge in prolactin provides maximum levels, available to brain and body, for several hours after birth. This pattern of release may be important in optimising maternal behaviours at this time, as well as ensuring successful lactation.

Prolactin in sexual behaviour

Prolactin has important influences on sexual arousal and mating behaviour in mammals. In humans, prolactin levels rise during sexual activity (masturbation) and peak at orgasm in men and women. In contrast to oxytocin and A/NA, whose levels drop steeply post-orgasm, prolactin levels remain elevated for at least 1 hour afterwards (Exton *et al.* 1999; Kruger *et al.* 2002). In this situation, prolactin's libido-reducing effects may contribute to the post-coital drop in sexual interest.

In female rats, prolactin surges can also be induced by cervical stimulation (Freeman *et al.* 2000) which may also stimulate the prolactin surge in human birth (Fernandes *et al.* 1995; Fernandes *et al.* 1999). However, prolactin suppresses stereotypical male sexual behaviour in rats and sheep (Freeman *et al.* 2000).

Prolactin therefore has a pattern of release during sexual activity that parallels that of late labour and birth, with a prolonged release post-orgasm and post-natally. Prolactin's involvement in both birth and sexual activity further underlines the close physiological and hormonal parallels in both reproductive acts.

Summary: the ecstatic hormones

The research presented demonstrates that labour and birth, and sexual activity leading to orgasm, have physiological and hormonal parallels. The involvement of A/NA in both activities reflects the necessity of safety during both crucial reproductive acts.

Conclusion

This chapter has argued that labour and birth are intrinsically sexual experiences, based on labouring women's physiology, anatomy, subjective experiences and personal reports. Recognising the sexual dimensions of birth will help all of those involved in the care of labouring woman to appreciate the need for extreme sensitivity, not only in physical and verbal interactions, but also in the atmosphere that they create and maintain for those under their care. Conditions that enhance a labouring woman's sense of privacy and safety and help her to feel unobserved are likely to reduce her A/NA levels, thereby optimising her labour progress and possibly benefitting the blood supply to her baby.

The physiological parallels discussed in this chapter would further suggest that an optimal birthing atmosphere is one that would be optimal for sexual activity. Practically, this emphasises the guardian role of the midwife and her importance in protecting the privacy of the labour room as far as possible. Dim lighting, low sounds, and limiting extraneous conversation will also contribute to a private atmosphere in labour.

This chapter also presents anecdotal evidence that sexual activity during labour may benefit the labouring woman by easing pain and enhancing progress without the side-effects associated with other labour analgesia and stimulants. This may be a welcome perspective for some women and their partners, and could be usefully discussed in antenatal classes. More formal studies by midwives, students and others of the use of sexual activity in labour should also be encouraged.

References

Alehagen S, Wijma B, Wijma K *et al.* (2005) Fear, pain and stress hormones during childbirth. *Journal Psychosomatic Obstetrics and Gynaecology* 26(3): 153–65.

Andrews BJ (1999) Rx For Whelping and Ceasarians. *Showsight Magazine*, March 1999.

Andrews ZB (2005) Neuroendocrine regulation of prolactin secretion during late pregnancy: easing the transition into lactation. *Journal of Neuroendocrinology* 17(7): 466–73.

Argiolas A (1999) Neuropeptides and sexual behaviour. *Neuroscience Biobehavioral Review* 23(8): 1127–42.

Argiolas A, Melis MR (2003) The neurophysiology of the sexual cycle. *Journal of Endocrinology Investigations* 26(Suppl 3): 20–2.

Ariel Drori S (2005) *Combining the feminine orgasm in the childbirth process.* http://www.leida.co.il/shiraz/show_top.asp?link=2.

Bacigalupo G, Riese S, Rosendahl H *et al.* (1990) Quantitative relationships between pain intensities during labor and beta-endorphin and cortisol concentrations in plasma. Decline of the hormone concentrations in the early postpartum period. *Journal of Perinatal Medicine* 18(4): 289–96.

Baker JP (2001) *Prenatal Yoga and Natural Childbirth.* Berkeley, North Atlantic Books.

Ben-Jonathan N, Hugo ER, Brandebourg TD *et al.* (2006) Focus on prolactin as a metabolic hormone. *Trends Endocrinology Metabolism* 17(3): 110–6.

Blanks AM, Thornton S (2003) The role of oxytocin in parturition. *British Journal of Obstetrics and Gynaecology* 110(Suppl 20): 46–51.

Bodnar RJ (2007) Endogenous opiates and behavior: 2006. *Peptides* 28(12): 2435–513.

Brinsmead M, Smith R, Singh B *et al.* (1985) Peripartum concentrations of beta endorphin and cortisol and maternal mood states. *Australian and New Zealand Journal of Obstetrics and Gynaecology* 25(3): 194–7.

Buckley SJ (2004) Undisturbed birth: nature's hormonal blueprint for safety, ease and ecstasy. *MIDIRS Midwifery Digest* 14(2): 203–9.

Buckley SJ (2009) Undisturbed birth: mother nature's blueprint for safety, ease and ecstasy. *Gentle Birth, Gentle Mothering: A Doctors Guide to Natural Childbirth and Early Parenting Choices.* Brisbane, Celestial Arts.

Buhimschi CS (2004) Endocrinology of lactation. *Obstetrics and Gynaecology Clinics of North America* 31(4): 963–79, xii.

Burleson MH, Trevathan WR, Todd M *et al.* (2007) In the mood for love or vice versa? Exploring the relations among sexual activity, physical affection, affect, and stress in the daily lives of mid-aged women. *Archives of Sex Behaviours* 36(3): 357–68.

Carmichael MS, Humbert R, Dixen J *et al.* (1987) Plasma oxytocin increases in the human sexual response. *Journal of Clinical Endocrinology Metabolism* 64(1): 27–31.

Carter AM, Olin T (1972) Effect of adrenergic stimulation and blockade on the uteroplacental circulation and uterine activity in the rabbit. *Journal of Reproductive Fertility* 29(2): 251–60.

Csaba G, Tekes K (2005) Is the brain hormonally imprintable? *Brain Development* 27(7): 465–71.

Davis-Floyd R (2003) *Birth as an American Rite of Passage.* Berkeley, University of California Press.

Exton MS, Bindert A, Scheller F *et al.* (1999) Cardiovascular and endocrine alterations after masturbation-induced orgasm in women. *Psychosomatic Medicine* 61(3): 280–9.

Ferguson J (1941) A study of the motility of the intact uterus at term. *Surgery Gynaecology and Obstetrics* 73: 359–66.

Fernandes PA, Boroditsky RS, Roberts GK *et al.* (1999) The acute release of maternal prolactin by instrumental cervical dilatation simulates the second stage of labor. *Journal for the Society of Gynaecological Investigations* 6(1): 22–6.

Fernandes PA, Szelazek JT, Reid GJ *et al.* (1995) Phasic maternal prolactin secretion during spontaneous labor is associated with cervical dilatation and second-stage uterine activity. *Journal of the Society of Gynecological Investigations* 2(4): 597–601.

Ferris CF, Kulkarni P, Harder JA *et al.* (2005) Pup suckling is more rewarding than cocaine: evidence from functional magnetic resonance imaging and three-dimensional computational analysis. *Journal of Neuroscience* 25(1): 149–56.

Florence R (2002) *Lambing FAQ: What do I Have to do for a 'Normal' Birth?*

Foley KM, Kourides IA, Inturrise CE *et al.* (1979) Beta-endorphin: analgesic and hormonal effects in humans. *Proceedings of the National Academy of Science USA* 76(10): 5377–81.

Franceschini R, Venturini PL, Cataldi A *et al.* (1989) Plasma beta-endorphin concentrations during suckling in lactating women. *British Journal of Obstetrics and Gynaecology* 96(6): 711–3.

Fraser J (2008) Birthrape (Poem). *The Mother Magazine*, (26): 15.

Freeman ME, Kanyicska B, Lerant A *et al.* (2000) Prolactin: structure, function, and regulation of secretion. *Physiological Review* 80(4): 1523–631.

Freeze R (2008), PhD thesis *Born Free: Unassisted Birth in North America.* University of Iowa, Iowa city, April 08.

Fuchs AR, Romero R, Keefe D *et al.* (1991) Oxytocin secretion and human parturition: pulse frequency and duration increase during spontaneous labor in women. *American Journal of Obstetrics and Gynaecology* 165(5 Pt 1): 1515–23.

Gamble JA, Creedy DK (2001) Women's preference for a cesarean section: incidence and associated factors. *Birth* 28(2): 101–10.

Gaskin IM (2002) *Spiritual Midwifery.* Summertown, TN, The Book Publishing Company.

Gaskin IM (2003) *Ina May's Guide to Childbirth.* New York, Bantam, 161.

Gimpl G, Fahrenholz F (2001) The oxytocin receptor system: structure, function, and regulation. *Physiological Review* 81(2): 629–83.

Goffin V, Bouchard B, Ormandy CJ *et al.* (1998) Prolactin: a hormone at the crossroads of neuroimmunoendocrinology. *Annals of New York Academy of Science* 840: 498–509.

Goldstein A, Hansteen RW (1977) Evidence against involvement of endorphins in sexual arousal and orgasm in man. *Archives of General Psychiatry* 34(10): 1179–80.

Grattan DR (2001) The actions of prolactin in the brain during pregnancy and lactation. *Progress in Brain Research* 133: 153–71.

Griesemer L (1998) *Unassisted Homebirth: An Act of Love*. San Francisco, Terra Publishing.

Gutkowska J, Jankowski M, McCann SM *et al.* (2000) Oxytocin is a cardiovascular hormone. *Brazilian Journal of Medical and Biological Research* 33(6): 625–33.

Harris J, Stanford PM, Oakes SR *et al.* (2004) Prolactin and the prolactin receptor: new targets of an old hormone. *Annals of Medicine* 36(6): 414–25.

Hofmeyr GJ, Gulmezoglu AM, Nikodema VC *et al.* (1995) Labor experience and beta-endorphin levels. *International Journal of Gynaecology and Obstetrics* 50(3): 299–300.

Hull EM, Dominguez JM (2007) Sexual behavior in male rodents. *Hormones and Behaviour* 52(1): 45–55.

Insel TR (2003) Is social attachment an addictive disorder? *Physiology and Behavior* 79(3): 351–7.

Jones C (1997) *The Secret Life of the Expectant Mother*. Secaucus, Citadel Press.

Kinsey A (1953) *Sexual Behavior in the Human Female*. Philadelphia, Saunders.

Kinsley CH, Lambert KG (2006) The maternal brain. *Scientific American* 294(1): 72–9, p. 73.

Kitzinger S (1984) *The Experience of Childbirth*. Hammondworth, Penguin, 22.

Kitzinger S (2006) *Birth Crisis*. London, Routlege.

Kruger T, Exton MS, Pawlak C *et al.* (1998) Neuroendocrine and cardiovascular response to sexual arousal and orgasm in men. *Psychoneuroendocrinology* 23(4): 401–11.

Kruger TH, Haake P, Hartmann U *et al.* (2002) Orgasm-induced prolactin secretion: feedback control of sexual drive? *Neuroscience and Biobehavioral Review* 26(1): 31–44.

Kruger TH, Haake P, Chereath D *et al.* (2003) Specificity of the neuroendocrine response to orgasm during sexual arousal in men. *Journal of Endocrinology* 177(1): 57–64.

Laatikainen TJ (1991) Corticotropin-releasing hormone and opioid peptides in reproduction and stress. *Annals of Medicine* 23(5): 489–96.

Lederman RP, Lederman E, McCann DS *et al.* (1978) The relationship of maternal anxiety, plasma catecholamines, and plasma cortisol to progress in labor. *American Journal of Obstetrics and Gynecology* 132(5): 495–500.

Lederman RP, Lederman E, McCann DS *et al.* (1985) Anxiety and epinephrine in multiparous women in labor: relationship to duration of labor and fetal heart rate pattern. *American Journal of Obstetrics and Gynecology* 153(8): 870–7.

Lin SH, Kiyohara T, Sun B *et al.* (2003) Maternal behavior: activation of the central oxytocin receptor system in parturient rats? *Neuroreport* 14(11): 1439–44, p. 1444.

Lundeberg T, Uvnas-Moberg K, Agren G *et al.* (1994) Anti-nociceptive effects of oxytocin in rats and mice. *Neuroscience Letter* 170(1): 153–7.

Mahomed K, Gulmezoglu AM, Nikodem VC *et al.* (1995) Labor experience, maternal mood and cortisol and catecholamine levels in low-risk primiparous women. *Journal of Psychosomatic Obstetrics and Gynaecology* 16(4): 181–6.

Matthiesen AS, Ransjo-Arvidson AB, Nissen E *et al.* (2001) Postpartum maternal oxytocin release by newborns: effects of infant hand massage and sucking. *Birth* 28(1): 13–9.

McCarthy MM, Altemus M (1997) Central nervous system actions of oxytocin and modulation of behavior in humans. *Molecular Medicine Today* 3(6): 269–75.

McCracken L (2000) *Resexualizing Childbirth: A Collection of Essays.* Vancouver, Birthlove.

Mehl L (1980) Psychophysiological aspects of childbirth. In Feher L. (ed) *The Psychology of Birth: The Foundation of Human Personality.* London, Souvenir Press.

Miller T (2003) *Looking After New-born and Orphan Fawns.*

Mills R (1982) Birth Reborn. UK, BBC television.

Moran M (1997) *Pleasurable Husband/Wife Childbirth: The Real Consummation of Married Love.* New York, Terra Publishing.

Moran M (1981) *Birth and the Dialogue of Love.* New York, Terra Publishing.

Morgan LA (2003) *The Power of Pleasurable Childbirth: Safety, Simplicity and Satisfaction Are All Within Our Reach.* Writers Club Press.

Morishima HO, Pedersen H, Finster M *et al.* (1978) The influence of maternal psychological stress on the fetus. *American Journal of Obstetrics and Gynecology* 131(3): 286–90.

Morishima HO, Yeh MN, James LS *et al.* (1979) Reduced uterine blood flow and fetal hypoxemia with acute maternal stress: experimental observation in the pregnant baboon. *American Journal of Obstetrics and Gynecology* 134(3): 270–5.

Murphy MR, Seckl JR, Burton S *et al.* (1987) Changes in oxytocin and vasopressin secretion during sexual activity in men. *Journal of Clinical Endocrinology and Metabolism* 65(4): 738–41.

Myers RE (1975) Maternal psychological stress and fetal asphyxia: a study in the monkey. *American Journal of Obstetrics and Gynecology* 122(1): 47–59.

Myers GG, Krapohl AJ, Peterson RD *et al.* (1972) New method for measuring lag time between human uterine contraction and the effect on fetal heart rate. *American Journal of Obstetrics and Gynecology* 112(1): 39–45.

Naaktgeboren C (1989) The biology of childbirth. In Chalmers I, Enkin M, Keirse MN (eds) *Effective Care in Pregnancy and Childbirth,* Vol. 2. Oxford, Oxford University Press, 795–804, p. 801.

Nestler EJ, Hyman SE, Malenka SE *et al.* (2001) Neuropeptides and Purines. *Molecular Neuropharmacology: A Foundation for Clinical Neuroscience.* New York, McGraw-Hill, 213–34.

Newnham JP, Dennett PM, Ferron SA *et al.* (1984) A study of the relationship between circulating beta-endorphin-like immunoreactivity and post partum 'blues'. *Clinical Endocrinology (Oxford)* 20(2): 169–77.

Newton N (1955) *Maternal Emotions: A Study of Women's Feelings Toward Menstruation, Pregnancy, Childbirth, Breastfeeding and Other Aspects of Their Femininity.* New York, Harper and Brothers, 89.

Newton N (1971) Trebly sensuous woman. *Psychology Today* 98: 68–71.

Newton N, Foshee D, Newton M *et al.* (1966a) Experimental inhibition of labor through environmental disturbance. *Obstetrics and Gynecology* 27(3): 371–7.

Newton N, Foshee D, Newton M *et al.* (1966b) Parturient mice: effect of environment on labor. *Science* 151(717): 1560–1.

Nissen E, Lilja G, Widstrom AM *et al.* (1995) Elevation of oxytocin levels early post partum in women. *Acta Obstetrica Gynecologae Scandanavia* 74(7): 530–3.

Numan M (2006) Hypothalamic neural circuits regulating maternal responsiveness toward infants. *Behavioral and Cognative Neuroscience Review* 5(4): 163–90.

Odent M (1987) The fetus ejection reflex. *Birth* 14(2): 104–5.

Odent M (2001) *The Scientification of Love*. London, Free Association Books.

Pancheri P, Zichella L, Fraioli F *et al.* (1985) ACTH, beta-endorphin and met-enkephalin: peripheral modifications during the stress of human labor. *Psychoneuroendocrinology* 10(3): 289–301.

Panksepp J, Nelson E, Siviy S *et al.* (1994) Brain opioids and mother-infant social motivation. *Acta Paediatric Supplement* 397: 40–6.

Pascali-Bonaro D (2007) *Orgasmic Birth* (Film).

Press JZ, Klein MC, Kaczorowski J *et al.* (2007) Does cesarean section reduce postpartum urinary incontinence? A systematic review. *Birth* 34(3): 228–37.

Raisanen I, Paatero H, Salminen S *et al.* (1984) Pain and plasma beta-endorphin level during labor. *Obstetrics and Gynecology* 64(6): 783–6.

Read GD (1949) Observations on a series of labours; with special reference to physiological delivery. *Lancet* 1(18): 721–6.

Ribeiro SC, Kennedy SE, Smith YR *et al.* (2005) Interface of physical and emotional stress regulation through the endogenous opioid system and mu-opioid receptors. *Progress in Neuropsychopharmacol Biological Psychiatry* 29(8): 1264–80, p. 1267.

Rigg LA, Yen SS (1977) Multiphasic prolactin secretion during parturition in human subjects. *American Journal of Obstetrics and Gynecology* 128(2): 215–8.

Roman-Ponce H, Thatcher WW, Caton D *et al.* (1978) Effects of thermal stress and epinephrine on uterine blood flow in ewes. *Journal of Animal Science* 46(1): 167–74.

Rosenfeld CR, Barton MD, Meschia G *et al.* (1976) Effects of epinephrine on distribution of blood flow in the pregnant ewe. *American Journal of Obstetrics and Gynecology* 124(2): 156–63.

Seaman J (2000) *A Clear Road to Birth (DVD)*.

Segal S, Csavoy AN, Datta S *et al.* (1998) The tocolytic effect of catecholamines in the gravid rat uterus. *Anesthesia and Analgesia* 87(4): 864–9.

Shanley L (2008a) *Orgasmic Childbirth*. www.unassistedchildbirth.com/sensual/orgasmic.html (accessed 26/03/08).

Shanley L (2008b) *Pain Relief with Unassisted Birth*. www.unassistedchildbirth.com/uc/pain.html (accessed 26/03/08).

Shanley L (2008c) *Sensual Pregnancy and Birth*. www.unassistedchildbirth.com/sensual/ (accessed 26/03/08).

Shanley LK (1994) *Unassisted Childbirth*. Westport CT, Bergin & Garvey, 69.

Shnider SM, Wright RG, Levinson G *et al*. (1979) Uterine blood flow and plasma norepinephrine changes during maternal stress in the pregnant ewe. *Anesthesiology* 50(6): 524–7.

Simkin P, Klaus P (2004) *When Survivors Give Birth: Understanding and Healing the Effects of Early Sexual Abuse on Childbearing Women*. Seattle, Classic Day Publishing.

Stefos T, Sotiriadis A, Tsirkas P *et al*. (2001) Maternal prolactin secretion during labor. The role of dopamine. *Acta Obstetrica Gynecologae Scandanavia* 80(1): 34–8.

Tew M (1998) *Safer Childbirth? A Critical History of Maternity Care*. London, Free Association Books.

Thackare H, Nicholson HD, Whittington K *et al*. (2006) Oxytocin – its role in male reproduction and new potential therapeutic uses. *Human Reproduction Update* 12(4): 437–48.

Torner L, Neumann ID (2002) The brain prolactin system: involvement in stress response adaptations in lactation. *Stress* 5(4): 249–57.

Uvnas-Moberg K (1989) Physiological and psychological effects of oxytocin and prolactin in connection with motherhood with special reference to food intake and the endocrine system of the gut. *Acta Physiogical Scandanavia Supplement* 583: 41–8.

Uvnas-Moberg K (2003) *The Oxytocin Factor*. Cambridge, Da Capo Press.

Volpe A, Mazza V, De Renzo GC *et al*. (1982) Prolactin and certain obstetric stress conditions. *International Journal of Biological Research Pregnancy* 3(4): 161–6.

Wessel H (1963) *Natural Childbirth and the Christian Family*. New York, Harper and Rowe.

Young LJ, Lim MM, Gingrich B *et al*. (2001) Cellular mechanisms of social attachment. *Hormones and Behaviour* 40(2): 133–8.

Ziegler TE (2000) Hormones associated with non-maternal infant care: a review of mammalian and avian studies. *Folia Primatolgica (Basel)* 71(1–2): 6–21.

Chapter 13
Spirituality and Labour Care

Jenny Hall

> ... the birth of a child not only marks the transition of a new soul into the universe, but the journey of a woman into motherhood, of a man into fatherhood and of the family into a new design which enables continuation of a personal and community growth. The circle of life is renewed, and communities rejoice.
>
> (Wickham 2001, www.withwoman.co.uk)

Introduction

The powerful nature of birth has been recognised since the earliest literature. As recorded in ancient religious and philosophical writings, birth is seen to have a spiritual significance with participants in the creation and wonder of new life. Ancient philosophers, Socrates and Plato, used the symbolism of birth and midwives in their writings (Mullin 2002). Birth indicated to them a powerful message about life that we could all learn from.

Davis-Floyd (2003) has described the clear link between birth and death and from the earliest times, midwives, as the local wise women, had a role in both, providing care at both ends of the spectrum. Birth can thus be viewed as a part of the continuum of life with the potential to be transformative for all concerned, as indicated by Sara Wickham's (2001) quote at the start of this chapter. For many women, the journey into motherhood is viewed as the most important learning experience (Belenky *et al.* 1996) or as a 'peak' time (Bergum 1989) in their lives. The act of birth is also on a continuum with pregnancy and all that has gone before and the post-natal period and all that goes after. It is a time of rituals that relate to the place, culture and societies where birth happens (Sweet & de Vries 2006). What occurs in labour is affected by the culture, the values, upbringing, education, religion, society, family and many other factors in which a woman lives or has grown (Ayers-Gould 2000). The woman will bring all these with her to her labour and it is important to remember that they may all have an influence.

Women speak about birth in a number of ways, but their stories often indicate spiritual meaning and beliefs that may be different from our own (Hebblethwaite 1984; Gaskin 2002; LaChance 2002; Milan 2003; Clark Callister 2004; Semenic *et al.* 2004). Flandermeyer (2008: 122) writes that spiritual meaning 'fosters renewed hope and leads to peace of mind that enables people to accept and live with otherwise insolvable problems'. Spiritual meaning can also be understood as 'the subjective significance of a pivotal life event such as childbirth' (Clark Callister *et al.* 1996: 67). Many women write about childbirth as being a life-changing, powerful event that catalyses the transition to motherhood. In some cultures this time of transformation is regarded as a rite of passage – a move to a new social status (Balin 1988; Ayers-Gold 2000) as mothers, honoured and revered (Kitzinger 2000a). This transformation, power and sacredness can lead women to consider the events of labour as having a spiritual nature. Ayers-Gold (2000) writes of a 'transcendence of a hope and a dream into a real, living being' and 'the creation of life'. For those with a religious belief, Baumiller (2002) suggests that giving birth may bring women closer to the Higher Being they believe in. It is strange, therefore, that there continues to be limited research carried out to explore the spiritual significance of birth to women, though nursing literature on spiritual issues is considerable, especially in relation to life-threatening disease or end-of-life care.

In Europe, a commitment has been made to ensure that care throughout the lifecycle has a 'holistic' focus (European Forum of National Nursing and Midwifery Associations 2004). In addition, the International Confederation of Midwives (ICM) (2007) states that 'midwifery care is holistic in nature, grounded in an understanding of the social, emotional, cultural, spiritual, psychological and physical experiences of women and based on the best available evidence' and that 'childbearing is a profound experience, which carries significant meaning to the woman, her family and the community'. In the United Kingdom, current maternity care policy encourages viewing the pregnant woman as central to care, as an individual and as a whole person (Department of Health 2004; Nursing Midwifery Council 2004). Holistic practice is often discussed without identification of what this means. A whole person approach implies addressing all aspects of a person's life, as indicated by the ICM above, as well as understanding the interaction between them. This tends to be in direct conflict with the 'technocratic' paradigm (Davis-Floyd 2001) currently present in the developed world maternity services. The framework of holism under which midwifery is meant to be taught includes the spiritual nature of persons and therefore midwives require education in relation to spirituality (Hall & Mitchell 2008). How this should take place is debated, especially in relation to the evidence underpinning spirituality (Mitchell & Hall 2008). The aim of this chapter is to consider the evidence that is currently available and to provide a suggested framework under which midwives may offer spiritual care.

Definitions

Holistic care: 'Multidimensional, person-centred care' that includes reference to physical, psychological, spiritual and social aspects. (Greenstreet 2006, p. 25).

Spirituality: 'Spirituality is a personal search for meaning and purpose in life, which may or may not be related to religion. It entails connection to self-chosen and/or religious beliefs, values and practices that give meaning to life, thereby inspiring and motivating individuals to achieve their optimal being. This connection brings faith, hope, peace, and empowerment. The results are joy, forgiveness of oneself and others, awareness and acceptance of hardship and mortality, a heightened sense of physical and emotional well-being and the ability to transcend beyond the infirmities of existence' Tanyi (2002, p. 506).

Spiritual care: 'To be able to assess the spiritual needs of the client and to be able to meet those needs' (Hall 2001, p. 4) .

Religion: Is 'a system of faith and worship which expresses an underlying spirituality. This faith is frequently interpreted in terms of particular rules, regulations, customs and practices, as well as the belief content of the named religion' (Speck 1998).

Culture: Is a 'particular group's values, beliefs, norms and practices that are learned and shared and that guide thinking, decision, and actions in a patterned way' (Leininger 1985, p. 209).

Women's views

Evidence of the spiritual nature of birth comes from women themselves. Stories they relate of their birthing experience tell of their beliefs in the power of the labour experience, its sacred nature and the transformation that takes place (Balin 1988; Klassen 2001; Gaskin 2002; Semenic *et al.* 2004). For example, Meg in Klassen's study (2001) states:

> I saw it, I felt it, I experienced a spirit-type thing moving through me, changing my perceptions of things with seeing people, hearing the

noises [in a] funny [way]. I know it was probably physical . . . your body going through physical changes, but something was making that happen. My body was being altered so that it could work with something that was greater than it. (p. 91)

Heather relates:

The experience itself is so different from anything you ever experience except when you're having birth, so in that respect, I think it's a spiritual experience, just as any other rites of passage . . . it's an experience that you never forget . . . [It's] spiritual and significant . . . because of the feelings that you have, the lessons that you learn, the insights in relation to the experience. (p. 94)

Research that asks women about their views of the spiritual nature of labour and birth is limited. Recent studies have been specifically related to women's views of spiritual issues in relation to pregnancy (Carver & Ward 2007; Jesse *et al.* 2007) or complicated pregnancies (Price *et al.* 2007). In a study carried out as part of BSc studies O'Shea (1998) interviewed women who had just had their first baby. They were from different nationalities and three of them had given birth at home. O'Shea had investigated whether childbirth is a spiritual experience and concluded that this was true for all the participants, whatever beliefs the women had. Carver and Ward's (2007) study considered the views of seven women, five of whom thought spirituality was important to them in pregnancy. For each of these women, their expression of this was individual. They did not have expectations that health carers would be in a position to meet their spiritual needs but they did expect respect for their beliefs. To enable this, it is clear that midwives need to know women to be able to know how women express their individual spirituality and to be able to respect this individuality in labour.

The women who had religious faith in Klassen's study (2001) believed in a deity who was 'an empowering partner . . . who had faith in themselves and in birth' (p. 77). Religious belief may thus provide women with significant support. The influence of religious belief on birth has been investigated by a few studies (Sered 1991; Clark Callister *et al.* 1996; Cioffi 2004; Semenic *et al.* 2004). It leads to the introduction of religious rituals and behaviours that may be unusual to the midwife caring for the family. In Sered's (1991) study of the experience of Jewish women, she concluded that this group did not view their birth experiences as 'peak incidents' or of 'religious significance' but as part of the 'continuation of their lives'. Sered suggests that the effect of the Jewish law regarding birth as 'polluting' was to deny women the ability to express the experience in spiritual terms. For this group, men have the responsibility during childbirth to undertake most of the rituals and prayers. This is in contrast to the Semenic *et al.* (2004) study of orthodox Jewish women living in Canada, where it was the women who spoke of spiritual and meaningful qualities of their birth experiences. The differences between the studies may be related to the different cultures in which they were carried out.

A number of resources provide information about the care of women in labour of particular religious and cultural groups, such as Schott and Henley (1996), Sheikh and Gatrad (2000), Hollins (2006) and the **NHS** Education for Scotland (2006). It is wise for midwives to be aware of the religious and cultural groups in their community and the role these beliefs may play on labour. However, even though a woman may belong to such groups, there is a potential that she may not practice or agree with the doctrine. Midwifery care should involve asking if the belief is significant to her and what impact this will have on her wishes for labour and birth.

Jesse *et al.*'s (2007) study focused on a population of 130 low-income African-American and Caucasian women, asking 'How does your faith or spirituality affect your pregnancy if at all'? Forty-seven percent of the women felt spirituality was significant to them during pregnancy while 45% did not. Though not related to labour, and recognising the continuum of pregnancy and birth, this study indicates that nearly half of the women may regard birth as having spiritual significance. Midwives should therefore take this into account when caring for women and their families.

Birth environment

It has been suggested that the environment of labour is significant in enabling a woman to find a safe place to give birth and that privacy, security and not being disturbed are essential (Ayers-Gold 2000; Odent 2002). She should feel safe within the environment, but also with those present 'if she is to be able truly to let go of who she is and open herself up to what she will become' (Hall & Taylor 2004). In this setting, the woman should have the freedom to practise any rituals or ceremonies that are significant for her beliefs (Hall & Taylor 2004). In Klassen's (2001) study, most of the women stated that 'birth could be an empowering spiritual process and that home birth was the best way to allow such spirituality to be manifested' (p. 82). For others, a spiritually safer place will be in hospital. However, Sered's (1991) study indicated that Jewish couples tended to carry out ceremonies prior to going into hospital. Even in societies where religion is central to culture, it appears that women feel more comfortable about carrying out rituals outside of the institution. Kahn (1995) has suggested that it is not possible to have a spiritual experience in hospital environments. However, women could be encouraged to find ways to 'prepare' the space spiritually within a hospital setting (Stockley 1986; England & Horowitz 1998; Ayers-Gould 2000; Gaskin 2002).

Much has been written about the contrasts between the institutional environment and the comfortable atmosphere of most homes (Lavender & Kingdon 2006: 336–7, Newburn & Singh 2003). Though there has been an increasing effort 'to create "softer"places in hospital', the philosophy of the carers within that environment is also significant (Page 2002). The aim to increase the number of smaller, midwifery-led units, as described by Walsh (2007) recognises that women and midwives feel more comfortable in a more personal environment.

Connection and relationship

The lead up to labour and birth is a time of preparation for women and their partners. It has been noted that the process of pregnancy includes establishing connections with other women who are in the same position or who have already given birth (Kahn 1995; O'Shea 1998; Gaskin 2002; LaChance 2002). This may be through connecting more deeply with the woman's own mother, as 'now they too know' (Baumiller 2002), though this may be potentially difficult if the relationship has previously been poor (Raphael-Leff 1991). Women may also form deeper connections in relation to their religious faith, or other beliefs, or by understanding their own family histories (Burkhardt 1994). Such connecting relationships have been seen as spiritually significant to women.

The most important connection the woman will make during pregnancy will be with her unborn child. The relationship where they are joined physically together, yet remain as two separate beings (Bergum 1989), is on a number of levels – physically, psychologically and spiritually – as the woman comes to terms with the pregnancy. Sered's (1991) study relating to Jewish women showed that for many the spiritual experience was in the developing relationship with their new baby during pregnancy instead of during labour. An important role for the midwife is to enable the woman to make these 'connections' with her baby, both during pregnancy and afterwards (Walsh 2006; Hall 2006). This may be through encouraging the woman to communicate with her unborn child in pregnancy (Robertson 2005; Verny & Weintraub 2005) and also in labour (Walsh 2006).

The process of pregnancy and birth is also a potentially transformative time for the partner. Deeper 'connections' may take place with the woman as they evolve into a family (O'Shea 1998). The experience of each partner will be individual to each situation. Awareness of the couple's relationships prior to the birth will enable the midwife to assess if the presence of the partner is appropriate throughout labour

(Gaskin 2002). Stories have been related of how the presence of some may detract the woman from being able to give birth effectively (Klassen 2001; Gaskin 2002). In some cultures, men are expected to stay away from the birth (Semenic *et al.* 2004) as it is 'women's work' or men may have particular rituals to undertake (Sered 1991). Midwives should make an effort antenatally to get to know the principles and expectations that the family has for the time around labour.

Women may also form deep connecting relationships with a primary midwife during the antenatal period. In an ideal situation, a large majority of women would probably prefer to 'know' the midwife who would care for them in labour, to know they have formed a relationship that is safe and trusting. (Halldorsdottir & Karlsdottir 1996; Morrison *et al.* 1999; Hodnett *et al.* 2007). Women may make considerable efforts to ensure that this takes place, by financially paying for an independent midwife or moving to a part of the country where this could be guaranteed. Some countries already have such schemes in place that enable midwives to care for women individually (Crabtree 2004). However, it is significant that a common philosophy of care, attitude of the carers and a comfortable environment such as in birth centres may mean women have less need to 'know' the person who cares for them in labour (Waldenström 1998).

The role of the midwife in developing a relationship with a woman in labour is significant to spiritual care. Making a woman feel safe, secure and cared for in labour is part of the skill of midwifery care. This may be more significant spiritually in a home birth situation, where the woman may feel safe enough to practise rituals and where midwives may feel more able to practise autonomously and intuitively, though this has also been noted by Walsh (2006) in his study of a birth centre. The skill of intuition is viewed as a significant part of spiritual care (Davis-Floyd & Davis 1997; Gaskin 2002) and it appears it is achieved when effective relationships have developed. It is also suggested that caring is an instinctive feeling, aided by self-knowledge of being cared for by others (Clarke & Wheeler 1992). Women appear to value intuitive skill and to recognise when midwives are using it (Halldorsdottir & Karlsdottir 1996; Downe *et al.* 2006). Further, when it is not perceived to be used, it appears that the women's confidence is affected (Berg *et al.* 1996).

A further issue in the caring relationship that appears to be of value is that of 'presence' (Hall & Taylor 2004). In nursing care it has been described in four ways by Osterman and Schwartz-Barcott (1996):

1. Absent presence: The nurse is physically in the room with the patient, but totally self-absorbed and not connected.
2. Partial presence: The nurse is physically present, but putting all her energy on a task instead of the patient.

3. Full presence: The nurse is physically and psychologically present and each patient interaction is 'personalised'.
4. Transcendent presence, or 'spiritual' presence: The nurse 'centres' herself, which could be understood as coming from a 'spiritual source'. The presence of the carer is felt as peaceful, comforting and harmonious. The ability to care appears to be boundless and she is able to recognise a 'oneness' or unity with the person being cared for.

'Patients ... intuitively seem to know whether the practitioner is authentically there or merely going through the motions of caring' (Covington 2005). In more simple terms, Wright (2001) highlights the difference between those carers with 'clear eyes' – who are focused on the individual – and those with 'glassy eyes' –who are distracted by other things. Further, Burkhardt (1998) writes of the need for the carer to actively 'let go' of the needs and worries of the person she has just been with in order to be able to be completely 'present' with the next person. This is a challenge in busy labour units where midwives may not have the opportunity to give one-to-one care.

Coping with labour

As indicated above, labour is a physical event that profoundly affects the woman's body and emotional processes. Ayers-Gold (2000) writes of the 'empowering and life-giving' nature of the pain of labour. Leap and Anderson (2004) write of labour pain being part of the rite of passage and offering relief to women 'is to deny them their transformation and their triumph, and ultimately to diminish them, both as strong women and as mothers' (p. 37). How she copes with the depth of the feelings and emotions involved will be personal. This may involve strategies that involve pharmacological relief, labour in water, or complementary therapies. The choices a woman makes will relate to her cultural roots and the society in which she is residing.

In Klassen's study, many women used prayer as a method of coping with labour. Some used the chanting of sacred texts or phrases, while others positively focused on their previous experience of birth or their own births (p. 79). These women had chosen to give birth at home and were open to experiencing the labour as a source of personal growth.

Effective care involves being able to judge and meet the needs of the woman. It is a balance between knowing 'she can do it' and appropriately giving support and comfort. To some women the use of an epidural will enable her to achieve a very positive birth. It is not always possible to judge how women will perceive the experience of birth, as illustrated in Clare's story below.

Case study: Clare's story

Clare was pregnant with her first child. She attended local National Child-birth Trust (NCT) classes and felt very positive about how she would cope in labour. She prepared a birth plan with her partner and planned the strategies they would use to cope. They were both very excited about the experience when she started labour. The actual time of the labour was only 1 hour and she gave birth naturally, without using any of the strategies they had planned. When she went home and was visited by her midwife she expressed her great disappointment with the whole experience, feeling she had been 'cheated' of the experience she had wanted. She was especially upset that 'she would not have a story to tell' to the others in her class.

For Clare, despite the labour being natural, the feelings of disappointment related to her expectations clouded her view emotionally and spiritually.

Complicated labour and birth

Research in relation to women's experience of complicated pregnancy demonstrates that women turned to spiritual resources to help them cope with their fears and anxieties (Price *et al.* 2007). Generally, these women believed spirituality was central to their humanity and was a source of health. It follows that women with more complicated labours may require support in order to use their spiritual resources to cope.

The effect of an unexpectedly difficult or traumatic time in labour can make women view the experience of birth very differently. For those women with particular spiritual beliefs, they may find resources in their beliefs that have positive effects, such as reducing stress (Jesse & Reed 2004). However, for some, strong beliefs may also have more negative effects if they do not achieve their expectations. In Klassen's study, Kathryn (p. 51) did not consider her labour and birth as spiritual, but felt it was more grounded in the physical nature. For her, the baby gave her spiritual meaning. Tessa in Klassen's study (p. 47) talked of her closeness to the 'other side' during birth in relation to her 'openness' at the point of transition. This 'openness' may be related to stories of out-of-body experiences or transpersonal events taking place during labour (Powell Kennedy 2002; Lahood 2007).

Sered's study (1991) of the religious experience of some Jewish women in birth discovered that it was when things went wrong that they turned to God for help. In relation to a complicated pregnancy, a study has shown that some women used spiritual belief and practices to enable them to cope with the experience (Price *et al.* 2007). Price *et al.*'s (2007) review of the literature in relation to spirituality and complicated pregnancy identified that women used prayer and other spiritual practices as coping strategies.

Third stage of labour

To some women and some cultural groups, the third stage of labour is viewed as sacred (Schneiderman 1998; Guthrie 1999; Spencer Lemon 2002; Wickham 2002). Sara Wickham suggests that the current 'disposal' of the placenta and waste products is a phenomenon of recent origin. She suggests that in ancient times the placenta would have been treated with respect. Sheila Kitzinger (2000b, pp. 144–6) describes how traditional cultures demonstrate the value placed in the placenta.

Particular rituals may take place in relation to the third stage and midwives should discuss these in the antenatal period to aid the family in facilitating the process. This is illustrated in Janet Schneiderman's article (1998) showing the diversity of cultural practices. In Klassen's study (p. 79) reverence of the third stage was expressed through the burial of the placenta, while others chose practices such as 'lotus birth' (Wickham 2002; Buckley 2005). Burial at the third stage has become more common in the developed world, with 'ceremonies' conducted at the time of burial. Practical issues relate to the transfer of the placenta from the hospital, if birth has taken place outside the home environment and ensuring that burial takes place at sufficient depth to comply with local laws and regulations. 'Lotus birth' involves leaving the umbilical cord intact following the birth of the placenta and keeping it attached until the cord falls off naturally at any time between 3 and 10 days (Buckley 2005). The use of herbs, oils and salt to help dry and keep the placenta sweet smelling is suggested (Wickham 2002; Buckley 2005). Wickham (2002) also highlights the advantages of this procedure to the mother and child relationship as the baby is less likely to be disturbed or handled by others. Other women celebrate the placenta through placentaphagy (eating the placenta) or inviting others to do this at a 'placenta party'. Though this is common behaviour amongst other mammals, it has only become a more regular occurrence for women in the developed worlds since the 1970s. Originally it was encouraged as a preventative measure against post-natal depressive illness, but more recently it was done as a celebration of the significance of the placenta.

Spirituality of the unborn

As labour leads to the birth of a new person, midwives should also consider the spiritual nature of the unborn child. Wickham (2001, p. 5) suggests that 'Holistic midwives understand the newly born baby is a unique and fully grown soul'. This entails understanding the cultural and religious care needs expressed by the parents. There is a likelihood that the experience of birth will affect the baby spiritually (Hall 2006) and Michel Odent (2002) suggests that the increasing intervention rates will affect future generations. Therefore, consideration should be given as to how labour and birth are carried out in relation to the environment of birth, the use of induction or augmentation, epidural anaesthesia and Caesarean section which, Odent (2002) concludes, have an effect on the release of the hormones that enable a woman to love her child.

Each woman and her family may also have views on the spiritual values of the child, which will be influenced by her beliefs and her culture (Hall 2006). This could affect how deeply she has made a connection with her baby during pregnancy, though those with more complicated pregnancies or labours may try not to become attached until the baby is perceived to be safe (McGeary 1994).

Implications

The above discussion demonstrates that there is, currently, a need to carry out more research into women's and midwives' perception of the spirituality of childbirth. Current research examines women's embodied sense of self (Parratt 2008), midwives' views of spirituality (Linhares 2005) and indigenous experiences of women (Sweet 2008). It is clear that there needs to be more research in order to know how spiritual care in labour should be carried out. Further philosophical discussion should be encouraged to assist in understanding the nature of spirituality in relation to the unborn (Hall 2006) and the implications for care during labour.

The issues raised above clearly identify areas where midwifery practice could be altered to enable more effective spiritual care. Individualisation of care will enhance spiritual care by aiming to meet the holistic needs of a woman and her family. This entails time as the midwife needs to dedicate effort in 'getting to know' the woman and her desires and needs. The evidence shows that women would like stronger relationships with their midwives and generally would prefer to know the person who will be the main caregiver in labour. Providing a known carer is more likely to ensure that appropriate relationships are established, to enable the woman to explore spiritual rituals and practices around childbirth, if they so desire. It will help women to find meaning and purpose in the event. In the antenatal period, midwives could ask questions to open up the area of spirituality. For example,

- How do you feel about the pregnancy? Can you describe positive and negative thoughts/feelings you have about it?
- Do you have a belief that is meaningful to you? Might they affect your choices for intervention or screening? Does your partner have the same beliefs or are there others who you turn to for support?
- What religions are represented in the midwife's community? Does the midwife know what their beliefs are about pregnancy, abortion, antenatal testing, labour, death of a baby and post-natal care of the infant? To give culturally and ethically sensitive care, it is important to find out the answers to these questions.
- Do you pray or meditate?
- Are there cultural or religious traditions you would like to carry out at the birth or after?
- Are there religious leaders or other individuals whom you would like to see the baby at birth?
- What can be done about organisation and structures to help women have spiritual care? How can the structures where you work be improved to enable facilitation of spiritual care?

The midwives Klassen spoke to (p. 80) 'felt largely that their role was not to impose a spiritual perspective on birth, but to be there to help with the birth, and let a woman practice and interpret her spirituality as she saw fit'. The more culturally and religiously diverse populations are, the greater the need to individualise care.

Some of the following could be suggested to women and their families, if they have an interest in exploring spirituality during pregnancy and birth.

Box 13.1 Suggestions to celebrate pregnancy and birth (Wickham 2001; Hall 2007, p. 223)

- Meditation to communicate with the unborn
- Journaling during pregnancy
- Special food for labour
- Music
- Candle ceremonies
- Massage oils
- Mantras or prayers
- A birth box to celebrate the event
- Connecting with other women
- Walking in a special place
- Creating a meaningful symbol

The way midwives are educated is significant in relation to spiritual care. It suggests that students should explore spiritual issues from a personal perspective to enable them to understand the concepts in greater depth (Mitchell & Hall 2008). However, the evidence in this area is limited and requires more research. The increasing diversity of populations requires more understanding of the cultural nature of labour and birth. Educational systems, therefore, should reflect the local populations in order for midwives to become grounded in the needs of these women.

Conclusion

As labour is a significant time in women's lives, it is clear that midwives should make an effort to ensure that everything is in place to enable this to be as meaningful as possible. Women-centred, holistic care involves asking questions that will help this care to be provided to the best of the midwives' ability. It is clear that current policies and structures militate against this, with a culture of technology and focusing on the physical nature of the birth experience above all else. Conversely, in areas where midwives are able to practise autonomously and have some control over the comfort of the environment, the experience of the women is meaningful and powerful (Klassen 2001; Gaskin 2002; Walsh 2006). In order to re-establish birth as a positive spiritual event midwives should take more responsibility for the environments they work in and practices they carry out. Women need midwives to be there for them, and what midwives do will have an effect for the lifetime of that woman and her baby. As Wickham (2001, p. 6) states,

> Birth is a beautiful and wondrous rite of passage for everyone concerned. As a midwife I feel privileged to witness this miracle on a regular basis; every day is a birthday, and every birth can also be an enlightening and empowering expression of a woman and her family's spirituality.

References

Ayers-Gould JN (2000) Spirituality in birth: creating sacred space within the medical model. *International Journal Childbirth Education* 15: 14–7.

Balin J (1988) The sacred dimensions of pregnancy and birth. *Qualitative Sociology* 11: 275–301.

Baumiller R (2002) Spiritual development during a first pregnancy. *International Journal of Childbirth Education* 17: 7.

Belenky M, Clinchy B, Goldberger M, Mattuck Tarule J (1996) *Women's Ways of Knowing: The Development of Self, Voice and Mind*, 10th anniversary edition. New York, Basic Books.

Berg M, Lundgren I, Hermansson E *et al.* (1996) Women's experience of the encounter with the midwife during childbirth. *Midwifery* 12: 11–5.

Bergum V (1989) *Woman to Mother: A Transformation*. Granby, Bergin & Garvey.

Buckley S (2005) *Lotus Birth: A Ritual for our Times*, available from: http:// sarahjbuckley.com/articles/lotus-birth.htm (accessed 31/12/07).

Burkhardt MA (1994) Becoming and connecting: elements of spirituality for women. *Holistic Nursing Practice* 8: 12–21.

Burkhardt MA (1998) Reintegrating spirituality into healthcare. *Alternative Therapies* 4: 127–8.

Carver N, Ward B (2007) Spirituality in pregnancy: a diversity of experiences and needs. *British Journal of Midwifery* 15(5): 294–6.

Cioffi J (2004) Caring for women from culturally diverse backgrounds: Mid-wives' experiences. *Journal of Midwifery and Women's Health* 49: 437–42.

Clark Callister L (2004) Making meaning: women's birth narratives. *Journal of Obstetric, Gynaecologic and Neonatal Nursing* 33(4): 508–18.

Clark Callister L, Vehvilainen-Julkunen K, Lauri S (1996) Cultural perceptions of childbirth: a cross-cultural comparison of childbearing women. *Journal of Holistic Nursing* 14(1): 66–78.

Clarke JB, Wheeler SJ (1992) A view of the phenomenon of caring in nursing practice. *Journal of Advanced Nursing* 17: 1283–90.

Covington H (2005) Caring presence: providing a safe space for patients. *Holistic Nursing Practice* 19(4): 169–72.

Crabtree S (2004) Midwives constructing 'normal birth'. In Downe S (ed) *Normal Childbirth: Evidence and Debate*. Edinburgh, Churchill Livingstone.

Davis-Floyd R (2001) The technocratic, humanistic and holistic paradigms of childbirth. *International Journal of Gynaecology and Obstetrics* 75: S5–S23.

Davis-Floyd R (2003) Windows in space and time: a personal perspective on birth and death. *Birth: Issues in Perinatal Care* 30(4): 272–7.

Davis-Floyd R, Davis E (1997) Intuition as authoritative knowledge in midwifery and homebirth. In Davis-Floyd R, Sargent C (eds) *Childbirth and Authoritative Knowledge*. London, University of California Press.

Department of Health (2004) *The Children's National Service Framework [online]*, available from www.doh.gov/nsf/children/externalwg.htm (accessed 2009).

Downe S, Simpson L, Trafford K (2006) Expert intrapartum maternity care: a metasynthesis. *Journal of Advanced Nursing* 57(2): 127–40.

England P, Horowitz R (1998) *Birthing from Within*. Albuquerque, Partera Press.

European Forum of National Nursing and Midwifery Associations (2004) *Health21 – The Nursing and Midwifery Contribution*, available from http:// www.euro.who.int/efnnma/work/20040322_1 (accessed 25/11/07).

Flandermeyer P (2008) In response to: Easley R (2007) harmony: a concept analysis. *Journal of Advanced Nursing* 59(5): 551–6.

Gaskin IM (2002) *Spiritual Midwifery*. Cambridge, Summertown.

Greenstreet W (ed) (2006) *Integrating Spirituality in Health and Social Care: Perspectives and Practical Approaches*. Oxford, Radcliffe.

Guthrie P (1999) *Many Cultures Revere Placenta, By-product of Childbirth Tides of Life: An International Women's Holistic Health Resource Group*, available from http://www.tidesoflife.com/placenta.htm (accessed 31/12/07).

Hall J (2001) *Midwifery Mind and Spirit: Emerging Issues of Care*. Oxford, Books for Midwives.

Hall J (2006) Spirituality at the beginning of life. *Journal of Clinical Nursing* 15: 804–10.

Hall J (2007) Creativity, spirituality and birth. In Davies L (ed) *The Art and Soul of Midwifery: Creativity in Practice, Education and Research*. Edinburgh, Churchill Livingstone.

Hall J, Mitchell M (2008) Exploring student midwives creative expression of the meaning of birth. *Thinking Skills and Creativity* 3 (1): 1–14 available from: http://www.sciencedirect.com/science?_ob=ArticleURL&_udi=B7XN8-4PRRBYN-1&_user=5939061&_rdoc=1&_fmt=&_orig=search&_sort=d&_docanchor=&view=c&_searchStrId=1044450164&_rerunOrigin=google&_acct=C000009959&_version=1&_urlVersion=0&_userid=5939061&md5=3c2e4c17225f0f2d01cae02b33add772 (accessed 25/09/07).

Hall J, Taylor M (2004) Birth and spirituality. In Downe S (ed) *Normal Childbirth: Evidence and Debate*. Edinburgh, Churchill Livingstone.

Halldorsdottir S, Karlsdottir SI (1996) Empowerment or discouragement: women's experience of caring and uncaring encounters during childbirth. *Health Care Women International* 17: 361–79.

Hebblethwaite M (1984) *Motherhood and God*. London, Geoffrey Chapman.

Hodnett ED, Gates S, Hofmeyr GJ, Sakala C (2007) Continuous support for women during childbirth. *Cochrane Database of Systematic Reviews* (1) The Cochrane Collaboration. Published by John Wiley & Sons, Ltd. Date of Most Recent Substantive Amendment: 9 May 2003.

Hollins S (2006) *Religions, Culture and Healthcare*. Oxford, Radcliffe Publishing.

International Confederation of Midwives (2007) *Philosophy and Model of Midwifery Care*, available from: http://www.internationalmidwives.org/index.php?module=ContentExpress&func=display&ceid=59&bid=22&btitle=ICM%20Documents&meid=52 (accessed 02/04/07).

Jesse E, Reed P (2004) Effects of spirituality and psychosocial well-being on health risk behaviours in Appalachian pregnant women. *Journal of Obstetrics, Gynaecological Neonatal Nursing* 33(6): 739–47.

Jesse DE, Schoneboom C, Blanchard A (2007) The effect of faith or spirituality in pregnancy: a content analysis. *Journal of Holistic Nursing* 25(3): 151–8.

Kahn RP (1995) *Bearing Meaning: The Language of Birth*. Champaign, University of Illinois Press.

Kitzinger S (2000a) Some cultural perspectives of birth. *British Journal of Midwifery* 8: 746–50.

Kitzinger S (2000b) *Rediscovering Birth*. Boston, Little Brown and Co.

Klassen PE (2001) *Blessed Events: Religion and Home Birth in America*. Princeton, Princeton University Press.

LaChance CW (2002) *The Way of the Mother: The Lost Journey of the Feminine*. London, Vega.

Lahood G (2007) rumour of angels and heavenly midwives: anthroplogy of transpersonal events and childbirth. *Women and Birth* 20: 3–10.

Lavender T and Kingdon C (2006) keeping birth normal. In Page LA, McAndlish R (eds) *The New Midwifery: Science and Sensitivity in Practice*, 2nd edition. Edinburgh, Churchill Livingstone.

Leap N, Anderson T (2004) The role of pain in normal birth and the empowerment of women. In Downe S (ed) *Normal Childbirth: Evidence and Debate*. Edinburgh, Churchill Livingstone.

Leininger M (1985) Transcultural care diversity and universality: a theory of nursing. *Nursing and Health Care* 9: (4): 209–12.

Linhares CH (2005, July-August) Spirituality in midwifery and childbirth: a literature review (Abstract). Proceedings from the International Confederation of Midwives, Brisbane.

McGeary K (1994) The influence of guarding on the developing mother–unborn child relationship. In Field PA, Marck PB (eds) *Uncertain Motherhood: Negotiating the Risks of the Childbearing Years*. London, Sage Publication, 139–62.

Milan M (2003) Childbirth as healing: three women's experience of independent midwife care. *Complementary Therapies in Nursing and Midwifery* 9: 140–6.

Mitchell M, Hall J (2007) Teaching spirituality to student midwives: a creative approach. *Nurse Education in Practice* 7(6): 416–24.

Morrison S, percival P, Haucky Y, McMurray A (1999) Birthing at home: the resolution of expectations. *Midwifery* 15: 32–9.

Mullin A (2002) Pregnant bodies, pregnant minds. *Feminist Theory* 3(1): 27–44.

Newburn M, Singh D (2003) *Creating a Better Birth Environment: Women's Views about the Design and Facilities in Maternity Units: A National Survey. An Audit Toolkit*. London, National Childbirth Trust.

NHS Education for Scotland (2006) *Multi-Faith Resource for Healthcare Staff*, available from http://www.nes.scot.nhs.uk/documents/publications/classa/multifaith/Interactive%20master.pdf (accessed 20/11/07).

Nursing Midwifery Council (2004) *Midwives Rules and Code of Practice*. London, NMC.

Odent M (2002) *The Scientification of Love*, 2nd edition. London, Free Association.

O'Shea M (1998) *An exploratory study of women's experience of childbirth specifically identifying the spiritual dimension*. Unpublished thesis, BSc Midwifery Studies, The Nightingale Institute, King's College London.

Osterman P, Schwartz-Barcott D (1996) Presence: four ways of being there. *Nursing Forum* 31: 23–30.

Page L (2002) Building for a better birth. *British Journal of Midwifery* 10: 536–8.

Parratt J (2008) Territories of the self and spiritual practices during childbirth. In Fahy K, Foureur C, Hastie C (ed) *Birth Territory and Midwifery Guardianship*. London, Elsevier Science, 39–58.

Powell Kennedy H (2002) Altered consciousness during childbirth: potential clues to post traumatic stress disorder? *Journal of Midwifery and Woman's Health* 47: 380–2.

Price S, Lake M, Breen G, Carson G, Quinn C, O'Connor T (2007) The spiritual experience of high risk pregnancy. *Journal of Obstetrics, Gynaecological and Neonatal Nursing* 36: 63–70.

Raphael-Leff J (1991) *Psychological Processes of Childbearing*. London, Chapman & Hall.

Robertson T (2005) *Communicating with your Unborn Child*, available from: http://www.birthintuitive.com/communication.html (accessed 17/11/05).

Schneiderman J (1998) Rituals of placental disposal. *Maternal and Child Nursing* 23(3): 142–3.

Schott J, Henley A (1996) *Culture, Religion & Childbearing: A Handbook for Health Professionals*. Cheshire, Books for Midwives Press.

Semenic SE, Clark Callister L, Feldman P (2004) Giving birth: the voices of orthodox Jewish women living in Canada. *Journal of Obstetric, Gynaecologic, and Neonatal Nursing* 33(1): 80–7.

Sered SS (1991) Childbirth as a religious experience? Voices from an Israeli hospital. *Journal of Feminist Studies in Religion* 7: 7–18.

Sheikh A, Gatrad R (eds) (2000) *Caring for Muslim Patients*. Oxford, Radcliffe Publishing.

Speck P (1998) The meaning of spirituality in illness. In Cobb M, Robshaw V (eds) *The Spiritual Challenge of Healthcare*. Edinburgh, Churchill Livingstone.

Spencer Lemon B (2002) Exploring Latino rituals in birthing: understanding the need to bury the placenta AWHONN lifelines. *Association of Women's Health, Obstetric and Neonatal Nurses but 'AWHONN Lifelines* 6(5): 443–5.

Stockley S (1986) Psychic and spiritual aspects of pregnancy, birth and life. In Claxton R (ed) *Birth Matters*. London, Unwin, 75–98.

Sweet L (2008) Breastfeeding advocacy . *Who is responsible? Women & Birth* 21(4): 139–40.

Sweet M, de Vries DJ (2006) Birth rituals, wellbeing and transformation. *The International Journal of Healing and Caring* 6(2): 1–8 [Online], available from: http://www.wholistichealingresearch.com/may_2006_v6_n2.html.

Tanyi RA (2002) Towards clarification of the meaning of spirituality. *Journal of Advanced Nursing* 39(5): 500–9.

Verny TR, Weintraub P (2005) *The Womb – Your Child's First School Mothering 132*, available from: http://www.mothering.com/articles/pregnancy_birth/birth_preparation/womb.html (accessed 24/07/08).

Waldenström U (1998) Continuity of carer and satisfaction. *Midwifery* 14(4): 207–13.

Walsh D (2006) Nesting' and 'Matrescence' as distinctive features of a free-standing birth centre in the UK. *Midwifery* 22(3): 228–39.

Walsh D (2007) *Improving Maternity Services. Small is Beautiful – Lessons from a Birth Centre*. Oxford, Radcliffe Publishing.

Wickham S (2001) *Reclaiming Spirituality in Birth*, available from: http://www.withwoman.co.uk/contents/info/spiritualbirth.html (accessed 20/10/07).

Wickham S (2002) *The Internal Grandmother*, available from: http://www.withwoman.co.uk/contents/info/lotus.html (accessed 20/10/07).

Wright S (2001) Presence of mind. *Nursing Standard* 15(42): 22–3.

Chapter 14
How Midwives Should Organise
to Provide Intrapartum Care

Chris McCourt

Introduction

As we have seen in Chapter 1 of this book, the norms of place of birth shifted dramatically in the last century from a situation where almost all births, worldwide, occurred in women's homes, to one where almost all births in resource-rich 'developed' nations and increasing numbers in 'developing' nations took place in hospitals. This chapter, therefore, focuses on how midwives should organise to provide care as well as possible when labour and birth take place mainly in hospital settings. The discussion leaves aside the considerable and continuing debates about 'where to be born' (Tew 1995; Macfarlane & Mugford 1984), which is dealt with in Chapter 1. Given that in countries such as the United Kingdom, over 95% of women at the time of writing give birth in hospital[1], the challenge to be discussed is how care can best be organised to facilitate labour and birth that is optimal in this setting. Optimality can be related to broad concepts of safety that include not only clinical safety but also cultural and psychosocial safety, since all these different components of safety are fundamental to positive outcomes – a healthy outcome for mother and baby in the widest sense.

A number of critiques have focused on the characteristics of modern hospital organisation and their underlying design (Foucault 1976, 1980; Martin 1989; Arney 1982; McCourt in press). Being organised to provide care on a large scale, but also being influenced by prevailing cultural and social norms developing in Western countries in the modern era (McCourt in press, Downe and Walsh in this volume), hospitals were modelled and developed along the lines of factory production, as epitomised by the Ford motor factory and Taylorist principles (Martin 1989; McCourt in press). This chapter discusses organisational and workforce measures that have been tried to address some of the problems thrown up by the prevailing models of hospital care, and attempts to reform their operation. Implementing organisational change, to introduce new models or to reform existing ones inevitably presents the need to address what is often referred to as 'organisational culture' so this chapter also discusses cultural issues that may influence the nature and experience of birth in hospital, the ways in which midwives work when providing hospital-based intrapartum care, and the ability to bring about constructive change. To explore such issues, the chapter looks first at evidence on women's views and experiences of hospital birth, and on this basis goes on to explore the evidence on organisational forms and reforms that may be effective in helping to optimise hospital birth, and appropriate models of midwifery care for women giving birth in hospital.

What are women's views of hospital birth?

Despite notable exceptions, most women in 'Western' countries now take it for granted that birth takes place in a hospital. As Tew noted in her historical statistical analysis of birth outcomes data for the United Kingdom in the 20th century, from about 1970 in the United Kingdom, women were firmly advised that hospital birth was the safest choice and that home birth was risky, or even positively dangerous. The change had deeper roots of course, which are discussed elsewhere (see Chapter 1 in this volume) and the epidemiological historian Loudon (2002) noted that early in the 20th century in the United Kingdom, women began to choose hospital birth because they were advised that it offered the safety of medical care, as well as advantages such as access to pain relief. Loudon highlighted that as early as the 19th century, very clear observational evidence on the relatively high risks of hospital birth prior to 1930 was not explored or acted on by professionals, and not made apparent to the women, who understandably, therefore, associated the shift to hospital birth with ideas of medical and social progress. In the decades from the inception of a national health service (NHS) (1948 in the United Kingdom) to the 1970s, access to hospital beds was also understood very much as a hard-won right for ordinary people. Women were encouraged to view hospital birth as progressive, clean and safe and home birth (or birth in general practitioner-led small units) as old-fashioned, unhygienic and unsafe (Macfarlane & Mugford 1984; Tew 1995; Allison 1996). Similar processes have been observed in recent years for women in 'non-Western' countries where access to hospital birth has remained more limited, particularly in rural areas. Women living within reach of hospitals tend to accept hospitals births for a range of reasons, including the view that it is more modern, safe and hygienic (Van Hollen 2003; El–Nemer *et al.* 2006) despite their personal and sociocultural views which may include many reservations about giving birth in hospital.

As a consequence, many women (even in non-Western countries) hold the view that birth should take place in a hospital for safety reasons, and some also hold preferences around hygiene and now see hospital as a more 'normal' and appropriate location for labour and birth. Nonetheless, women are often making trade-offs between these basic assumptions and their personal, social and cultural views about the problems of labouring and giving birth in hospital.

Most of the evidence about women's views of hospital birth, in Western countries, comes from general studies of women's views of maternity or labour and birth care since, as most women give birth in hospital, it is rare for studies to focus specifically on views of hospital birth. National surveys (such as the NHS Survey 2005) tend to show that while the majority of women report satisfaction with birth care, a significant minority express very strong concerns about the care they receive. The following quote, from the NHS survey, illustrates the degree to which a negative experience may affect women emotionally:

1729: More support. Never saw the same person twice and was always made to feel like I was wasting their time. I know they are busy but they made the birth of my child a nightmare that even eight months later it makes me want to cry when thinking about it.

(NHS 2005, p. 61)

1791: I felt as if we were on a conveyer belt, and left to it pretty much once my son had been born.

(NHS 2005, p. 61)

Findings like these have been illuminated in greater depth in a number of smaller qualitative studies of birth. For the significant minority of women who have negative experiences, their feelings are of major importance, and will last and may even increase in their emotional significance with time (Simkin 1991; Waldenstrom 2004a). Additionally, studies focused on the birth experiences of more socially disadvantaged or minority ethnic women tend to show particular problems with quality and access to care (McCourt *et al.* 2000; Harper-Bulman & McCourt 2002).

The UK National Survey conducted by the National Perinatal Epidemiology Unit (NPEU), with a random sample of women giving birth in 2006 (Redshaw *et al.* 2007) analysed and reported data for hospital births and home births separately. Both the closed-question responses (tick box) and open text-box comments in this survey indicated the importance of professional support in labour to the women. As with other studies, the nature of the support was also important, with some women making clear the importance of simply being listened to. The following quotes, for example, illustrate the degree to which some staff may not be supporting women in a responsive manner:

> My midwife didn't believe I was in labour.

> The midwife that delivered my baby did everything by the book but I feel she didn't listen to me. When I went into the last stage of labour she wasn't even in the room, she'd left to get some pethidine which was administered too late.
>
> (Redshaw *et al.* 2007, p. 42)

Information and communication are key aspects of good quality support that have been highlighted in earlier studies (Garcia *et al.* 1998, McCourt *et al.* 2000) and continue to be raised, although the importance of good communication is more explicitly recognised in current policy (RCOG 2008). The 2006 NPEU survey indicated that while most women were satisfied that they were given information that they could understand, and were treated with respect, perhaps reflecting the growing professional awareness of information and communication issues, 11% of women reported that one or more midwives did not treat them with respect. Similarly, while very few women indeed had wholly negative views of their care by midwives or doctors, and the majority gave positive views, 20% of women had mixed views about their care from midwives.

The survey also indicated that, despite the evidence on the value of continuous support in labour, over half of the women and their birth partners had been left alone during their labour, and 18% reported having been worried by this. A further important area was choice, with only just over half of women indicating that they had choice in being able to move around and choose their positions, and only 15% reporting that they felt able to use alternative birth positions. Women's open responses indicated that they saw choices as depending on circumstances – medical problems often preventing some choices – but in some cases lack of choice led to feelings of lack of control, which studies have shown can lead to more negative perceptions and consequences of labour and birth (Green & Baston 2003). The following two quotes, from survey open responses illustrate that women with quite differing expectations of labour may be disappointed when organisational or professional (rather than clinical) considerations mean their choices cannot be supported:

> I was informed in labour that I was unable to have an epidural as all the anaesthetists were in theatre. The midwife then came in with pethidine. I felt a bit like I had no control.

> Luckily the first midwife I encountered finished her shift and I had a different midwife who was fantastic and respected my wishes to allow my labour to be as natural as possible. The first midwife almost forced me to consider an epidural and even got a chair to take me.
>
> (Redshaw *et al.* 2007, p. 41)

Clearly, not all choices are possible and medical complications may limit choice, and women appreciate and cope with this, but responses in this survey and many smaller studies highlight situations where lack of choice is governed primarily by organisational and institutional considerations. These are areas that could, and should, be changed (DH 2007).

Staff attitudes, forms and levels of support are often the most significant area of dissatisfaction (NHS 2005). Such studies also show that women tend to be more satisfied if they receive higher levels of choice and of continuity of care and carer (NHS 2005). However, the majority of women giving birth in hospital are attended by midwives they do not know, and many did not feel sufficiently well informed to make choices about the place of birth (NHS 2005). Overall, the NHS survey in 2005 indicated the main areas for improvement as being better support and staff attitude, better continuity of care, more personal treatment and more and better information (NHS 2005). Many women excuse lack of attention and support as they perceive staff to be very busy and often hard pressed, but poor staff attitudes are also a focus of concern. Staff who are excessively busy and working in stressful circumstances may, of course, find it difficult to provide a caring service. The following section will discuss ways in which labour and birth care in the hospital could improve these key indicators.

In Western countries, such as the United States and Canada, where midwifery care in labour is not the norm, the nature of hospital labour and birth care is different – for example, more technology-intensive labour is the norm and midwives or nurse midwives commonly attend women in labour but are required to call physicians for the birth. Nonetheless, studies highlight similar issues as being important to women. The first US national survey of women's experiences of childbearing (De Clercq *et al.* 2002), which used a stratified national sample, highlighted that while the majority of women also expressed satisfaction with their care, and felt well informed and involved, women showed relatively limited awareness of their rights relating to informed consent in labour and had limited knowledge of the benefits and risks of birth interventions and pain-relief methods. The study also highlighted relatively high rates of intervention on a routine rather than clinically selective basis, which appeared to be related to factors such as professional or organisational norms and convenience, such as continuous electronic fetal monitoring used in place of professional presence.

Studies from non-western contexts show great consistency across very differing circumstances in that women may perceive hospital care to be ideal because it is safe and modern, and staff professional, but may find staff attitudes uncaring and unsupportive (Van Hollen 2003; D'Ambruoso *et al.* 2005; El–Nemer *et al.* 2006). As a result, women may delay going to hospital until the second stage of labour, and access to hospital care is not necessarily a reflection of greater medical risk levels. Such trade-offs for women between perceived quality and perceived safety of care could be avoided with both better information about risks and benefits and a more humanistic approach to care in hospital.

A wide range of studies, both surveys and more in-depth qualitative studies, and in a range of social and national contexts, therefore, indicate that the quality and continuity of support given to women is of major importance to women's experiences, sense of control, satisfaction and well-being in labour. Key dimensions of good support include presence (Hodnett *et al.* 2008), information and communication (including being listened to and treated with respect) (Waldenstrom 2004b), choice, having a sense of control (Green & Baston 2003) and perceiving staff to be both caring and competent (Simkin 1991; McCourt *et al.* 2000; Wilkins 2000; McCourt 2006). While the majority of women are highly satisfied with their labour and birth care, or are understanding when care did not meet their expectations for particular reasons, the responses to qualitative studies illuminate how far quality of support can be compromised by the constraints of institutionally provided care.

How is intrapartum care currently organised in hospitals?

Although practice and organisation varies widely within as well as between different countries, there are nonetheless clear patterns of provision that characterise patterns of intrapartum care in obstetric units. The majority of hospitals that include maternity services generally have a unit with obstetric services, led by consultant obstetrician(s) but mainly staffed by midwives who provide the bulk of intrapartum care to women. The role of midwives varies internationally and in some countries, such as the United States, care is given by certified nurse-midwives, or obstetric nurses. In other countries, such as Australia, midwives have less clinical and professional autonomy than they do in the United Kingdom. In these contexts, midwives may provide much of the care throughout labour but are required to call on a physician or obstetrician to make decisions and to attend the birth itself. European and Nordic states' systems tend to vary between these two points (De Vries *et al.* 2001) while obstetric units in 'developing' countries in many cases employ nurses, with traditional midwives providing labour and birth care for rural women outside the formal health-care system.

The level of hierarchy and organisational forms of obstetric units also vary widely, but the most typical profile is of a relatively rigid and steep hierarchy, and organisational forms modelled on industrial production (Martin 1989; Arney 1982; McCourt in press). In many countries, midwives, despite their training, are below medical staff in the formal hierarchy, and there is also a clear hierarchy of roles within midwifery itself. In practice, researchers have noted that midwives often provide most of the care and operate most clinical decision-making, but significant ceremonial attention is given to maintaining the hierarchical organisational structure (Hunt & Symonds 1995; Kirkham 1999; Stevens 2003). Additionally, the adoption of an industrial model for the hospital unit and ward design means that professional staff are treated much in the manner of operatives (Martin 1989; Arney 1982) with the consequence that staff in a defined professional role have limited decision-making roles and are seen as substitutable for each other. Formal protocols or guidelines, as well as less formally acknowledged but equally established ways of working (which some might refer to as cultures or tacit rules and modes of practice), are intended to underpin this. In theory, when a hospital shift changes, and the individual staff change with it, care is expected to remain consistent.

As indicated in the previous section, successive studies of women's and their families' experiences of intrapartum care, and a number of government enquiries have revealed that in practice, care is experienced as highly fragmented and inconsistent. This may impact on quality of care in the more subtle (but important) senses of how it is experienced by service providers and users, but also on its quality in terms of the consistency, continuity and ultimate safety of clinical care. Recent reports such as the Confidential Enquiry into Maternal and Infant Health (Lewis 2004; CEMACH 2007) and the Healthcare Commission's reports into quality and safety of care (HCC 2006, 2008) have highlighted that fragmentation and problems of information flow and communication around decision-making are often at the root of major safety problems and adverse events, as well as affecting the quality of women's personal experience of birth.

The evidence has therefore indicated for some time an imperative need to reform the ways in which hospital maternity units are organised and operated to provide more optimal care. Following the UK Health Select Committee report on maternal and infant health in 1992 (HoC 1992) and subsequent policy reports and recommendations (DH 1993, 2004, 2007), considerable attention has been given in the United Kingdom (as in other countries) to reform. The following section looks at the evidence on reform attempts that have been systematically evaluated.

Evidence on reform

Staffing models

Hospital maternity units have tended to evolve operating with very large teams of midwives, organised on a ward basis or as multi-professional team 'under' an obstetric consultant. Additionally, more senior midwives typically take on the role of ward 'sister' or manager. This role includes the organisation of shifts and staffing rotas for midwives and ancillary staff, such as maternity-care assistants. In many cases, labour wards operated with a single set of obstetric-led clinical guidelines. The ward sister provided hands-on advice and oversight of care on the ward, with obstetricians being referred to in cases of medical need, although in many cases, there would be more routine obstetric interest and roles in oversight of care, including the use of obstetric ward rounds, where each ongoing case is reviewed. However, the 2007 Safer Childbirth Report (RCOG 2007) recommended a more selective or targeted approach, with consultant obstetrician presence to provide oversight of complicated births, and to be available for referral and consultation with midwives providing care. It emphasised the autonomy of midwives in the care of women with healthy pregnancy and labours, their responsibility and accountability for their own practice, their capacity to diagnose deviations from the norm and refer appropriately.

Another area highlighted in this and other reports (Lewis 2004; CEMACH 2007) is the importance of effective communication inter-professionally and within teams to the safety and quality of care. However, in many units, teams were so large that it is difficult to imagine how working in such a team involved any clear sense of team identity (Wraight *et al.* 1993). Teams might also be cross-ward based so that midwives could be moved from one area to another to cover changing work demands and staff shortages. Midwives, as much as women, expressed concerns about the lack of continuity and consistency in the way they worked, and their lack of autonomy in practice in a system which did not seem to support their capacity to fully utilise the clinical or interpersonal skills developed in their training (HoC 1992; ICM 2007). In the United Kingdom, midwives' training and rules clarify that they should be capable of making independent clinical decisions, and assessing cases where there is a need for referral owing to possible medical complications (UKCC 1998). Midwives are also educated to provide the full range of pain-relief options apart from initial administration of epidural and to support women in coping with pain.

During the 1990s, following calls for reform of ways of working, some small team projects were developed and evaluated. In Australia, for example, where midwives operated mainly in the hospital and with little autonomy, Rowley *et al.* (1995) conducted a randomised controlled trial (RCT) to compare hospital-based team midwifery with the usual care. In the United Kingdom, Flint and colleagues (Flint & Poulengeris 1987) developed a small team hospital-based project – the Know Your Midwife Project – where women would mainly receive their maternity care from a named midwife as part of a small team. Such teams tended to have a combined caseload of women, providing care antenatally, in labour and post-natally. Evaluations of these early hospital-based projects, both designed as RCTs, indicated that women were more satisfied with their care, and reliance on pharmacological pain relief was reduced but there were no significant differences in clinical interventions or outcomes (Rowley *et al.* 1995). Similarly, controlled studies of small-team midwifery introduced in Scottish hospitals (Hundley *et al.* 1994, 1995; Turnbull *et al.* 1996; Shields *et al.* 1998) indicated some limited differences in interventions, and increased satisfaction with care. During the 1990s in the United Kingdom, further development and evaluation projects following the Changing Childbirth report and recommendations (DH 1993) indicated only limited differences in outcomes and women's satisfaction with team midwifery, even in those projects where team midwives worked across community and hospital boundaries and the studies also highlighted some possible stressors for midwives (Green *et al.* 1998).

Green and colleagues' review of studies (1998) highlighted that in many cases schemes to introduce team midwifery took place in a way that created conflicts for midwives and increased demands on their flexibility without increasing their autonomy or capacity to work flexibly. Most were fitted onto existing hospital-based structures, without fundamental reform of those structures, and team midwives could be called upon to cover for gaps and shortfalls in the wider service while still attempting to provide all care for their caseload of women. Combined team caseloads meant that team midwives could only 'get to know' women to a limited extent, and would be on-call regularly to attend births for a relatively large pool of women. In some schemes, continuity of carer in pregnancy or post-natally was decreased in order to ensure women had 'met' all midwives in a team, to comply with targets for attendance by a 'known' midwife in labour (Green *et al.* 1998). The contradictions created for midwives were reflected in Sandall's (1997) large-scale survey of stress and burnout among midwives in the United Kingdom, which concluded that team midwives were more likely to be stressed or suffering 'burnout' than traditional community midwives, or midwives working with a personal caseload.

Several schemes to develop 'caseload' midwifery were also developed and evaluated in the United Kingdom in the 1990s (Benjamin *et al.* 2001; Page *et al.* 1999, 2001; Sandall *et al.* 2001). Key features of caseload midwifery schemes were that midwives held individual caseloads, though they worked with partners to provide backup, support and cover for births, and they tended to work across hospital–community boundaries and with mixed (high- and low-risk) caseloads of women. The organisational and structural implications of this different model proved to be more far reaching than some of the early studies anticipated, since they facilitated a higher level of autonomy and professional responsibility for the midwives involved (Stevens 2003; McCourt *et al.* 2006) and a different quality of relationship with women (Walsh 1999; Wilkins 2000; McCourt & Stevens 2009). Although few trials of caseload midwifery have been conducted, a series of controlled studies (McCourt *et al.* 1998; Benjamin *et al.* 2001; Page *et al.* 1999, 2001; Sandall *et al.* 2001) indicated significantly higher satisfaction among women, and lower rates of some birth interventions. Additionally, women reported feeling better informed and more able to make choices, and a higher number of women chose out-of-hospital births, or were able to remain flexible and make a decision during labour as to their preferred place of birth. A cluster RCT, based on general practitioner (GP) practices allocated to caseload or traditional community midwifery, conducted in North Staffordshire (2000), England, identified significant reduction in the rates of epidural analgesia and labour augmentation. However, the description of the model suggests that it did not share all the characteristics of other 'caseload midwifery' schemes, in terms of level of autonomy, and the satisfaction outcomes measured were not reported (NSCCRT 2000). This pattern of findings was confirmed in a Cochrane review of evidence on midwife-led models of care (Hatem *et al.* 2008) suggesting that the autonomy of midwives in this model, and its element of midwife-led care for those women who are low-risk, plus collaborative care for women of higher obstetric risk, may be an important factor in the greater differences found with caseload, as compared to team-based models of midwifery.

Few studies looked in depth at the experiences of the midwives involved. However, Stevens' (2003) ethnographic study of caseload midwives illuminated the degree of difference in style and orientation of the work, arising from the model and organisation of care. It appeared that once midwives acclimatised to working with a personal caseload of women, their focus shifted away from an institutional orientation to a more woman- or family- and community-centred approach to midwifery care. McCourt *et al.* (1998) suggested that this shift in orientation also reflected a professionalisation process (Sandall 1996) but one that could be described as more feminised and client-centred than the classic processes of professionalisation described by sociologists for the case of medicine (Friedson 1970; Witz 1992). McCourt *et al.* (2006), argued that this shift was partly one of organisational and consequent cultural changes that enabled midwives to develop and consolidate their expertise, decision-making, self-management and team-working capacities more fully, through enabling more direct learning from experience, and fostering a greater sense of personal and professional responsibility for decisions made. Although caseload models of midwifery practice may appear to be highly individual, with midwives practising more independently, in practice more autonomous working required and encouraged greater focus on communication and effective working with others, and midwives described peer support and peer review as particularly important aspects of their practice (McCourt *et al.* 2006; McCourt & Stevens 2009). Further research is needed on the experience of caseload models of practice but the studies undertaken to date indicate that this approach to work enables midwives to 'professionalise' their role and status in a way which builds on the opportunity to form positive relationships with women and with colleagues, rather than an exclusionary or exclusive model of practice (Walsh 1999; McCourt & Stevens in 2009). Midwives are able to develop an orientation which is focused on their accountability to the women, their community and professional role and relationships, rather than to an employing institution (Kirkham 1996). Such midwives may also develop a more post-modern orientation towards work and time which enables them to overcome the institutional constraints that have been described as features of hospital-based maternity care (McCourt in press; Stevens in press).

A further important feature of some of the team projects developed, and all the caseload midwifery schemes evaluated, was the introduction or re-establishment of midwife-led care. This involves acting as lead professional for women of low medical risk but also maintaining a co-ordinating role for women of high-risk, working collaboratively with other professionals (Hatem *et al.* 2008). Traditionally, midwife-led care had been the norm for most women worldwide. Doctors were called as needed, in cases of medical complications. The shift of intrapartum care for most women was also accompanied by a shift away from the norm of midwife-led care. Although with the formal regulation of midwives in 1902 in the United Kingdom, and in similar time periods in other countries, the sphere of midwifery care was defined as normal childbirth, and the sphere of obstetrics as complicated childbirth, such norms or boundaries have arguably shifted as hospital birth became the norm in most 'developed' countries. By the early 1980s in the United Kingdom, very few women giving birth in hospital experienced midwife-led care, this being largely confined to the 'domino' scheme (domiciliary in and out), where a small number of selected low-risk women received care from a community midwife, who accompanied them into hospital for intrapartum care, after initial labour assessment at home.

Following the Changing Childbirth recommendations, new models of care also re-introduced midwife-led care, and some caseload midwifery schemes reported development of more positive relationships with obstetricians (Stevens 2003) despite initial tensions and frictions in hospital settings within and between professional groups. Such changes were also accompanied in some hospital settings by the development of midwife-led (or low-risk) care pathways and clinical guidelines, agreement that midwives could conduct antenatal risk assessments at booking, referring women appropriately for medically-led care, and could admit and discharge low-risk women from hospital labour wards. In countries such as Canada, where midwifery was newly introduced and regulated during the 1990s, and in New Zealand, where a more independent model of midwifery was established, such midwifery-led features of care for low-risk women were established as part of the core definition and model of midwifery practice. In contrast, in countries such as Australia, midwife autonomy has remained limited, and reformed models of hospital intrapartum care remain team-based (Rowley *et al.* 1995; Biro *et al.* 2000; Homer *et al.* 2001).

Hatem *et al.*'s Cochrane review of midwife-led models of care (2008) indicates that compared with other models, midwife-led care shows reductions in some key birth interventions, and in the need for pain relief. Women evaluate their care more positively, and there is no evidence of increased clinical risk. Midwife-led care has been defined as care where 'the midwife is the lead professional in the planning, organisation and delivery of care given to a woman from initial booking to the post-natal period' (RCOG 2007). As a midwifery model of care is generally focused on pregnancy and birth as normal life events, and monitors pregnancy as being healthy unless indicated otherwise (Van Teijlingen 2005), midwife-led care also generally implies a somewhat different philosophy and approach to care compared with medically led or shared models of care. It also needs to be underpinned by appropriate organisation and staffing arrangements, as reflected in the Cochrane review which found that most models of midwife-led care followed a small team or caseload midwifery pattern. The overview found reductions in episiotomy (RR 0.82, 95% CI 0.77 to 0.88), and instrumental delivery (RR 0.86, 95% CI 0.78 to 0.96) and increased rates of spontaneous vaginal birth (RR 1.04, 95% CI 1.02 to 1.06), while no differences in infant outcomes were found. Women used less regional analgesia (epidural) (RR 0.81, 95% CI 0.73 to 0.91), and were more likely to experience no intrapartum analgesia or anaesthesia (RR 1.16, 95% CI 1.05 to 1.29). Women were also more likely to feel in control during labour and childbirth (RR 1.74, 95% CI 1.32 to 2.30), to be attended at birth by a known midwife (RR 7.84, 95% CI 4.15 to 14.81) and initiate breastfeeding (RR 1.35, 95% CI 1.03 to 1.76) (Hatem *et al.* 2008).

In looking at such evidence, it is difficult to unpick and separate out the effects of the organisational model of care (such as caseload midwifery) from the effects of midwife-led care per se, since the introduction of both have often overlapped. However, it can be argued that to try to isolate such effects is artificial and inappropriate, since these are complex packages or arrangements of care, and it seems unlikely that effective team or caseload midwifery models would operate without care for low-risk women being midwife-led. Indeed midwife-led care would be difficult to provide and sustain without such models of care being in place. Caseload midwives, for example, generally provide midwife-led care to those women on their caseload who are healthy and have low medical risks, while also providing continuing midwifery care to women with medical risks who may have an obstetrician as their lead professional. This helps to ensure that women with medical needs also receive good continuity of care and midwifery support. Additionally, just as caseload midwifery care does not imply midwives practising alone or in isolation from other midwives and professions, midwife-led care involves active consultation and co-operation with other professionals and services, as appropriate to each woman's needs and preferences.

Stevens' study of the experiences of conventional and caseload midwives in the United Kingdom highlighted that midwives working in hospital-based teams, or conventional community midwifery teams often do not experience the sense of teamwork that these models of care imply. The dysfunctional scenario observed in her ethnographic study, of midwives and other maternity professionals working alongside each other, but in tension, and with limited or difficult communication, has been highlighted in other studies of contemporary midwives' experiences. Hunter's (2004) and Deery's (2005) studies, for example, highlighted the degree to which the emotional labour of midwifery is concerned with inter- and intra-professional relationship difficulties, rather than working with women, as might be expected. In parallel, successive government reports have highlighted the safety implications of poor inter-professional relations and communication in maternity units (RCOG 2007). Kirkham, in a study of the culture of midwifery in England, found midwifery work was typified by lack of mutual support or positive role models. Guilt, self-blame and learned helplessness were coupled with considerable pressure to conform, a common characteristic of oppressed groups (Kirkham 1999). In contrast, positive working in hospital maternity environments has been identified as characterised by shared philosophies of care, positive inter-professional attitudes and relationships, underpinned by positive leadership and commitment to information sharing, peer networks and evidence-based practice (OWHC 2000).

Hospital- or community-based organisation of care?

With the shift to hospital births during the 20th century, the organisation of maternity services, as we have seen, also changed. What had once been a community-based form of care became located within the acute health sector, with most midwives in countries with regulated midwifery employed and managed within hospitals. In the UK NHS, midwives were initially employed as primary health-care workers. Community- and public-health services remained closely linked to wider public services provided by local authorities, until a major re-organisation in 1974, which brought the services under a hospital base. As this service re-organisation also followed closely on government reports advocating hospital birth for all (MoH 1970), the organisational and arguably the cultural basis of much of midwifery work was fundamentally changed. Following rising concerns about changes in the maternity services, the House of Commons (1992) select committee report on maternal and infant health advocated a return to managing maternal and infant health care within a broader social-policy model of health. However, the structural implications of its recommendations did not sit well with the prevalent political policy of the time and the remit of the expert maternity group convened to produce service recommendations did not include basic structural reform (McCourt *et al.* 1998; Kirkham 1999). The recommendations in the group's report, Changing Childbirth (DH 1993), led to the pilot projects and evaluations that have been discussed in this chapter, but in most cases these were modelled and piloted within an acute-sector model, with midwives being employed and managed as part of NHS Hospital Trusts. Like most hospital- and community-based midwives in the United Kingdom, midwives in the new models of practice were employed by hospitals, even where, as was the case with all caseload models, and a number of integrated team models, midwives began to work across and bridge hospital and community boundaries. Midwives in the one-to-one caseload practice scheme studied by Stevens (2003) worked seamlessly across community and hospital boundaries, since they followed the needs and choices of the women on their caseloads, but negotiating these was a major source of stress and conflict for the midwives. Such boundaries may be both practical and ideological (Hunter 2005). In contrast to this acute-sector model of maternity care, the thrust of government health policy has been to recommend a more primary care-based model of health care, with patients only referred to acute services based on clear preference and need. During the 1990s, the UK government developed Primary Care Trusts, able to commission health services on behalf of their local community, to underpin this shift. Additionally, a shift to a primary care base is supported by maternity policies such as the National Service Framework (2004) and its associated guidance Maternity Matters (2007), which also advocate that pregnant women should have a clear choice of in- or out-of-hospital birth.

However, there are very few instances of midwives in the United Kingdom being employed or managed as part of primary health care, and these tend to be as part of a specialised team or group, oriented towards areas of social deprivation, or individual midwives working within multidisciplinary Sure Start teams. One exception to this in the United Kingdom is the Albany Practice in London (Sandall *et al.* 2001), which contracts in to the health service as a group of independent practitioners, and is based in a primary care setting. Evaluation of this model has demonstrated excellent health outcomes, but the organisational model is unfamiliar within the UK health service and has not yet been taken up more widely. Examples of primary care-based midwifery in other countries include New Zealand, where midwives are self-employed practitioners contracting in to the public health service, in a manner comparable to GPs (family doctors). Midwifery in New Zealand also demonstrates a strong partnership orientation (Guilliland & Pairman 1995). In Canada, where midwifery was largely eliminated during the 20th century, its recent re-introduction and regulation has also been with a primary-care model of midwives based and largely working in the community, and accompanying women to hospital for births, according to the needs and choices of each woman they care for (De Vries *et al.* 2001). Such models of practice demonstrate that midwifery care can be provided to women having hospital births while organised as a primary care model, with a community base.

Economic and organisational implications of new models of care

Although a number of evaluations have been conducted of new or reformed models of midwifery, few studies have included detailed economic evaluation. In the United Kingdom, it was widely assumed that models piloted following the 1993 Changing Childbirth report were expensive, but little attention had been given to the hidden economic costs or inefficiencies of the established models of hospital-based care. McCourt and Page's evaluation of caseload midwifery (1996) included a detailed economic study (Piercy *et al.* 1996) which concluded that caseload midwifery care did not cost more than conventional maternity care, owing to savings produced by reduced lengths of stay in hospital, and a shift from care provided by doctors to that provided by midwives. This economic picture was maintained in a follow-up study during a period in which routine lengths of hospital post-natal stay fell considerably in the United Kingdom (Beake *et al.* 2001). Similarly, Hatem *et al.*'s Cochrane review indicated that where economic studies have been conducted, midwife-led models of care show economic benefits compared with shared or obstetrically led models. Any increase in midwifery costs are offset by reduced costs of hospital stays, interventions and medical staffing (Hatem *et al.* 2008).

Political, managerial and leadership skills

In her article drawing on a study of supervision within midwifery, Kirkham (1999) described the culture of midwifery in the United Kingdom as having been profoundly influenced by the history of its formalisation and regulation. Historical analyses such as Heagerty's (1997) have focused on the 1902 regulation of midwifery act as a historic compromise in which midwives not only agreed a division of labour with obstetricians, based on 'normal' versus complicated childbirth, but agreed to disciplinary regulation by other dominant professional groups. Drawing on Foucault's work, and wider critical theory perspectives, the move towards a regulated and hospital-based model of midwifery was analysed as a disciplinary project in which midwives became subject to the rigid and patriarchal structure on which institutions such as hospitals had been modelled (Kirkham 1999). In Foucault's (1980) theory of disciplinary power, groups and individuals who are subject to modern forms of surveillance, hierarchy and discipline develop a self-disciplining approach in which they modify their own and their peers' behaviour to conform with expected norms. Hunter's study of emotion work in midwifery (2004, 2005) found that boundary work and ideological conflict between senior and junior midwives in hospital practice tended to lead to bullying behaviour. Senior midwives attempted to maintain control by behaviours which junior midwives perceived as intimidating, rather than adopting more enabling approaches to development (Hunter 2005). As a result, many newly qualified midwives leave practice (Ball *et al.* 2002). Similar patterns of hierarchical and self-disciplinary control have been described for nursing (Davies 1995). Hunter's study identified hospital-based midwifery as following a pragmatic approach to providing care for large numbers 'aimed at standardisation of care, risk reduction, efficiency and effectiveness' (2004, p. 266) allowing little opportunity for being 'with woman'. This led to dissonance for the midwives with their philosophy of midwifery, and created emotional work and frustration, which was often resolved by a focus on getting through the work and on meeting organisational needs. However, it is debatable whether this dominant style of practice is truly 'effective', as evidenced by clinical, economic and satisfaction evaluations of alternative models of practice.

Studies of alternative models of midwifery, such as caseload or group practice, indicate that midwives are able to provide care with a high level of autonomy and responsibility. Such models of midwifery require less steep or formal organisational hierarchies and structures, since professionals are accountable for their practice and to the women in their care. In contrast to common assumptions, a style of practice which is more individualised, in the sense of orientation towards the needs of individuals, is highly socially oriented since it requires and facilitates the development of skills in working with others, both peers and clients and their communities. An appropriate management approach, therefore, is facilitative rather than directive, supported by evidence-based guidelines for practice, peer review and reflection (Stevens & McCourt 2001). In Stevens' ethnographic study of midwives, those in new models of practice, accountable for their caseload, reported enhanced learning from experience and development of skills in self-management, decision-making and working co-operatively with others. They perceived their ability to work effectively with other professionals as being improved, and this perception was shared by obstetricians and senior colleagues (Stevens 2003).

The skills required of senior colleagues in such a practice context are primarily those of leadership rather than hierarchical forms of management. The Ontario Women's Health Council study of maternity units, which achieved more optimal rates of Caesarean birth, identified a set of key features which are supported by wider evidence and which may help to support more optimal hospital birth experiences. Critical success factors included a positive institutional attitude towards childbirth, effective organisation, availability and sharing of knowledge and information, and commitment to the importance of connections (OWHC 2000). Key features of these four critical success factors were having a shared philosophy that supported birth as a normal physiological process, plus a commitment to one-to-one supportive care during active labour, strong leadership and effective multidisciplinary teams, and working hard to ensure connections that worked well, including continuity of care, peer networking and discussion and access to evidence.

Conclusion

This chapter has discussed women's views and experiences of giving birth in hospital, some of the challenges of providing care in hospital settings that meets their needs and expectations, and models of midwifery practice that have the potential to facilitate a more optimal hospital birth experience. Although the UK government has reaffirmed the choice for women in where they give birth, the majority of women in economically 'developed' countries give birth in hospital, and women with medical complications or more complex pregnancies equally need good quality care. Studies of women's intrapartum experience show that they value care that is both competent and kind, that offers good support, physically and psychologically, and that a positive sense of control is associated with well-being. Despite such evidence being developed over time, and measures taken to 'humanise' intrapartum care in hospitals, it remains difficult to provide care which meets these parameters, and women in many settings continue to describe care that is variable, with many, but not all, midwives providing an excellent standard of care, often in the face of considerable pressures of time and role conflict.

Studies of midwives indicate that many experience stress generated by conflicting demands and ideologies and the imperative to provide standardised care for large numbers of women, working within a hierarchical system, while also rapidly forming positive and supportive relationships, and offering choice and individualised care. The re-introduction of midwife-led care in many hospital settings has had positive outcomes for women, and may also help to support midwifery philosophies of practice. Models of care which enable midwives to hold a defined area of responsibility, such as caseload practice, or more specialised roles, have been shown to facilitate greater autonomy and satisfaction for midwives as well as for women, and positive clinical outcomes. However, midwives in such schemes continued to experience difficulties working in an institutional system whose structure is at odds with the development of women- and community centred care, and which does not effectively support professional autonomy for midwives, positive working relationships and collaboration with peers and other professionals. Ideally, the organisation and management of midwifery care should operate from a community base, with midwives being able to work across hospital and community boundaries, according to the needs and choices of the women in their care. A primary care-based model of midwifery, which incorporates the choice of birth in hospital, may help to resolve the contradictions described here of the system, process and outcomes for midwives and for women, their families and communities.

Notes

1 The NPEU survey of maternity care in 2007, using a random sample of all births in 2006 showed that just over 3% of births took place at home, and a quarter of these were unintended. The remaining 97% were in hospitals or midwife-led units (Redshaw *et al.* 2007). Numbers of births in stand-alone (out of hospital) midwife-led units remain very small, with 1.9% of births in this survey reported as being in birth centres separate from hospital. The NHS Maternity Statistics for 2003–4 give a home-birth rate of 2%. Rates of births in free-standing midwife-led units were not clearly recorded (ONS 2005).

References

Allison J (1996) *Delivered at Home*. London, RCM Press.

Arney WR (1982) *Power and the Profession of Obstetrics*. London, The University of Chicago Press.

Ball L, Curtis P, Kirkham M (2002) *Why Do Midwives Leave?* London, Royal College of Midwives.

Beake S, McCourt C, Page L (eds) (2001) *Evaluation of One-to-One Midwifery: Second Cohort Study*. London, Thames Valley University.

Benjamin Y, Walsh D, Taub N (2001) A comparison of partnership caseload midwifery care with conventional team midwifery care: labour and birth outcomes. *Midwifery* 17, 234–40.

Biro M, Waldenstrom U, Pannifex J (2000) Team midwifery care in a tertiary level obstetric service: a randomised controlled trial. *Birth* 27 (3): 168–73.

CEMACH (2007) *Saving Mothers' Lives. Reviewing Maternal Deaths to Make Motherhood Safer 2003-2005*. The Seventh Report of the Confidential Enquiries into Maternal Deaths in the United Kingdom. London, Confidential Enquiry Into Maternal and Child Health, December 2.

D'Ambruoso L, Abbey M, Hussein J (2005) Please understand when I cry out in pain: women's accounts of maternity services during labour and delivery in Ghana. *BMC Public Health* 5: 140.

Davies C (1995) *Gender and the Professional Predicament in Nursing*. Buckingham, Open University Press.

De Clercq ER, Sakala C, Corry MP, Applebaum S, Risher P (2002) *Listening to Mothers: Report of the First National U.S. Survey of Women's Childbearing Experiences*. New York, Maternity Center Association, October.

Deery R (2005) An action research study exploring midwives' support needs and the effect of group clinical supervision. *Midwifery* 21: 161–76.

DH (Department of Health) (1993) *Changing Childbirth: Report of the Expert Maternity Group*. London, HMSO.

DH (Department of Health) (2004) *National Services Framework for Children, Young People and Maternity Services*. London, The Stationery Office.

DH (Department of Health) (2007) *Maternity Matters: Choice, Access and Continuity of Care in a Safe Service*. London, The Stationery Office.

De Vries R, Benoit C, van Teijlingen E, Wrede S (2001) *Birth by Design: Pregnancy, Maternity Care, and Midwifery in North America and Europe*. London, Routledge.

El–Nemer A, Downe S, Small N (2006) She would help me from the heart: an ethnography of Egyptian women in labour. *Social Science and Medicine*. 62 (1): 81–92.

Flint C, Poulengeris P (1987) *The 'Know Your Midwife' Report*. London, available from 46 Peckermans Wood.

Foucault M (1976) *The Birth of the Clinic: An Archaeology of Medical Perception*. London, Tavistock Publications.

Foucault M (1980) *Power/Knowledge. Selected Interviews and Other Writings by Michel Foucault 1972–1977*. London, The Harvester Press.

Friedson E (1970) *Professional Dominance: The Social Structure of Medical Care*. New York, Athenson Press.

Garcia J, Redshaw M, Fitzsimons B, Keene J (1998) *First Class Delivery: A National Survey of Women's Views of Maternity Care*. London, Audit Commission.

Green JM, Baston HA (2003) Feeling in control during labor: concepts, correlates, and consequences. *Birth* 30 (4): 235–47.

Green JM, Curtis P, Price H, Renfrew M (1998) *Continuing to Care, the Organization of Midwifery Services in the UK: A Structured Review of the Evidence*. Cheshire, Books for Midwives Press.

Guilliland K, Pairman K (1995) *The Midwifery Partnership: A Model for Practice*. New Zealand, Victoria University of Wellington.

Harper-Bulman K, McCourt C (2002) Somali refugee women's views and experiences of maternity care in West London. *Critical Public Health* 12 (4): 365–80.

Hatem M, Sandall J, Devane D, Soltani H, Gates S (2008) Midwife-led versus other models of care for childbearing women. *Cochrane Database of Systematic Reviews* Issue (1). Art. No.: CD004667. DOI: 10.1002/14651858.CD004667.

HCC (Commission for Healthcare Audit and Inspection) (2006) *Investigation into 10 Maternal Deaths at, or Following Delivery at, Northwick Park Hospital, North West London Hospitals NHS Trust, between April 2002 and April 2005*. London, HCC, August 2006.

HCC (Commission for Healthcare Audit and Inspection) (2008) *Towards Better Births. A Review of Maternity Services in England*. London, HCC.

Heagerty B (1997) Willing handmaidens of science? The struggle over the new midwife in early 20th century England. In Kirkham M, Perkins E (ed) *Reflections on Midwifery*. London, Balliere-Tindall.

Hodnett ED, Gates S, Hofmeyr GJ, Sakala C (2008) Continuous support for women during childbirth. *Cochrane Database Systematic Reviews* Issue (1).

Homer CS, Davis GK, Brodie PM, Sheehan A, Barclay LM, Wills J, Chapman MG (2001) Collaboration in maternity care: a randomized controlled trial comparing community–based continuity of care with standard hospital care. *British Journal of Obstetrics and Gynaecology* 108: 16–22.

House of Commons (1992) *Second Report on the Maternity Services by the Health Services Select Committee (Winterton Report)*. London, HMSO.

Hundley VA, Cruickshank FM, Lang GD *et al.* (1994) Midwife managed delivery unit: a randomised controlled comparison with consultant led care. *British Medical Journal* 309: 1400–4.

Hundley VA, Cruickshank FM, Milne JM *et al.* (1995) Satisfaction and continuity of care: staff views of care in a midwife-managed delivery unit. *Midwifery* 11: 163–73.

Hunter B (2004) Conflicting ideologies as a source of emotion work in midwifery. *Midwifery* 20: 261–72.

Hunter B (2005) Emotion work and boundary maintenance in hospital–based midwifery. *Midwifery* 21: 253–66.

Hunt S, Symonds A (1995) *The Social Meaning of Midwifery*. Basingstoke, MacMillan.

International Confederation of Midwives (2007) Philosophy and Model of Midwifery Care, available from: http://www.internationalmidwives.org/index.php?module=ContentExpress&func=display&ceid=59&bid=22&btitle=ICM%20Documents&meid=52 (accessed 02/04/07).

Kirkham M (1996) Professionalisation past and present: with women or with the powers that be? In Kroll D (ed) *Midwifery Care for the Future: Meeting the Challenge*. London, Balliere-Tindall.

Kirkham M (1999) The culture of midwifery in the National Health Service in England. *Journal of Advanced Nursing* 30 (3): 732–9.

Lewis G (ed) (2004) *Why Mothers Die 2000–2002: Sixth Report of the Confidential Enquiries into Maternal Deaths in the United Kingdom.* London, RCOG Press.

Loudon I (2002) *Death in Childbirth: an International Study of Maternal Care and Maternal Mortality.* Oxford, Clarendon Press.

Macfarlane A, Mugford M (1984) *Birth Counts: Statistics of Pregnancy and Childbirth.* London, United Kingdom, Stationery Office Books.

Martin E (1989) *The Woman in the Body.* Milton Keynes, Open University Press.

Maternity Advisory Committee (1970) *Domiciliary and Maternity Bed Needs: The Peel Report.* London, HMSO.

McCourt C (2006) Becoming a parent. In Page L, McCandlish R (ed) *The New Midwifery: Science and Sensitivity in Practice*, 2nd edition. Oxford, Churchill Livingstone.

McCourt C. *Time and Childbirth.* Oxford, Berghahn, in press.

McCourt C, Hirst J, Page L (2000) Caring. In Page L (ed) *The New Midwifery: Science and Sensitivity in Practice.* Edinburgh, Churchill Livingstone.

McCourt C, Page L, Hewison J, Vail A (1998) Evaluation of one-to-one midwifery: women's responses to care. *Birth* 25 (2): 73–80.

McCourt C, Stevens T (2009) Relationship and reciprocity in caseload midwifery. In Hunter B, Deery R (eds) *Emotions in Midwifery and Reproduction.* Hampshire, Macmillan.

McCourt C, Stevens T, Sandall J, Brodie P (2006) Working with women: continuity of carer in practice. In Page L, McCandlish R (eds) *The New Midwifery: Science and Sensitivity in Practice*, 2nd edition. Oxford, Churchill Livingstone.

National Service Framework (2004) *The Children's National Service Framework* [online], available from: www.doh.gov/nsf/children/externalwg.htm (accessed 03/09).

NHS (2005) *NHS Maternity Services Quantitative Research.* Edinburgh, TNS System Three.

North Staffordshire Changing Childbirth Research Team (2000) A randomised study of midwifery caseload care and traditional 'shared-care'. *Midwifery* 16: 295–302.

ONS (2005) *NHS Maternity Statistics, England: 2003–2004.* London, Office for National Statistics, March 2005.

Ontario Women's Health Council (2000) Ontario Women's Health Council caesarean section best practices project impact and analysis, available at www.womenshealthcouncil.com/ (accessed 03/09).

Page L, Beake S, Vail A, Mccourt C, Hewison J (2001) Clinical outcomes of one-to-one midwifery practice. *British Journal of Midwifery* 9: 700–6.

Page L, Mccourt, C, Beake, S, Vail A (1999) Clinical interventions and outcomes of one-to-one midwifery practice. *Journal of Public Health Medicine* 21: 243–8.

Piercy J, Wilson D, Chapman P (1996) *Evaluation of One-to-One Midwifery Practice.* York Health Economics Consortium, University of York.

RCOG (2008) *Standards for Maternity Care. Report of a Working Party.* London, RCOG Press.

Redshaw M, Rowe R, Hockley C, Brocklehurst P (2007) *Recorded Delivery: A National Survey of Women's Experience of Maternity Care.* Oxford, National Perinatal Epidemiology Unit, March 2007.

Royal College of Anaesthetists, Royal College of Midwives, Royal College of Obstetricians and Gynaecologists, Royal College of Paediatrics and Child Health (2007) *Safer Childbirth. Minimum Standards for the Organisation and Delivery of Care in Labour*. London, RCOG Press.

Rowley M, Brinsmead M, Wlodarczyk J (1995) Continuity of care by a midwife team versus routine care during pregnancy and birth: a randomised trial. *Medical Journal of Australia* 163: 289–93.

Sandall J (1996) Continuity of midwifery care in England: a new professional project? *Gender, Work & Organisation* 3 (4): 215–26.

Sandall J (1997) Midwives burnout and continuity of care. *British Journal of Midwifery* 5, 106–11.

Sandall J, Davies J, Warwick C (2001) *Evaluation of the Albany Midwifery Practice: Final Report March 2001*. London, King's College London.

Shields N, Turnbull D, Reid AH, Mcginley M, Smith LN (1998) Satisfaction with midwife-managed care in different time pediods: a randomized controlled trial of 1299 women. *Midwifery* 14: 85–93.

Simkin P (1991) Just another day in a woman's life? Women's long term perceptions of their first birth experience. Part 1. *Birth* 18: 203–10.

Stevens T (2003) *Midwife to midwife: a study of caseload midwifery*. PhD thesis, Thames Valley University, London.

Stevens T. Time and Caseload Midwifery, Chapter 5 in: McCourt C. (ed) Childbirth, *Midwifery and Concepts of Time*. Berghahn Books, Oxford/NewYork, In Press.

Stevens T, McCourt C (2001) One-to-one midwifery practice part 4: sustaining the model. *British Journal of Midwifery* 10 (3): 174–9.

Tew M (1995) *Safer Childbirth? A Critical History of Maternity Care*. London, Chapman and Hall.

Turnbull D, Holmes A, Shields N *et al.* (1996) Randomised, controlled trial of efficacy of midwife–managed care. *Lancet* 384: 213–8.

United Kingdom Central Council (1998) *Midwives Code of Conduct*. London, UKCC.

Van Hollen C (2003) *Birth on the Threshold. Childbirth and Modernity in South India*. Berkeley, University of California Press.

Van Teijlingen E (2005) A critical analysis of the medical model as used in the study of pregnancy and childbirth. Sociological Research Online 10 (2), available from www.scoresonline.org.uk/10/2/teijlingen/ (accessed 03/09).

Waldenstrom U (2004a) Why do some women change their opinion about childbirth over time? *Birth* 31 (2): 102–7.

Waldenstrom U (2004b) A negative birth experience: prevalence and risk factors in a national sample. *Birth* 31 (1): 17–27.

Walsh D (1999) An ethnographic study of women's experience of partnership caseload midwifery practice: the professional as friend. *Midwifery* 15: 165–76.

Wilkins R (2000) Poor relations: the paucity of the professional paradigm. In Kirkham M (ed) *The Midwife–Mother Relationship*. Basingstoke, Macmillan.

Witz A (1992) *Professions and Patriarchy*. London, Routledge.

Wraight A, Ball J, Seccombe I, Stock J (1993) Mapping Team Midwifery: A Report to the Department of Health. IMS Report Series, Vol. 242. Brighton, Institute of Manpower Studies.

Chapter 15
Feminisms and Intrapartum Care

Mary Stewart

Introduction

I imagine that some people may have seen the title of this chapter in the list of contents and wondered what feminisms have to do with intrapartum care. There are many ways of 'being feminist' and yet I am still astonished at the number of strong women who say to me 'oh but I'm not a feminist' as though this is something of which one might be ashamed. I think that this may be because the concept of feminism is not always well understood. Undoubtedly, some people think that changes in the law, such as the Equal Pay Act of 1970 and the Sex Discrimination Act of 1975 mean that feminism, as a political force, is no longer necessary. Other people may think that feminism is only of interest to militant lesbians. Yet another group of people believe that feminism has no relevance to men. However, I believe that all of these standpoints are misguided. I passionately believe that feminist thought forms the basis of holistic midwifery care. More than that, I feel equally passionately that if midwives are not engaged with politics and feminisms on some level then they do themselves and childbearing women a disservice. Feminisms, both collectively and separately, are concerned with exposing issues of power and social inequality and feminist research is politically motivated (Paliadelis *et al.* 2007). A feminist worldview challenges us to find humanistic models for understanding the experiences of individuals and their families (Anderson *et al.* 2000). Finally, there is a growing body of research evidence which demonstrates that identifying with feminism and feminist ideologies is beneficial for girls and women because it is associated with, among other things, higher self-esteem, greater academic achievement and better physical and mental well-being (Yoder *et al.* 2007). Given these simple facts it seems reasonable to ask whether a midwife could or should identify as non-feminist.

The aim of this chapter is to briefly summarise the key concepts of feminist theory. The literature on feminisms is rich and varied and it is impossible to do more than touch on some of its main features here, but I want to strongly urge readers to explore this for themselves. I have included a list at the end of this chapter with some suggestions for further reading. I will review some of the debates that feminists have had, and continue to have, about childbirth and the maternity services. My main focus, however, is on current norms of intrapartum care and, in particular, the concept of surveillance as a system of controlling both women and midwives. I will argue that surveillance is an example of a biomedical, patriarchal discourse that is the antithesis of good midwifery care. Finally, I will discuss the notion of woman-centred care and I will suggest that, while this is a well-intentioned ideal, the concept needs to be reframed as feminist care.

Feminisms

Perhaps the first point I need to make is to explain why I use the term 'feminisms' i.e. a plural rather than a singular noun. There are many strands within feminist thought, including liberal, standpoint, socialist, radical and even eco-feminism. However, all share an underlying concern for and desire to improve the lot of women in society (Hunt 2004). There is generally a shared agreement that Western society is intrinsically patriarchal, hierarchical and unequal. Patriarchy can be defined as an ideology that justifies and perpetuates male dominance and, within patriarchal social systems, power, benefits and burdens are unevenly distributed such that men, their values and characteristics are valued more highly than women (Rafael 1996; Kirkley 2000).

Feminists are therefore driven by an awareness that men are more socially and politically powerful than women, that they have more control within society and that they make more of the decisions that influence people's lives. Of course, this broad approach is somewhat simplistic. As Hooks (2000) notes, all men are not equal. Race and class are factors which may determine the extent to which an individual is discriminated against. Nonetheless, it is generally true that women are disadvantaged socially, economically and politically in comparison to men (Ramazanoğlu & Holland 2002), leading to feminists' concern with sexual politics and the transformation of patriarchy (Weedon 1997). This concern should not, however, be equated with an assumption that feminists are 'anti-men'. It is beliefs such as these that, not surprisingly, give feminisms a bad name but they are beliefs based on a lack of understanding. Speaking for myself, I have four brothers, five nephews, and close male friends all of whom I love unconditionally but I am also aware that they are, at a profound level, at an advantage simply because they were born male in a society and culture where gender is important and where masculinity is valued over and above femininity. (Of course, notions of masculinity and femininity are themselves only social constructions. This is not the place to deconstruct those concepts but for a fuller discussion you might wish to read the work of Tamsin Wilton listed at the end of this chapter).

Feminists believe that patriarchy has been used as a tool for controlling, silencing and oppressing women, and for allowing men's voices and opinions to dominate. Feminist research and practice is rooted in women's experience (Ramazanoğlu & Holland 2002). It strives to focus on women's lives, making them visible and giving them voice and, from a political perspective, aims to alleviate oppression and marginalisation (Roberts 1981; Hooks 1989; Stanley & Wise 1990; Huntington & Gilmour 2001; Letherby 2003; Grbich 2007). The purpose of taking a feminist stance is to present an alternative account of the world where women's voices are heard and valued and to question and challenge patriarchal assumptions (Letherby 2003). Feminist theory is more than just an academic, intellectual concern; it is grounded in political activism and a wish to achieve change in order to improve things not just for women but for society as a whole (Skeggs 1994). It is, as Stanley (1990: 12) points out, a matter of praxis, that is, 'understand the world and then change it'. (As an aside, it is worth pointing out that the reference list I give at the end of this chapter includes the first name of each author, rather than the more traditional practice of listing only family name and initials. This is a seemingly small but important feminist technique for acknowledging and celebrating the number of women, as well as men, who have contributed to my writing.)

A final point I want to make here is the fundamental importance that I and most feminists attach to the avoidance of binary absolutes. It is unhelpful and inaccurate to suggest, for example, that feminist thought can provide all the answers or that alternative perspectives are, by definition, flawed. Similarly, I do not want to fall into the easy, but lazy and incorrect trap that casts the medical profession and obstetricians as misguided villains or suggest that midwives always have women's best interests at heart. A feminist world view encourages us to avoid binaries (Turris 2005), because these always lead to one group being privileged at the expense of another or to simplistic notions that one world view is right and the opposing point of view is wrong, whereas life and truth are inevitably more complex. What I offer here is one person's opinion, based on a considerable body of literature and many years experience but I believe and hope that some of my own opinions will develop and, quite possibly, change as I continue to learn. You will inevitably have your own opinions and some of these may differ fundamentally from my own but both perspectives can be equally valid and each has a right to be heard.

A feminist critique of contemporary birth

Just as there are several schools of feminist thought, so feminists do not all share the same beliefs about childbirth and what it means for women and society. It is interesting to trace some of the ideas that were put forward by some of the 'second-wave' feminists[1] as these completely oppose the thought that is more contemporary. As Davis-Floyd (2003) points out, a number of these feminists embraced technological hospital birth as a welcome step towards what they hoped would be true equality of the sexes. These women rejected the stereotype of motherhood as the defining feature of woman's lives and home as the appropriate domain of women. Many of them sought out anaesthetised birth as they believed it gave them greater power and autonomy over their bodies. At its most extreme, some feminists such as Firestone (1970) argued that the sexes could only be truly equal through the development of technology that enabled extrauterine gestation.

However, at a similar period of history, other women were beginning to unite and question the increasing use of technology in childbirth, creating an alternative 'feminist re-endorsement of motherhood' (Umansky 1996: 53). This formed part of a counterculture, first associated with hippies in the 1960s, with women reclaiming their right to give birth at home, without the use of any technology and an increasing recognition that childbirth could and should be an empowering experience (Kitzinger 1996; Kirkley 2000). One example of this counterculture with which many midwives are familiar is The Farm, founded by Ina May Gaskin and her friends in Tennessee (2002). Some people might argue that The Farm was of its time, and may find the photographs of men and women with long flowing hair amusing. However, it is hard to over-estimate the effect that such pioneers had on improving childbirth for women throughout the westernised world.

Many authors, feminist and others, use the term 'biomedical model' when discussing the impact of technology and obstetrics on contemporary birth. Biomedicalisation can be defined as the intensification of medicine in complex, multidirectional and techno-scientific ways (Clarke *et al.* 2003). Biomedicine is far more than a straightforward attempt to cure or prevent illness. It has become embedded in society, is interwoven into government policy, it underpins public health message and affects us all, as individuals and as a society: it would be hard to overstate its influence. However, biomedicine is also simply a discourse, that is, it is a system of communication. Several different and contradictory discourses may coexist within a society at any one time but some of these may become dominant or restricted, accepted or disallowed through their relationships with other powerful discourses. For example, many feminist writers have challenged the authority of biomedicine, which is rooted in 'scientific' knowledge and particular ways of knowing (Miller 1998). Moreover, it can be seen as highly gendered, and as a form of 'male' knowledge, supposedly based on science and rationality, that is valued over and above 'female' knowledge. There are countless examples of the gendered nature of knowledge across historical and cultural divides (Walby 1990; Witz 1992; Macdonald 1995; Kent 2000) and, more specifically, the extent to which male knowledge has come to define what is taken for 'truth' in the maternity services (Ehrenreich & English 1973; Jordan 1997; Wickham 2004). Most feminists remain sceptical about the supposed benefits of modern technology and highly critical of the power held by obstetricians (Kirkley 2000) and point to the way in which women have accrued knowledge about childbirth over many centuries. However, much of this knowledge has often been disregarded and devalued (Jordan 1997; Murphy-Lawless 1998).

The current biomedical discourse is prevailing, powerful and reductive (Foucault 1976) and presents itself as impartial, reflecting objective reality (Wilson 2001). However, the knowledge presented by the biomedical discourse, and which underpins much of the information provided within the maternity services is determined, not by its relationship with truth, but by and through its fit with other assertions that are held collectively to be true (Ceci 2004). For example, we live in a society that validates science above art, and where the randomised controlled trial is held to be the highest form of evidence. Given this cultural context, it is not surprising that individuals come to believe these assertions. As Kent (2000) points out the success of biomedicine within the context of birth has been because people have supported and reinforced these dominant values and ideas. This includes obstetricians who develop the technologies, but also midwives and women who may welcome its development and feel reassured by its use.

I am not trying to suggest that all technology is malign. As Doyal (1995) points out, all women need access to safe and effective medical care. She goes on to suggest that the rejection of obstetric technology is the prerogative of women living in developed Western cultures where childbirth is, by and large, safe. There is no doubt that some of the technological advances that have been made within the maternity services have prevented maternal and neonatal deaths. The point I am trying to make is to illustrate the dominance of masculinised biomedicine at the expense of other, more female but equally important forms of knowledge. A glance through most mainstream textbooks about childbirth, whether directed at midwives or pregnant women, suggests that there should be time constraints on the length of labour and indicates that labour is divided into stages, as if these are absolute facts whereas they are simply examples of the biomedical discourse. There is ample evidence to demonstrate that, where the condition of the woman and her baby is satisfactory, time limits on labour are both unnecessary and unhelpful (Albers *et al.* 1996; Enkin *et al.* 2000) and that the stages of labour are no more than artificial constructs (Walsh 2008) but these alternative discourses get drowned out by the dominant force of biomedicine.

If one of the key aims of feminist research is to give women a voice, it is important that there is a space for all accounts to be recorded, and for alternative discourses to be valued, even if some of these may be uncomfortable to hear, or may appear contradictory. Miller (1998) makes a helpful distinction between the different voices that may be heard. She uses the term 'public' to refer to accounts of pregnancy and childbirth that are created by medical and health professionals. She uses the term 'private' to refer to lay knowledge of childbirth that arises from informal interactions between women, their families, mothers and sisters and friends. However, she also uses the term 'personal' to represent women's accounts that do not fit with either public or private accounts and which may challenge or contradict both of these forms of knowledge. A feminist approach to intrapartum care requires midwives to recognise that all these accounts exist and that each represents some form of 'truth'.

Having highlighted the gendered nature of biomedicine, and its dominance in contemporary maternity care, I now move on to consider the issue of surveillance, as one discrete facet of biomedicine.

Biomedicine as a form of surveillance

Within the biomedical discourse of childbirth, labour all too easily becomes simply a process of surveillance: surveillance of women who are measured, timed and scrutinised to ensure they are labouring in line with a firmly held, but intrinsically flawed belief about the length of labour. I begin this section with a scenario that, although imaginary, is probably familiar to many midwives.

Karen, an experienced, well-intentioned midwife is caring for Helen, who is in advanced labour in hospital with her first baby. Helen begins to experience a slight urge to push but there are no external signs of full dilatation. It is 4 hours since the previous vaginal examination (VE) so, with Helen's consent, Karen does a VE and discovers that the cervix is fully dilated but the baby's head is still above the ischial spines. Karen is confident, based on her experience and her knowledge of physiology, that Helen will continue to labour well and push her baby out without any need for intervention or assistance but, rather than recording what she found, Karen writes in the clinical notes that the cervix is 9 cm dilated. Sure enough, 2 hours later Helen triumphantly gives birth to her baby.

This little vignette, which is acted out in labour wards throughout the westernised world, is a telling example of the power of the biomedical model of care and its main tool of surveillance. It is worth beginning by considering why the midwife felt the need to do a VE in the first place. Many midwives adhere, at least in principle, to a philosophy and practice that Tricia Anderson described so vividly as 'drinking tea intelligently' (Walsh 2004). Within this philosophy, the midwife uses her knowledge of normal physiology and her clinical experience alongside her knowledge of the woman she is with. She has a deep respect for and trust in the process of birth, as well as a belief that most women, given the right support, time and space, will give birth safely and well with little need of intervention. However, it is hard to practice in this way in a labour ward that is run on biomedical principles, driven by a need to measure, time and control. Such a system depends on a belief that it is possible to 'know', with a considerable amount of certainty, how labour will and should progress and various tools of surveillance, such as the partogram, VE and time limits on the length of labour are predicated on this assumption.

This approach to care can be allied with the concept of Fordism, that is, the concept of the moving assembly line within mass production (Björkman 1996). Walsh (2006) develops this concept to describe the work within a typical National Health Service (NHS) maternity unit, where women are processed using a mechanistic model, which has a timescale for completion of the process within a highly sophisticated regulatory framework. The Fordist model is also an example of what Hall describes as a monochronic culture, driven towards 'tasks, schedules and procedures' (Hall 1984, p. 34). Such cultures are equated with organisation and productivity, leading ultimately to a belief that time can be regulated by the clock ('clock time') that it is unilinear and needs to be imposed in order to ensure the smooth running of society. This approach to time can be seen as both 'male' and 'public' and is characteristic of bureaucracy, business and government. In contrast, time can be viewed as more temporal, 'female' and 'private', governed by the rhythms and laws of nature.

'Doing' is a key feature of the Fordist, monochronic approach to childbirth (Fahy 1998) and VE is one of the tasks that midwives might choose to do. It can be seen as a means of quality control and is a key aspect of the industrial model of birth that attempts to reduce, limit and control production time (Hillier 2003). Moreover, it is a tool of surveillance that is used to assess whether a woman's labour is progressing according to the prescribed norms of the biomedical discourse. In the scenario described above, the first reason Karen may have done the VE is simply to follow hospital protocol as one audit of national policies indicated that all hospital trusts have a policy of VE being undertaken every 4 hours (CSAG 1995). Given this fact, it is worth pondering that Karen may have done the VE because she felt under surveillance herself. There is evidence that midwives may do a VE to meet the demands and expectations of the labour ward coordinator, rather than because of any perceived clinical need. As one midwife commented:

> You know, you do a VE against your better judgement to keep your senior staff happy so they're off your back . . . .
>
> (Stewart 2008, p. 197)

Karen probably knows that there are many different ways of assessing progress in labour, such as observing the sounds a woman makes. However, VE fits within the prevailing and masculinised discourse that health professionals, in this case midwives and obstetricians, have access to a superior form of knowledge, and that it is always possible to objectively measure and assess the workings of the human body. Midwives are usually acutely aware that cervical dilatation can only ever provide a partial account of how labour is progressing and the information obtained from VE is also liable to change at any time. However, this is at odds with the discourse of biomedicine that makes claims for objective knowledge and truth.

As Bergeron (2007, p. 480) notes, within biomedicine, the unpredictable nature of childbirth has been addressed as 'so many medical *problems* for which medical *solutions* were offered rather than inherent components of a natural and awesome process for which women are biologically and physiologically ready' (italics in original). She goes on to point out that although women need to be supported emotionally and physically through labour and birth, this does not mean that the process needs to be taken over. That is, women do not need rescuing from the intensity of labour and birth but need security and reassurance. Bergeron (2007, p. 481) goes on to argue that 'Efficiency in childbirth has been achieved but at the expense of women's trust in the strength and physiological perfection of their bodies'.

So what would be an alternative response to the vignette described at the beginning of this section? Most midwives recognise that a woman who is beginning to experience an urge to push is probably approaching what is nominally called the 'second stage' of labour (and see Chapter 6 for a critique of this) and that her cervix is probably approaching full dilatation. A feminist approach to this scenario is to consider the woman as a person, an individual giving birth, with her own particular needs, fears and beliefs. The midwife will listen to what the woman is saying and, equally importantly, to what she is not saying. She will observe that woman's behaviour, watch the way her body is moving and listen to the sounds she is making. She will maintain quiet communication with the woman that is sensitive to the woman's need to focus in on herself but is alert to the woman's changing needs. The feminist approach is attuned to *this* woman's needs at *this* moment, rather than being driven by protocols or the expectations of colleagues. In this scenario, it *may* be appropriate to do a VE but this is a decision that is made based solely on the woman's needs and wishes, rather than being driven by hospital protocol. Even more importantly, all decisions are made *with* the woman, rather than *for* her. This leads me on to the final section of this chapter and a discussion of the concept and associated problems of matriarchal care.

Woman-centred care and the trap of matriarchy

Let us just return to consider why Karen, the midwife in the vignette, recorded a cervical dilatation of 9 cm when, in fact, she believed the cervix to be fully dilated. Whenever I discuss this scenario with colleagues, they nod in recognition and acknowledge that they, too, may work in this way. Many NHS labour wards still have polices that recommend obstetric intervention, often in the form of ventouse or forceps delivery, if a primiparous woman has not given birth within 60–90 minutes of active pushing. (For multiparous women, time limits may be as short as 30–60 minutes). These recommendations actually contradict the available evidence but still influence obstetric practice, demonstrating the excessive influence of biomedicine.

Midwives who alter the findings of VE illustrate the fact that they have access to a knowledge base (Albers *et al*. 1996; Enkin *et al*. 2000; NICE 2007) that contradicts the biomedical discourse and that demonstrates that labour may take longer than is acknowledged in many textbooks or hospital protocols. Of course some people might suggest that midwives who work in this way are lying about their findings. However, I think that it is unhelpful to use such emotionally loaded terminology, and inaccurate because, on one level, these midwives *are* speaking the truth, that is, they are articulating the fact that labour may take longer than expected and yet still be physiologically normal. The problem is that this knowledge is being used in a very subversive way which, while it may appear to protect a woman from intervention, actually does all midwives and women a disservice. Using midwifery knowledge in this hidden way means that the biomedical discourse remains unchallenged and fails to acknowledge wisdom and understanding that should be in the public domain.

This practice is also problematic and flawed on another level. The midwives I speak to are clearly kind and well-intentioned. They believe that they are protecting the woman from unnecessary intervention and may argue that they are working in a woman-centred way. This, I think, is the crux of the problem as, whenever I have witnessed this practice, or heard midwives talking about it, it is apparent that the midwife works alone. When she makes the choice to alter the findings of VE, the midwife does not appear to involve the woman in this decision. So, while she may argue that this is in the woman's best interests, the facts belie this.

Other authors have written about the ways in which midwives become part of the system and act out the biomedical discourse and patriarchal behaviour that takes little account of women's emotional, psychological or spiritual needs (Curtis *et al.* 2006). Less well described is a tendency I see among midwives to behave in a manner that can be best described as matriarchal. Within this model of care, midwives may be deeply kind and caring but, and this is the crucial point, it still represents an uneven balance of power. The midwives have the power to decide what information they divulge and share with women, and what to withhold. Midwives may argue that they alter their findings from VE in order to protect women. However, this cannot be seen as truly woman-centred care because, unless women are involved in this decision-making, the midwives exert their power in a manner that belies any sense of an equal relationship. It is the way in which midwives use their power both to protect and at the same time to exclude women that is so matriarchal. As Georges (2003) points out, it is not the role of the health professional to assume a position of control in which she or he decides what is best for the individual. Rather, from a feminist perspective, the role of the midwife is truly about 'being with' women, where each person communicates honestly: midwives and women; midwives and obstetricians, midwives with each other and with themselves.

I do not want to suggest that the concept of mothering or nurturing within the midwife–mother relationship is intrinsically flawed. Pregnancy and birth are a time of significant vulnerability and it is appropriate that women look to their midwives for advice and support. However, those in positions of less power may experience some relief at relinquishing control and this is a crucial aspect of the seductive nature and remarkable success of patriarchy. Matriarchy, whilst well-intentioned, mirrors some of the overbearing attitudes of patriarchy.

Conclusion

So where does all of this leave us as midwives? We have seen that feminists do not all share the same belief about the way pregnancy and birth could and should be and that this belief has changed over time. However, all feminists do share a belief that women's voices count and that all women have an equal right for their voice to be heard. It is an inevitable corollary of that belief that we, as individuals, may disagree with some of the voices. Perhaps one of the most important contributions that feminists make, and where it differs from the technocratic, patriarchal approach is that simple but important belief that other points of view exist and, moreover, that they count. Our role as midwives is not to tell women what to do or what they should believe. Rather, it is to support women so they can make these decisions for themselves and to support them even when we might not agree with the decision they make. To tell women what they should do can broadly be described as patriarchal. To talk about woman-centred care while failing to involve women in decision-making can be described as matriarchal care. Both are intrinsically problematic. Surely the only right way forward is to embrace the concept of feminist care, where women are absolute equals and partners and in control over their own bodies – what is done to them, when and how and by whom. It is time to change some of the ways we think and act for, as Irigaray (1998, p. 69) says:

> If we continue to speak this sameness, if we speak to each other as men have spoken for centuries, as they taught us to speak, we will fail each other.

Notes

1   The term *second-wave feminists* generally applies to feminist writing that began in the late 1960s and 1970s and challenged all forms of sexual discrimination. First-wave feminists, e.g. the suffragettes, set out to change fundamental laws, such as women's right to vote.

Further reading

Rich Adrienne (1986) *Of Woman Born: Motherhood as Experience and Institution.* New York, WW Norton & Co. This is a classic text. Adrienne Rich draws on her own experiences to highlight women's subordinate place within patriarchal culture. Passionate and polemic.

Murphy-Lawless, Jo (1998) *Reading Birth and Death: A History of Obstetric Thinking.* Cork, Cork University Press. This is a fabulous book. Jo Murphy-Lawless takes the reader on an erudite but fascinating journey, tracing the way in which the medical profession has taken control of pregnancy and birth, and wrested power from women. Although based on Irish history, the book is absolutely relevant for midwives working in westernised countries. An essential read.

Wilton T (2004) *Sexual (Dis)Orientation: Gender, Sex, Desire and Self-Fashioning.* London, Palgrave Macmillan.

References

Albers Leah L, Schiff Melissa, Gorwoda Julie G (1996) The length of active labor in normal pregnancies. *Obstetrics and Gynecology* 87(3): 355–9.

Anderson Gwen W, Black Rita, Rorty Mary V (2000) Nursing and genetics: a feminist critique moves us toward transdisciplinary teams. *Nursing Ethics* 7: 191–204.

Bergeron Veronique (2007) The ethics of caesarean section on maternal request: a feminist critique of the American College of Obstetricians and Gynecologists' position on patient-choice surgery. *Bioethics* 21(9): 478–87.

Björkman Torsten (1996) The Rationalisation Movement in perspective and some ergonomic implications. *Applied Ergonomics* 27(2): 111–7.

Ceci Christine (2004) Nursing, knowledge and power: a case analysis. *Social Science and Medicine* 59(9): 1879–89.

Clarke Adele, Shim Janet K, Mamo Laura, Fosket Jennifer Ruth, Fishman Jennifer R (2003) Biomedicalization: technoscientific transformations of health, illness and US biomedicine. *American Sociological Review* 68(2): 161–94.

Clinical Standards Advisory Group (1995) *Women in Normal Labour. Report of a CSAG Committee*. London, HMSO.

Curtis P, Ball M, Kirkham M (2006) Bullying and horizontal violence: cultural or individual phenomena? *British Journal of Midwifery* 14(4): 218–21.

Davis-Floyd Robbie E (2003) *Birth as an American Rite of Passage*, 2nd edition. Berkeley, University of California Press.

Doyal Lesley (1995) *What Makes Women Sick? Gender and the Political Economy of Health*. London, Macmillan.

Ehrenreich Barbara, English Deirdre (1973) *Witches, Midwives and Nurses*. London, Writers' and Readers' Publishing Co-operative.

Enkin Murray, Keirse Marc JNC, Neilson James *et al.* (2000) *Guide to Effective Care in Pregnancy and Childbirth*, 3rd edition. Oxford, Oxford University Press.

Fahy Kathleen (1998) Being a midwife or doing midwifery. *Australian Midwives' College Journal* 11(12): 11–6.

Firestone Shulamith (1970) *The Dialectic of Sex: The Case for Feminist Revolution*. New York, Morrow.

Foucault Michel (1976) *Birth of the Clinic: An Archaeology of Medical Perception*. London, Tavistock.

Gaskin Ina May (2002) *Spiritual Midwifery*, 4th edition. Summertown, Book Publishing Company.

Georges Jane M (2003) An emerging discourse: toward epistemic diversity in nursing. *Advances in Nursing Science* 26(1): 44–52.

Grbich Carol (2007) *Qualitative Data Analysis: An Introduction*. London, Sage Publications.

Hall Edward T (1984) *The Dance of Life: The Other Dimension of Time*. New York, Anchor Books.

Hillier Dawn (2003) *Childbirth in the Global Village: Implications for Midwifery Education and Practice*. London, Routledge.

Hooks Bell (1989) *Talking back: thinking feminist, thinking black*. Boston, MA, South End Press.

Hooks Bell (2000) *Feminist Theory: From Margin to Center*. London, Pluto Press.

Hunt Sheila (2004) *Poverty, Pregnancy and the Healthcare Professional*. Edinburgh, Books for Midwives.

Huntington Annette D, Gilmour Jean A (2001) Re-thinking representations, re-writing nursing texts: possibilities through feminist and Foucauldian thought. *Journal of Advanced Nursing* 35(6): 902–8.

Irigaray Luce (1998) When our lips speak together (Burke, Carolyn, translator). *SIGNS: Journal of Women in Culture and Society* 6: 69–79.

Jordan Brigitte (1997) Authoritative knowledge and its construction. In: Davis-Floyd Robbie, Sargent Carolyn F (eds) *Childbirth and Authoritative Knowledge: Cross-Cultural Perspectives*. Berkley, University of California Press, 55–79.

Kent Julie (2000) *Social Perspectives on Pregnancy and Childbirth for Midwives, Nurses and the Caring Professions*. Buckingham, Open University Press.

Kirkley Debra L (2000) Is motherhood good for women? A feminist exploration. *Journal of Obstetric, Gynecologic, and Neonatal Nursing* 29(5): 459–64.

Kitzinger Sheila (1996) Sheila Kitzinger's letter from Europe: birth speak. *Birth* 23(1): 46–7.

Letherby Gail (2003) *Feminist Research in Theory and Practice*. Buckingham, Open University Press.

Macdonald Keith M (1995) *The Sociology of the Professions*. London, Sage Publications.

Miller Tina (1998) Shifting layers of professional, lay and personal narratives: longitudinal childbirth research. In: Ribbens Jane, Edwards Rosalind (eds) *Feminist Dilemmas in Qualitative Research: Public Knowledge and Private Lives*. London, Sage, 58–71.

Murphy-Lawless Jo (1998) *Reading Birth and Death: A History of Obstetric Thinking*. Cork, Cork University Press.

National Institute of Health and Clinical Excellence (2007) *Intrapartum Care: Care of Healthy Women and Their Babies during Childbirth*. London, NICE.

Paliadelis Penny, Cruickshank Mary, Sheridan Alison (2007) Caring for each other: how do nurse managers 'manage' their role? *Journal of Nursing Management*. 15: 830–7.

Rafael Adeline RF (1996) Power and caring: a dialectic in nursing. *Advances in Nursing Science* 19(1): 3–17.

Ramazanoğlu Caroline, Holland Janet (2002) *Feminist Methodology: Challenges and Choices*. London, Sage Publications.

Roberts Helen (ed) (1981) *Doing Feminist Research*. London, Routledge and Kegan Paul.

Skeggs Beverley (1994) Situating the production of feminist ethnography. In Maynard Mary, Purvis June (eds) *Researching Women's Lives from a Feminist Perspective*. London, Taylor & Francis Ltd.

Stanley Liz (1990) Feminist praxis and the academic mode of production: an editorial introduction. In Stanley Liz (ed) *Feminist Praxis: Research, Theory and Epistemology in Feminist Sociology*. London, Routledge.

Stanley Liz, Wise Sue (1990) Method, methodology and epistemology in feminist research processes. In Stanley Liz (ed) *Feminist Praxis: Research, Theory and Epistemology in Feminist Sociology*. London, Routledge.

Stewart Mary (2008) *Midwives' discourses on vaginal examination in labour*. Unpublished PhD dissertation, University of the West of England, Bristol.

Turris Sheila A (2005) Unpacking the concept of patient satisfaction: a feminist analysis. *Journal of Advanced Nursing* 50(3): 293–8.

Umansky Lauri (1996) *Motherhood Reconceived: Feminism and the Legacy of the Sixties*. New York, NYU Press.

Walby Sylvia (1990) *Theorizing Patriarchy*. Oxford, Blackwell.

Walsh Denis (2004) Psychological barriers to labour. *British Journal of Midwifery* 12(7): 438.

Walsh Denis (2006) Subverting the assembly line: childbirth in a free-standing birth centre. *Social Science and Medicine* 62(6): 1330–40.

Walsh D (2008) Normal birth: a retrospective. *Midirs Essence On-Line Newsletter* (12): 1.

Weedon Chris (1997) *Feminist Practice and Poststructuralist Theory*. Oxford, Blackwell.

Wickham Sara (2004) Feminism and ways of knowing. In Stewart Mary (ed) *Pregnancy, Birth and Maternity Care: Feminist Perspectives*. Edinburgh, Elsevier, 157–68.

Wilson Helen V (2001) Power and partnership: a critical analysis of the surveillance discourses of child health nurses. *Journal of Advanced Nursing* 36(2): 294–301.

Witz Anne (1992) *Professions and Patriarchy*. London, Routledge.

Yoder Janice D, Perry Rachelle L, Saal Ellen I (2007) What good is a feminist identity? Women's feminist identification and role expectations for intimate and sexual relationships *Sex Roles* 57: 365–72.

Chapter 16
Towards Salutogenic Birth
in the 21st Century

Soo Downe

Introduction

This final chapter presents a possible approach to progressing many of the issues raised in the book. It is focused on a theory (*salutogenesis*) that suggests that what makes things work well for systems, individuals, bodies and processes might hold the key to positive change in a range of areas, including maternity care. The chapter specifically considers the implications of this for collaboration between professional groups.

Working with salutogenic connectivity: physiology, evidence and politics

Salutogenesis is a theory which was first proposed by Aaron Antonovsky (1987). Antonovsky began to develop his central ideas while he was undertaking research on the psychological impacts of being a concentration camp survivor. Most individuals in the study experienced the expected high levels of psychological pathology. However, some were remarkably positive about their lives, and about the world. Rather than seeing these individuals as inconvenient exceptions to the rule, Antonovsky began to explore how these people, who had been through so much, could be so resilient, and so positive. This question developed into an exploration of what Antonovsky termed the *Sense of Coherence* concept. This postulated that an individual who can see the world as manageable, comprehensible and meaningful was more likely to see their life as coherent, and to be able to cope with adverse events positively, no matter how extreme their experiences might be. Apart from this specific psychological theory, Antonovsky began to think about what would happen if we saw life generally in terms of how it goes right, rather than what makes it go wrong:

> A salutogenic orientation facilitates seeing things that experts in a given pathology might well fail to see ... it ... pressures one to think in systems terms ... it leads one to deal with (both) entropic (disorder-promoting) forces and ... negentropic (order-promoting) forces (Antonovsky 1993)

This statement has a strong resonance for health care in general, and for maternity care in particular. Indeed, in a challenge to a highly risk-averse approach to health care, Antonovsky asked the following question in relation to disability:

> We are all familiar with the concept of a risk factor. Can we not think of the concept of a salutary factor?
>
> (Antonovsky 1993)

This has implications for how we understand particular events that might be seen as pathological (such as pain in labour, a long gestation, a slow labour, or the early pushing urge, as addressed in various chapters of this book). It also has implications for systems of maternity care. Given that there is disquiet nationally and internationally about high levels of intervention, and about women's views and staff morale, a salutogenic approach might create the energy to make the changes that appear to be elusive at the moment. This would ask, how do some services and systems get it so right, and how can we learn from them? The next section addresses some of these issues in the context of inter-professional collaboration.

Respectful inter-professional collaboration

Since the critique of modern maternity-care provision in the 1960s and 1970s (see Chapter 1), it has become almost taken for granted that so-called medicalisation is bad, and that social, holistic or midwifery ways of doing birth are good. However, more recently, there has been a growing concern at this simplistic binary approach to seeing birth (Annandale & Clark 1996). This point of view casts midwives as always aligned to and with women, and correctly focused on normality, while doctors are driven by power, income, and/or risk-aversion, with no real interest in the well-being of mother and baby. The consequent polarisation between professional groups creates silos which work for women who fall wholly within them – women who are well and do not need an obstetrician, and those who are very ill, for whom midwifery is only supportive. However, most women are not sited in these camps exclusively. For those who need and/or want both midwifery and obstetric care, moving between professional boundaries can be very difficult and stressful. Indeed, there is increasing evidence that a lack of effective collaboration may be a factor in maternal and infant mortality and morbidity, as illustrated in the United Kingdom in the recent Health Commission report into maternal deaths at Northwick Park Hospital (Healthcare Commission 2005), and more recent general reports into maternity care from the Kings Fund (Smith & Dixon 2007) and the Healthcare Commission (2008).

As these reports have demonstrated, getting maternity care right is not just about the kinds of things that are done, but, fundamentally, about how caregivers think about maternity care and about women, and about how they work together to achieve the best outcome possible. One of the key factors promoting high levels of normal birth in the Ontario Women's Health Council report on low rates of Caesarean section in hospital settings (Ontario Women's Health Council 2006) was 'effective teams who liked each other'. This kind of authentic mutual regard and trust creates environments where care is not only of high quality, but continually improving, and where staff enjoy coming to work and working together. This transmits itself to women and families, and, in turn, back to the staff, in mutually reinforcing positive (virtuous) cycles. Salutogenesis (literally, the creation of well-being) can be seen to be operating here. In contrast, the reports mentioned above suggest that where vicious circles of distrust, disrespect and lack of mutual esteem operate, this can affect the whole system. If this is allowed to go to the extreme, it may be associated with the deaths of women and babies.

A good example of how lack of regard is reinforced by a lack of a common language is given by the study of Simpson and colleagues (Simpson *et al.* 2006). This research involved nurse-midwives and obstetric physicians. Rather unusually for the United States, the nurse-midwives had a degree of autonomy in the provision of maternity care. The study covered four hospitals, each with between 3000 and 6000 births, and it included 54 nurse-midwives, and 398 physicians. As the authors noted, 'Nurses and physicians shared the common goal of a healthy mother and baby but did not always agree on methods to achieve that goal ....'

The key areas of contention were the use of augmentation in labour, and interpretation of the outputs of routine electronic fetal monitoring. The data revealed an extensive inability of the two groups to come out of their silos and to discuss the basis of their two positions. This resulted in a lack of trust and respect, and covert resistance, in which the doctors tried to force the nurses to adhere to their orders, and the nurses tried tricks and techniques to avoid informing the doctors, or to subvert their orders:

> Some doctors are a disaster so I make sure I don't call them for delivery until the head is almost out. That way I can try to prevent a vacuum or forceps, I don't have to deal with fundal pressure and I don't have to stand there while they sew up the inevitable fourth degree laceration. The patient is much better off and they don't even know what a favor I've done for them (p. 552)

One of the doctors reported rather plaintively:

> Sometimes I feel downright unwelcome when I show up on the unit to check my patient without being called. The nurses say ... 'What are you doing here? I didn't call you.' (p. 552)

As another doctor noted (without moving from his entrenched position on the 'pit', or pitocin – the US term for syntocinon), this lack of mutual trust and regard had clear consequences for the care of women in labour:

> So it almost becomes like a battle where you think she [the nurse] should be doing this and she has other ideas but doesn't necessarily tell you. Instead of directing all your attention to the patient you end up having to worry about the pit. It doesn't serve the patient well where you're not working really together. (p. 549)

This kind of dysfunctional working has been noted in a survey of the attitudes of junior doctors based in the northwest of England to the midwives they worked with (Pinki *et al.* 2007), and in a study of midwives and labour ward nurses in the United States (Kennedy & Lyndon 2008).

The vicious circle of negative thinking about the 'Other' group is not unique to the health sector. As Kelly and Allison note in their exploration of complexity theory in action in organisations:

> Agents, frightened of losing their positions, adopt threatening postures and tell 'white' lies to protect themselves. Afraid to report the truth as they see it, they don't provide full and accurate information. Decisions, made in ignorance backfire, leading to mistrust. People learn not to trust their individual survival to others in the group. Mistrust amplifies the fear and the cycle intensifies
>
> (Kelly & Allison 1999, p. 54)

They go on to note that:

> The major hurdle is to remove the underlying fear of telling the truth (p. 56) and Before it can be effective, an organisation must dismantle its vicious cycles . . . . (p. 63)

Perpetuating vicious circles does not serve women, babies or maternity-care staff. As an alternative, a good basis for such working might be the longstanding definition of health offered by the World Health Organization (WHO) in the Alma Alta declaration over half a century ago, if it is applied to health care staff as well as to those the staff offer care for:

> Health is . . .
> . . . a complete state of physical, mental and social well-being, and not merely the absence of disease or infirmity
> (WHO 1978)

It is likely that most if not all professionals working in maternity care would agree with this as a basis to work from. The trick, then, is to create respectful, authentically mutual relationships within and between professional groups.

Conclusion: a vision for the 21st century – changing the world, one birth at a time

There are signs of change, and indications that individuals, politicians, governments and professional organisations are noticing and responding to the need to change the current conversation of maternity care. In countries such as Nepal and Brazil innovations based on community engagement and respectful engagement with staff and women have decreased unnecessary interventions (Misago *et al.* 2001) and lowered maternal mortality rates (Barker *et al.* 2007). In England, Scotland, Spain, South America, North America, Japan, the Middle East and Eastern Europe, there are movements for change that are variously targeted on normal birth, humanising birth, more home birth and mother-friendly birth. These movements are all concerned with the well-being of women and babies. To a greater or lesser extent, they are also concerned with the well-being of staff, and with increasing inter-professional dialogue to maximise the well-being of all concerned. A vision for the 21st century might be for a maternity care that combines a kind of expert practice that encompasses wisdom, skilled practice, and enacted vocation (Downe *et al.* 2007) and that works flexibly with the kind of evidence-based medicine proposed by Sackett and colleagues: best evidence (including that from randomised controlled trials (RCTs) and narratives, from experts, childbearing women and clinicians); clinical skills; and the values of the woman, her family and her maternity caregivers (Sackett *et al.* 2002).This approach could encompass a combination of the following, resulting in effective change and optimal practice:

- A coherent humanist realist philosophy
- Effective clinical and interpersonal skills
- Comprehensive knowledge
- Positive appreciative relationships
- Facilitative health system/organisational context
- Societal/community buy-in

The vision for the future that is presented in this book is one in which a wide range of ways of knowing and of responding to the needs of women, babies and families are accepted as legitimate, as long as they promote the well-being of those using the service, and of those providing it. This knowledge encompasses trials evidence, physiology, complexity, uncertainty, and salutogenic systems theory, observation and deduction, and narrative and story telling. The vision allows for a much more nuanced, subtle and flexible ontology of childbirth. In the end, it presents a call to every midwife, obstetrician, researcher, educationalist, manager, maternity services politician service commissioner, childbearing woman, family member and other stakeholder to consider and respond to Gandhi's call to action:

Be the change you want to see in the world.

References

Annandale E, Clark J (1996) What is gender? Feminist theory and the sociology of human reproduction. *Sociology of Health and Illness* 18: 17–44.

Antonovsky A (1987) *Unravelling the Mystery of Health: How People Manage Stress and Stay Well*. California, Jossey-Bass.

Antonovsky A (1993) The implications of salutogenesis: an outsiders view. In Turnbull AP, Patterson J, Behr SK (eds) *Cognitive Coping Families and Disability*, Chapter 8.

Barker CE, Bird CE, Pradhan A, Shakya G (2007) Support to the safe motherhood programme in Nepal: an integrated approach. *Reproductive Health Matters* 15(30): 81–90.

Downe S, Simpson L, Trafford K (2007) Expert intrapartum maternity care: a meta-synthesis. *Journal of Advanced Nursing* 57(2): 127–40.

Healthcare Commission (2005) *Review of Maternity Services Provided by North West London Hospitals NHS Trust*. London, Healthcare Commission.

Healthcare Commission (2008) *Towards Better Births: A Review of Maternity Services in England*. London, Healthcare Commission.

Kelly S, Allison MA (1999) *The Complexity Advantage: How the Science of Complexity Can Help Your Business Achieve Peak Performance*. New York, McGraw-Hill.

Kennedy HP, Lyndon A (2008) Tensions and teamwork in nursing and midwifery relationships. *Journal of Obstetric, Gynecologic, and Neonatal Nursing* 37(4): 426–35.

Misago C, Kendall C, Freitas P *et al.* (2001) From 'culture of dehumanization of childbirth' to 'childbirth as a transformative experience': changes in five municipalities in north-east Brazil. *International Journal of Gynaecology and Obstetrics* 75(Suppl 1): S67–S72.

Ontario Women's Health Council (2006) www.womenshealthcouncil.com/.

Pinki P, Sayasneh A, Lindow SW (2007) The working relationship between midwives and junior doctors: a questionnaire survey of Yorkshire trainees. *Obstetrics and Gynaecology* 27(4): 365–7.

Sackett DL, Straus SE, Richardson WS, Rosenberg W, Haynes RB (2002) *Evidence Based Medicine: How to Practice and Teach EBM*. Edinburgh, Churchill Livingstone.

Simpson KR, James, DC, Knox GE (2006). Nurse-physician communication during labor and birth: Implications for patient safety. *Journal of Obstetric, Gynecologic, and Neonatal Nursing* 35(4): 547–56.

Smith & Dixon (2007) *The Safety of Maternity Services in England*. London, Kings Fund.

WHO (1978) *Alma Alta Declaration*. Copenhagen, WHO Regional Office for Europe.

Index

Page numbers in *italics* represent figures, those in **bold** represent tables.